D0983819

PRACTICAL
GASTROINTESTINAL
ENDOSCOPY

Practical Gastrointestinal Endoscopy

Peter B. Cotton
MD, FRCP
Medical Director, Digestive Disease Center
Assistant Dean, International Programs
Medical University of South Carolina
Charleston, SC 29425, USA

Christopher B. Williams
MA, BM, BCh, FRCP
Endoscopy Unit
St Mark's Hospital for Colorectal and
Intestinal Disorders
Harrow, London HA1 3UJ, UK

FOURTH EDITION

Presented with the compliments of
Astra Pharmaceuticals Ltd

Blackwell
Science

The views expressed in this publication are not
necessarily those of Astra Pharmaceuticals Ltd

© 1980, 1982, 1990, 1996 by
Blackwell Science Ltd
Editorial Offices:
Osney Mead, Oxford OX2 0EL
25 John Street, London WC1N 2BL
23 Ainslie Place, Edinburgh EH3 6AJ
238 Main Street, Cambridge
  Massachusetts 02142, USA
54 University Street, Carlton
  Victoria 3053, Australia

Other Editorial Offices:
Arnette Blackwell SA
  224, Boulevard Saint Germain
  75007 Paris, France

Blackwell Wissenschafts-Verlag GmbH
  Kurfürstendamm 57
  10707 Berlin, Germany

  Zehetnergasse 6
  A-1140 Wien
  Austria

All rights reserved. No part of
this publication may be reproduced,
stored in a retrieval system, or
transmitted, in any form or by any
means, electronic, mechanical,
photocopying, recording or otherwise,
except as permitted by the UK
Copyright, Designs and Patents Act
1988, without the prior permission
of the copyright owner.

First published 1980
Reprinted 1981
Second edition 1982
Reprinted 1984, 1985, 1987, 1988
Third edition 1990
Reprinted 1991
Fourth edition 1996

Italian editions 1980, 1986
German edition 1985
French edition 1986

Set by Excel Typesetters Co.,
Hong Kong.
Printed in Great Britain
at the Alden Press, Oxford and bound
by Hartnolls Ltd, Bodmin, Cornwall

The Blackwell Science logo is a trade
mark of Blackwell Science Ltd,
registered at the United Kingdom
Trade Marks Registry

DISTRIBUTORS

Marston Book Services Ltd
PO Box 269
Abingdon
Oxon OX14 4YN
(*Orders*: Tel: 01235 465500
        Fax: 01235 465555)

USA
Blackwell Science, Inc.
238 Main Street
Cambridge, MA 02142
(*Orders:* Tel: 800 215-1000
        617 876-7000
        Fax: 617 492-5263)

Canada
Copp Clark Ltd
2775 Matheson Blvd East
Mississauga, Ontario
Canada, L4W 4P7
(*Orders:* Tel: 800 263-4374
        905 238-6074)

Australia
Blackwell Science Pty Ltd
54 University Street
Carlton, Victoria 3053
(*Orders:* Tel: 03 9347 0300
        Fax: 03 9349 3016)

A catalogue record for this title
is available from the British Library

ISBN 0-86542-851-4

Library of Congress
Cataloging-in-Publication Data

Cotton, Peter B.
    Practical gastrointestinal
endoscopy / Peter B. Cotton,
    Christopher B. Williams.—4th ed.
        p.   cm.
    Includes bibliographical
references and index.
    ISBN 0-86542-851-4
    1. Gastroscopy. I. Williams,
Christopher B. (Christopher
Beverley) II. Title.
    [DNLM: 1. Gastrointestinal
Diseases—diagnosis.
2. Endoscopy.
  WI 141 C851p   1996]
  RC804. G3C68   1996
  616.3'307545—dc20
  DNLM/DLC
  for Library of Congress   95-25737
                              CIP

Contents

Preface to the Fourth Edition

The biggest development in gastrointestinal (GI) endoscopy since the third edition of this book undoubtedly has been the explosive impact of laparoscopic surgery. This has many specific implications for endoscopists (e.g. a changing role for endoscopic retrograde cholangiopancreatography (ERCP) in the context of laparoscopic cholecystectomy), but also an important effect on the relationship between medical and surgical gastroenterology. We have chosen not to discuss laparoscopy in detail, nor endoscopic ultrasonography, which is rapidly becoming accepted as a legitimate clinical tool. Books on these techniques are proliferating, and we will continue to confine ourselves to flexible GI endoscopy. This field is maturing—maybe we are also.

The pace of technical development has slowed somewhat. There have been a few important new ideas, such as variceal banding and metal stents, but most changes have been incremental. It is difficult to keep up to date with all of these details as our discipline expands — and our brains contract. Therefore, we asked several friends to criticize sections of this edition in draft, and are enormously grateful to Joseph Leung, Rob Hawes, David Fleischer, John Morris and Marilyn Schaffner for their helpful suggestions; others have been generous with unusual illustrations. We have chosen to continue with English spelling, and, for simplicity of presentation, we still refer to all patients and doctors as 'he' and nurses as 'she'. We have maintained the practical 'cookbook' approach which has made earlier editions popular, and have somewhat reduced the emphasis on areas which are mainly of interest to unit directors, e.g. design, management and teaching arrangements. There are now many comprehensive and specialized reference sources, some of which are noted at the end of each chapter and in the general reading section. We recommend reading appropriate journals (especially *Gastrointestinal Endoscopy* and *Endoscopy*), the *Annual of Gastrointestinal Endoscopy* (Current Science, London), which we have edited with Guido Tytgat since 1988, and the quarterly series of *Gastrointestinal Endoscopy Clinics of North America* (WB Saunders, Philadelphia), edited by Michael Sivak.

A welcome change in the 1990s is the accelerating interest in scientific evaluation of endoscopic interventions, both diagnostic and therapeutic. The quality of endoscopic research and publication is improving; case reports and case series are giving way to prospective and controlled trials. Endoscopy training should now include exposure to the fundamental principles of clinical epidemiology and statistics, and the essential strength of prospective databases. We hope that our approach is consistent with these critical goals.

Sincere thanks are due to our families, colleagues and friends, on both sides of the Atlantic. The chapters on ERCP are dedicated (by PBC) to the memory of Howard Shapiro, special friend and teacher. We are grateful for the courtesy, patience and skills of our secretaries, Rita Oden, Robyn Lopez and Anna McNeil, and the Blackwell Science publishing team, especially Andrew Robinson, Helen Harvey, Catherine Jones and Graeme Chambers.

Peter B. Cotton
Christopher B. Williams

Preface to the First Edition

The human gut is long and tortuous. Diagnosis and localization of its afflictions relied for many decades on barium radiology, which provides indirect data in black and white. Man is by nature inquisitive and direct inspection in colour is instinctively preferable and probably more accurate. Rigid open-ended instruments allow direct visual examination (and biopsy sampling) of only the proximal 40 cm and distal 25 cm of the gut. Semiflexible lens gastroscopes were introduced in the 1930s and 1940s and used by a few experts; examinations were uncomfortable and incomplete, and biopsy facilities were poor.

The situation has changed dramatically since the late 1960s with the introduction of fully flexible and manoeuvrable endoscopes. Upper gastrointestinal (GI) endoscopy is now a routine procedure which has superseded the barium meal as the primary diagnostic tool. Duodenoscopy allows direct cannulation of the papilla of Vater for cholangiography and pancreatography (ERCP). The whole colon can be examined, and methods are available for small intestinal endoscopy. Tissue specimens can be removed from all of these areas under direct vision, using biopsy forceps, cytology brushes and snare loops.

A further revolution occurred in the late 1970s with the arrival of endoscopic therapy. Transendoscopic snare removal has revolutionized the management of polyps, and flexible endoscopes now allow removal of foreign bodies, sphincterotomy for gallstones, insertion of stents, dilatation of strictures, and direct attack on bleeding lesions and tumours.

GI endoscopy is a skill which requires motivation, determination and dexterity. Patients may suffer if examinations are not performed correctly, and endoscopic techniques themselves may fall into disrepute if results are suboptimal or unnecessary complications occur. The speed of development and the consequent clinical demand for endoscopy initially outstripped the evolution of training facilities. Many of the present 'experts' (including the authors) were self-taught, but instruction and experience of endoscopy should now be an integral part of GI training programmes.

This volume attempts to provide a basic framework for this process, and includes some 'tricks of the trade' which we find helpful.

1980
Peter B. Cotton
Christopher B. Williams

Basic Endoscopic Equipment

1

The modern era of endoscopy began with the development of fibreoptic instruments in the 1960s. For most purposes these are being supplanted by video chip endoscopes in the 1990s. Details of instruments for specific purposes, accessories and precise methods for management are outlined in other chapters. This chapter serves to introduce the true beginner to some principles which are common to all endoscopes and procedures.

Flexible endoscopes are complex (Fig. 1.1). Basically, they consist of a control head and a flexible shaft with a manoeuvrable tip. The head is connected to a light source via an 'umbilical' cord, through which pass other tubes transmitting air, water and suction, etc. The suction channel is used for the passage of diagnostic tools (e.g. biopsy forceps) and therapeutic devices.

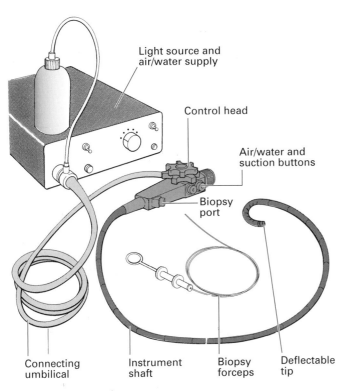

Light source and air/water supply

Control head

Air/water and suction buttons

Biopsy port

Connecting umbilical

Instrument shaft

Biopsy forceps

Deflectable tip

Fig. 1.1 Fibreoptic endoscope system.

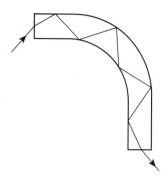

Fig. 1.2 Total internal reflection of light down a glass fibre.

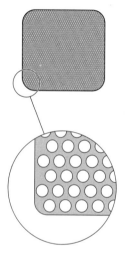

Fig. 1.3 Fibre bundle showing the 'packing fraction' or dead space between fibres.

Fibreoptic instruments and video-endoscopes

Fibreoptic instruments

These are based on optical viewing bundles, well described as a 'highly flexible piece of illuminated spaghetti'. The viewing bundle of a standard fibre-endoscope is 2–3 mm in diameter and contains 20000–40000 fine glass fibres, each close to 10 μm in diameter. Light focused onto the face of each fibre is transmitted by repeated internal reflections (Fig. 1.2). Faithful transmission of an image depends upon the spatial orientation of the individual fibres being the same at both ends of the bundle (a 'coherent' bundle). Each individual glass fibre is coated with glass of a lower optical densit to prevent leakage of light from within the fibre, since the coating does not transmit light. This coating and the space between the fibres causes a dark 'packing fraction', which is responsible for the fine mesh frequently apparent in the fibreoptic image (Fig. 1.3). For this reason, the image quality of a fibreoptic bundle, though excellent, can never equal that of a rigid lens system. However, fibreoptic bundles are extremely flexible, and an image can be transmitted even when tied in a knot. In most modern instruments the distal lens which focuses the image onto the bundle is fixed, and a pin-hole aperture gives a depth of focus from 10–15 cm down to about 3 mm. The image reconstructed at the top of the bundle is transmitted to the eye via a focusing lens, adjustable to compensate for individual differences in refraction.

Video-endoscopes

These are mechanically similar to fibre-endoscopes, with a charged couple device (CCD) 'chip' and supporting electronics mounted at the tip, to and fro wiring replacing the optical bundle and further electronics and switches occupying the site of the ocular lens on the upper part of the control head. Removing any need to hold the instrument close to the endoscopist's eye has hygienic advantages (avoidance of splash contamination) and also gives the opportunity for radical changes of instrument design and handling techniques in the future.

The subtleties of different CCD systems in design and performance are beyond the scope of this book. However, in essence, a CCD chip is an array of 33000–100000 individual photo cells (known as picture elements or pixels) receiving photons reflected back from the mucosal surface and producing electrons in proportion to the light received. In common with all other television systems the individual receptors of the CCD respond only to degrees of light and dark, and not to colour. 'Colour' CCDs have extra pixels to allow for an overlay of multiple primary colour filter stripes, making the pixels under a particu-

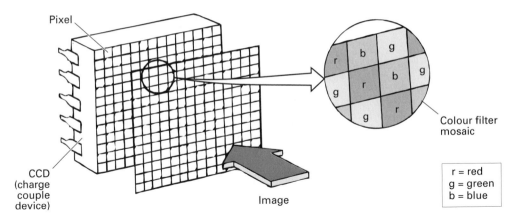

Fig. 1.4 Static red, green and blue filters in the 'colour' chip.

lar stripe respond only to light of that particular colour (Fig. 1.4). 'Black and white' (or, more correctly, sequential system) CCDs can be made smaller, or potentially of higher resolution, by the expedient of illuminating *all* the pixels with intermittent primary colour strobe-effect lighting produced by rotating a colour filter wheel within the light source (Fig. 1.5). The sequential primary colour images (in the gut mostly red, some green and little blue) are stored transiently in banks of memory chips in the processor and fed out sequentially to the red/blue/green electron guns of the TV monitor. The large numbers of chips and sophisticated computer 'image-processing' technology used to optimize the underlying single CCD output account for the excellence of the image produced by sequential CCD systems (and the high price involved), as well as the relatively large processor.

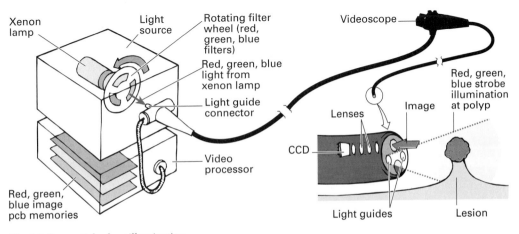

Fig. 1.5 Sequential colour illumination.

Video-endoscope or fibre-endoscope?

The screen-image quality of present video-endoscopes equals that of present fibrescopes in both colour and resolution. Video-endoscopy scores greatly by the fact that everyone can view the image simultaneously, with a clarity previously restricted to the endoscopist alone (teaching side-arms and add-on television cameras introduce optical interference and reduce quality). Whereas optical fibre technology is near its maximum theoretical performance (since below the 6–8 μm fibre diameter approached in modern bundles there is massive loss of light transmission), there is no reason why the 10 μm pixel size of present CCDs should not be reduced to around 1 μm. This means that future CCDs can be smaller, but also that the greatly increased numbers of pixels will increase resolution and allow the use of high-definition TV monitors. The objection that video-endoscopes introduce 'artificial colour' values is untenable since: (i) they can be shown in technical studies to give a remarkably faithful rendering of test charts; (ii) the visual assessment of lesions depends little on absolute colour values; and (iii) there is the inescapable fact that individual perception of colour varies significantly — the extreme example being colour blindness. In terms of hard-copy imaging there is also a clear advantage in employing only the ocular lens system at the instrument tip without the degrading effects of transmission down an optical bundle and through a secondary lens system. Of crucial importance is the fact that the digital signal simplifies image recording and manipulation, and opens the way for new methods of image enhancement, transmission and analysis.

For the fibre-endoscopist, the mechanical transition to handling video-endoscopes whilst viewing the TV monitor is mastered in a few minutes. Thereafter, most endoscopists tend to work this way instinctively, even with fibre-endoscopes if a video camera attachment is available. The ease of stance, brighter view and the natural visual field (combining a macular view of the image and peripheral view of the patient and the endoscopy room) make video-endoscopes extremely relaxing to use, and facilitates communication with patients and assistants. The mechanical manipulation of endoscope controls and subtle management of its shaft, including de-looping or rotatory movements, are also significantly easier with video-endoscopes, since the manipulating left hand can move freely without relationship to the endoscopist's eye. Although in individual practice no user of fibre-endoscopes need feel disadvantaged, the bonus for larger institutions or teaching hospitals of the shared view, including the ability for experienced endoscopists to see precisely the same image as obtained by an apprentice, scores highly in favour of using video-endoscopes.

For these many reasons, video-endoscopes have taken over a majority position in gastrointestinal (GI) endoscopic units.

Fibreoptic instruments will retain some role, by virtue of their simplicity and small-diameter capability, for instances where portability is relevant, as well as in other special circumstances.

Illumination

This is provided from an external high-intensity source through one or more light-carrying bundles. Since these light bundles do not transmit a spatial image, the fibres within them need not be 'coherent' and are randomly arranged. Because light intensity is reduced at any optical interface, light bundles run uninterruptedly from the tip of the instrument through its connecting 'umbilical' cord directly to the point of focus of the lamp. These may be xenon arc (300 W) or halogen-filled tungsten filament lamps (150 W). Light is focused by a parabolic mirror onto the face of the bundle, and the transmitted intensity is controlled by filters and/or a mechanical diaphragm. The light sources made by different companies are not always interchangeable; adapters may be provided, but involve a further optical interface and some loss of light. Small sources are mobile and relatively cheap and provide sufficient illumination for simple observation and standard photography. Large light sources are necessary for optimal photography and television application when using fibrescopes or video-endoscopes.

Instrument tip

Control of the instrument tip depends upon pull wires attached at the tip just beneath its outer protective shaft, and passing back through the length of the instrument shaft to the angling controls

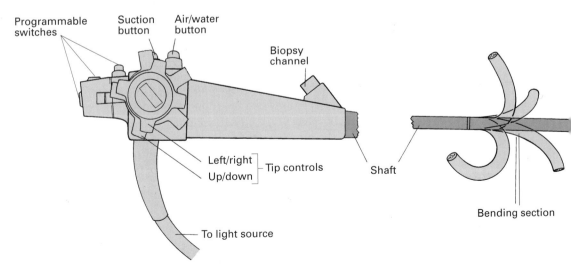

Fig. 1.6 Basic design—control head and bending section.

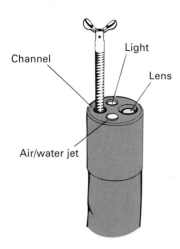

Fig. 1.7 The tip of a forward-viewing endoscope.

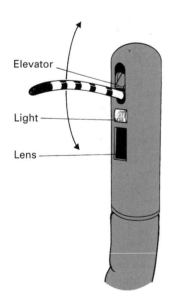

Fig. 1.8 A side-viewer with cannula protruding from the elevator.

in the control head (Fig. 1.6). The two angling wheels/knobs (for up/down and right/left movement) incorporate a friction braking system, so that the tip can be fixed temporarily in any desired position; angling with the brakes on causes no damage. The instrument shaft is torque stable so that rotatory 'corkscrewing' movements applied to the head are transmitted to the tip—if the shaft is relatively straight at the time.

Instrument channels

An 'operating' channel (usually 2–4 mm in diameter) allows the passage of fine flexible accessories (e.g. biopsy forceps, cytology brushes, sclerotherapy needles, diathermy snares) from a port on the endoscope control head (see Fig. 1.6) through the shaft and into the field of view (Fig. 1.7). In some instruments (especially those with lateral-viewing optics), the tip of the channel incorporates a small deflectable elevator or bridge, which permits some directional control of the forceps and other accessories independent of the instrument tip (Fig. 1.8); this elevator or bridge is controlled by a further thumb lever. The operating channel is also used for aspiration in single-channel instruments; an external suction pump is connected to the 'umbilical' cord of the instrument near the light source and suction is diverted into the instrument channel by pressing the suction valve.

The channel size varies with the instrument purpose. 'Therapeutic' endoscopes with large channels allow better suction and larger accessories. Twin-channel endoscopes exist for specialized applications. An ancillary small channel transmits air to distend the organ being examined; the air is supplied from a pump in the light source and is controlled by another valve (see Fig. 1.6). The air system also pressurizes the water bottle so that a jet of water can be squirted across the distal lens to clean it. In colonoscopes there is a separate proximal opening for the water channel, to allow high-pressure flushing with a syringe.

Different instruments

The basic design principles apply to most endoscopes, but specific instruments differ in length, size, stiffness, sophistication and distal lens orientation. Most GI endoscopy is performed with instruments providing *direct forward vision* (Fig. 1.7), via a 90–130° wide-angle lens (the angle being measured across the diagonal of square image endoscopes). However, there are circumstances in which it is preferable to view *laterally* (Fig. 1.8) — particularly for endoscopic retrograde cholangiopancreatography (see Chapter 6). Oblique and even movable lens instruments have been developed, but are no longer popular. The overall diameter of an endoscope is a compromise between engineering ideals and patient tolerance. The shaft must contain and protect many bundles, wires and tubes, all of which are stronger and more efficient when larger. A colonoscope can reasonably approach 15 mm in diameter to provide resilience and torque stability, but this size is acceptable in the upper gut only for specialized therapeutic instruments. Most routine upper GI endoscopes are between 8 and 11 mm in diameter. Smaller endoscopes are available; they are better tolerated by all patients and have specific application in children. However, smaller instruments inevitably involve some compromise in durability, image quality and biopsy size. All modern endoscopes can be completely immersed for cleaning and disinfection; non-immersible instruments are obsolete.

Several companies now produce a full range of endoscopes at comparable prices. However, since light sources and other accessories produced by different companies are not always interchangeable, most endoscopy units concentrate for convenience on equipment from only one manufacturer. Endoscopes are delicate and some breakages are inevitable. Only close communication, repair and back-up arrangements with an efficient company and its agents can maintain an endoscopy service. The quality of this support varies with different companies (and countries), and is often the critical factor affecting the choice of manufacturer.

Accessories

Tissue-sampling devices

Tissue sampling is a crucial part of endoscopy. Forceps consist of a pair of sharpened cups (Fig. 1.9), a spiral metal cable and a control handle (Fig. 1.10). The maximum diameter is limited by the size of the operating channel, and the length of the cups by the radius of curvature through which they must pass in the instrument tip. This may be acute in side-viewing instruments with forceps elevators. When it is necessary to take biopsy specimens from a lesion which can only be approached tangentially (e.g. the wall of the oesophagus), forceps with a central spike may be helpful; however, these present a significant puncture hazard, and should probably not be used to avoid accidental infectious inoculation of endoscopy staff. Cytology brushes have a covering plastic sleeve to protect the specimen during withdrawal (Fig. 1.11). Other diagnostic and therapeutic devices will be described in the relevant chapters.

Suction traps

Suction traps, such as those used for collecting samples of sputum during bronchial aspiration, are equally useful for

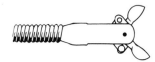

Fig. 1.9 Biopsy cups open.

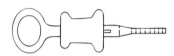

Fig. 1.10 Control handle for forceps.

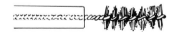

Fig. 1.11 Cytology brush with outer sleeve.

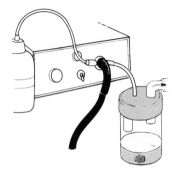

Fig. 1.12 A suction trap to collect fluid specimens.

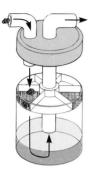

Fig. 1.13 A filtered suction trap is better for tissue specimens.

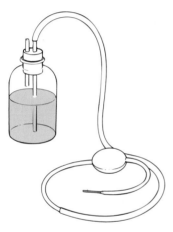

Fig. 1.14 A rubber bulb for flushing through the instrumentation channel.

taking samples of intestinal secretions and bile. When fitted temporarily into the suction line (Fig. 1.12) they allow the collection of samples for microbiology, chemistry and 'salvage' cytology. Solid or snare-loop specimens can also be retrieved in an ingenious filtered suction trap available commercially (Fig. 1.13).

Fluid-flushing devices

Flushing fluids through the channel may be necessary to provide optimal views of lesions, particularly in the presence of food residue or acute bleeding. With standard endoscopes, this can be done with a syringe, manual bulb (Fig. 1.14) or a pulsatile electric pump, with a suitable nozzle through the biopsy port. Some therapeutic instruments have an in-built forward-facing flushing channel at the tip. For more precise aiming, a simple Teflon tube can be passed down the instrument channel to clear mucus or blood from areas of interest with a jet of water, or to highlight mucosal detail by 'dye spraying' (using a nozzle-tipped catheter).

Overtubes (sleeves)

These are flexible hoses (24–45 cm long, depending on the indication) designed to fit over the endoscope shaft (Fig. 1.15). Sophisticated low-friction versions are produced but suitable alternatives can be made from plastic hose; the internal diameter needs to be tailored to the size of the endoscope. The wall should be as thin as possible (to minimize patient discomfort) but should have sufficient strength not to kink and to maintain its shape when the endoscope is removed. The top end of the tube should have a flange which abuts against the mouthguard, or some device which can be gripped by the assistant (to prevent it from disappearing into the mouth or anus). Overtubes are mainly used when repeated intubation is anticipated, e.g. for change of endoscopes, removal of multiple polyps, variceal banding or use of muzzle-loaded forceps and biopsy capsules. The endoscope is passed in the usual way, with the overtube at the top of the shaft. Once the endoscope is in position, the overtube is lubricated and slid over the shaft. It is then simple to remove and to replace the endoscope without significant patient

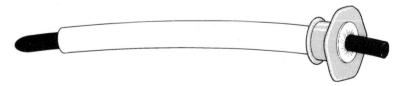

Fig. 1.15 An overtube with toothguard over a rubber lavage tube.

discomfort. Alternatively, the upper GI overtube can be passed first, sitting snugly on a large dilator (or lavage tube) (Fig. 1.15). The dilator is then withdrawn, leaving the overtube in place; this protects the airway and allows the passage of endoscopes without additional patient discomfort.

Longer and larger overtubes are used for the removal of sharp foreign bodies from the stomach and, by some practitioners, windowed overtubes have been found useful during variceal injection sclerotherapy, especially during active bleeding. They can be used also as stiffening devices during colonoscopy and enteroscopy. The use of colonic (split) overtubes is described in Chapter 9.

Electrosurgery equipment

Details are given in Chapter 10.

Teaching attachments

Sharing an image from a fibrescope requires a 'clip-on' side-arm teaching attachment, or a 'video converter', essentially a small CCD chip camera which is applied to the eyepiece of the fibrescope, and transmits the image to a TV monitor (for both the primary operator and assistants).

Use and maintenance

Handling, storage and security

Endoscopes are expensive and complex tools. They should be stored safely, hanging vertically in cupboards through which air can circulate. Care must be taken whilst carrying instruments, since the rigid optics are easily damaged if left to dangle or knocked against a hard surface. The head, tip and umbilical connector should all be held (Fig. 1.16).

Instrument checking

Instruments must be checked before use. The nurse assistant will normally set up the system with the water bottle and other accessories suitably cleaned and disinfected. However, the endoscopist must check that the equipment is ready and safe for use, that the controls are all functional (including tip deflection and air/water/suction channel) and that the image is clear, before starting the procedure.

Channel blockage

Blockage of the air/water (or suction) channel is one of the most

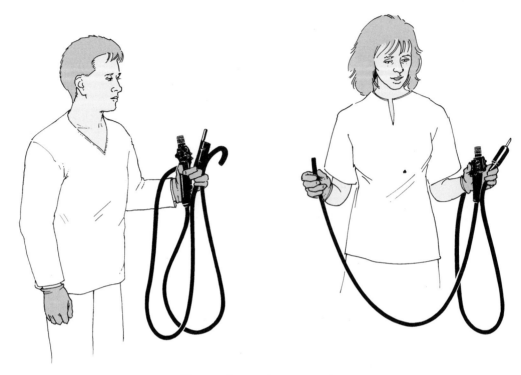

Fig. 1.16 Carry endoscopes carefully to avoid knocks to the optics in the control head and tip.

common endoscope problems. When blockage occurs, the various systems and connections (instrument umbilical, water bottle cap or tube, etc.) must be checked, including the tightness and the presence of rubber O-rings where relevant. It is usually possible to clear the different channels by flushing with a syringe and a suitable soft plastic introducer or micropipette tip. Water can be injected down any channel and, since water is not compressed, more force can be applied than with air. Remember that a small syringe (1–5 ml) generates more pressure than a large one, whereas a large one (50 ml) generates more suction. The air or suction connections at the umbilical, or the water tube within the water bottle can be syringed until water emerges from the instrument tip. Care should be taken to cover or depress the relevant control valves while syringing. Another method for unclogging the suction channel is to remove the valve, and apply suction directly at the port.

Irreversible air-channel blockages are invariably due to coagulated residue inside or just above the small-angled tube inserted at the instrument tip and held in place by a small grub screw covered with soft mastic. If irrigation with a small syringe and fine needle is ineffective, as a last resort this angled tube can be removed with a very small screwdriver and cleaned with a fine wire. The best way to avoid such blockages is to insist on scrupulous cleaning regimens (see Chapter 3).

Maintenance

The life of an endoscope is almost completely determined by the quality of maintenance. Details of cleaning and disinfection are given in Chapter 3. Close collaboration with hospital bioengineering departments and servicing engineers is essential, but most of the important work is done in the unit by the GI staff— for example regular 'leakage testing' of immersible endoscopes. It is important to maintain complex accessories (e.g. electrosurgical equipment) in a safe condition, properly calibrated and adjusted. Repairs and maintenance must be properly documented. A case can be made for returning some instruments to the manufacturers for detailed inspection and 'tightening up' from time to time. Some large endoscopy units may find it cost-effective to employ their own biomedical technician.

Further reading

Sivak M. *Gastroenterologic Endoscopy*. Philadelphia: WB Saunders, 1987.
Zuccaro G. Video endoscopy and the charge-coupled device. In Sivak M, ed. *Gastrointestinal Endoscopy Clinics of North America*, Vol. 2(2). Philadelphia: WB Saunders, 1992.

2 The Endoscopy Unit and Staff

Most endoscopists, especially beginners, focus on the individual procedures and not on the extensive infrastructure which is now necessary for efficient and safe activity. Ageing experts can remember when they started with one instrument, a makeshift room and a hijacked assistant. Now many of us work in units with multiple procedure rooms full of complex electronic equipment, with space dedicated to preparation, recovery and reporting, in collaboration with teams of specially trained support staff. Endoscopy is a sophisticated industry. More and more units resemble operating room suites—but with a human touch. Endoscopists are also learning (often painfully) some of the imperatives of surgical practice, such as efficient scheduling, disinfection and safe anaesthesia.

Setting up and running an endoscopy unit is a complex topic, of particular interest to directors and nurse managers, with an expanding literature. Some basic principles are mentioned here briefly.

Staff and management

Endoscopy units nowadays are complex organizations, with many people of different backgrounds and training. Understanding and motivating the team is a fascinating challenge. Procedures are performed by many different types of doctor, including gastroenterologists, surgeons, internists (general physicians), some family practitioners and radiologists. There are also many different types of supporting staff. Most of the endoscopy assistants are nurses, whose primary role is to care for the patients' comfort and safety before, during and after the procedures. Nurses, nursing aides and technicians are responsible for cleaning, disinfection and maintenance of endoscopy equipment and accessories. Other staff handle reception, documentation and billing duties. All of the staff need to be specially trained, and fully orientated.

The endoscopy team has to liaise effectively with many other people and services within the hospital or clinic (e.g. the departments of radiology, pathology, anaesthesia and bioengineering) and outside (e.g. referring doctors and equipment manufacturers).

The unit must have a designated *medical director*, responsible for overall policies and results. The director is assisted by an *endoscopy nurse manager* (or head nurse) who helps formulate policies, and is responsible for implementing them on a day-today basis. The ramifications of this role are considerable, and the contribution is often undervalued by colleagues and institutions. Policies should be developed into a *procedure manual*, covering many of the aspects discussed in Chapter 3, relating particularly to patient and staff safety.

Team morale and quality of service are dependent upon mutual respect and good communications amongst the staff. The mission — improving the quality of patient care — requires constant study and nurture.

The endoscopy unit

Like a hotel, or large Victorian household, the endoscopy unit should have a smart public face ('upstairs'), and a more functional back hall ('downstairs'). From the patient's perspective, endoscopy consists of reception, preparation, procedure, recovery and discharge. Enabling these activities are a series of other functions, which include scheduling, cleaning, preparation, maintenance and storage of equipment, reporting and archiving, and staff management (Table 2.1).

Many questions have to be addressed when planning endoscopy facilities.

Where should the unit be, and how independent?

Gastrointestinal (GI) endoscopy certainly now requires dedicated space; how independent it should be of other hospital or clinic activities will depend upon its size, and the institutional layout. Ideally, a hospital unit should be suitable for out-patients and in-patients, and be easily accessible both day and night. However, there is a size of institution above which it makes sense to have two GI endoscopy areas — a high-volume, easy access, patient-friendly unit for out-patients, and a smaller higher tech facility to service patients in the wards and intensive

Patient-related	Support
Reception	Scheduling
Preparation	Equipment inventory
Procedure	Disinfection
Recovery	Resuscitation
Discharge	Reporting
	Statistics
	Storage
	Staff management

Table 2.1 Endoscopy unit functions.

care units. Here is another analogy with surgery, which has main operating rooms and out-patient day surgery units.

If endoscopy is located in an out-patient (or day surgery) area, it may seem tidy to share space and staff with other disciplines for reception and recovery functions. The efficiency of such shared arrangements depends much upon the quality of staff interrelations and the stability of patient volume. The risk of having support space dedicated only to endoscopy is that it will become inadequate; sharing space carries the risk of encroachment from others. Some units find it convenient to share facilities with other endoscopic interventions, such as bronchoscopy (since the needs for recovery space and dedicated disinfection methods are similar). However, generic 'departments of endoscopy', including other techniques such as cystoscopy and arthoscopy, are culturally awkward and have not become popular.

Procedure rooms

The number of endoscopy rooms required depends on many factors. These include the volume and spectrum of procedures, sedation practice, efficiency of scheduling, quality of technical support and the presence or absence of trainees.

The spectrum of procedural complexity has a major impact on time, equipment and staff usage. We use a simple relative value scale to reflect this variability for audit purposes (Table 2.2). The point value is doubled for any procedure done outside normal working hours. Keeping track of the total points gives a better measure of workload than a simple tally of examinations. This is essential when attempting to justify increases in staff and facilities.

Translating these concepts into room requirements and scheduling is a complex exercise. How many procedures can a room handle? Whilst most endoscopists will say that they can complete simple upper procedures in 20 min, colons in 45 min and ERCPs in under an hour, analysis of actual logs shows that many factors combine to increase the time between consecutive patients, and to reduce the total throughput. Patients and

Procedure	Points
Diagnostic upper endoscopy	1
Therapeutic upper, diagnostic colon	2
Therapeutic colon, diagnostic ERCP	3
Therapeutic ERCP	6
(Flexible sigmoidoscopy	0.5

ERCP, endoscopic retrograde cholangiopancreatography.

Table 2.2 Relative value scale for endoscopic workload.

doctors arrive late, sedation may be slow, instruments or accessories may need additional attention, and teaching can be time-consuming.

The total number of procedure rooms needed in a unit is determined mainly by the volume of the 'standard' procedures (i.e. uppers and colons), which constitute the bulk of the workload. The *maximum* capacity of a room is approximately 1600 standard procedures per year—if these are equally split between uppers and colons, and if a third of each are therapeutic, that is a total of 3200 units, as defined above. This assumes 250 working days per year, and 8 h work days. It is best to aim at about 75% of maximum room capacity, allowing for inevitable fluctuations in workload and necessary flexibility. Therefore, a good working rule for a 'routine' room is about 1200 standard procedures per year. Sigmoidoscopy is performed without sedation; with sufficient instruments, staff and efficient scheduling, one room could easily accommodate 3000 sigmoidoscopy procedures per year. However, by its nature, sigmoidoscopy is often done 'on demand' during a clinic visit, so that scheduling is usually haphazard. ERCP demands a dedicated room (whether in the main endoscopy unit or elsewhere). Six procedures can take a whole day, especially when teaching is involved. One ERCP room will accommodate about 1000 procedures per year.

Procedure room design

Endoscopy procedures vary in complexity. Some require more staff and equipment, and rooms therefore need to be larger. However, all procedure rooms share many common design features. Rectangular rooms often work better than square ones. They must be wide enough to enable the trolley (stretcher) to be spun around its axis. The precise layout is determined by many factors, including the endoscope umbilical and its associated equipment (light source, processor, monitors, etc.). Functional planning of the endoscopy room with avoidance of cross-traffic is crucial to efficient work. Geographical spheres of activity should be defined for doctors, nurses and trainees, with their relevant equipment in the appropriate sector (Fig. 2.1).

The room should contain large sinks to accommodate contaminated accessories (and for initial cleaning of endoscopes if this is done in the procedure room), adequate work surfaces, storage cupboards and power points. The floor should be washable and smooth; anaesthetic considerations may dictate the need for antistatic flooring. Any windows should have blackout curtains and blinds. General room lights should be dimmable, with spotlights over the worktops. The endoscopist and nurses should be able to turn the main room light on and off without moving from their working positions (e.g. with a ceiling pull switch) and have easy access to intercom, telephone and alarm systems. Door

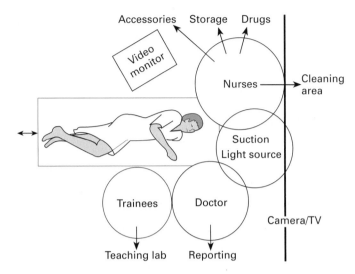

Fig. 2.1 Functional planning — spheres of activity.

openings should be 3.5 m (4 ft) wide, to facilitate moving patient stretchers (or beds) and occasional large pieces of equipment.

Procedure rooms should have piped oxygen and suction (two outlets) and an alarm system. Resuscitation equipment must be available nearby. Fixed examination tables are unnecessary (except with full X-ray equipment). Patient trolleys (stretchers) are convenient for examination and recovery; it should be possible to tilt the top into a head-down position and it is convenient if the height of the trolley can be adjusted.

Patients often enter the examination rooms without sedation. The hardware may look frightening, and should preferably be hidden from immediate view by appropriate planning or a curtain. The ambience should be cheerful rather than clinical, and should resemble a modern kitchen rather than an operating room. Piped music may be appreciated. There must be appropriate arrangements for maintaining a reasonable temperature and for extracting odours, both clinical and chemical.

Efficiency of utilization would be improved if all procedure rooms could be 'generic', i.e. used for all types of procedure. There is no need to separate upper examinations from colonoscopies, since the room requirements are similar. However, some procedures require other sophisticated heavy (and expensive) equipment which cannot easily be moved or duplicated—especially X-ray machines and lasers. Thus, it is usual to have several generic 'standard' rooms, a smaller number of dedicated 'specialized' high tech rooms plus one or more small simpler rooms for flexible sigmoidoscopy where appropriate.

Standard procedure rooms. These do not have to be large. A floor area of 15–20 m² (50–65 ft²) is adequate if the layout is functional.

Specialized procedure rooms. Specialized rooms are larger because of the additional staff and extra bulky equipment, especially for radiology, endoscopic ultrasound and lasers. Some endoscopy units have developed close to (or even within) radiology departments, with such good working relationships that access to radiology procedure rooms is available 'on demand' for fluoroscopy and ERCP. However, casual arrangements are vulnerable, and are easily outgrown. Fluoroscopic screening must be available quickly and predictably for many endoscopic procedures, especially dilatations. C-arm fluoroscopy units are now relatively inexpensive, and can be used with a radiolucent-topped patient stretcher. ERCP is a complex procedure with substantial benefits and risks. To do it without optimal equipment (and staff support) is inappropriate. Units providing an ERCP service—say more than 300 procedures per year — need modern fully independent X-ray equipment, which can also be used for other fluoroscopic procedures. Fortunately, digital equipment has now simplified this issue and eliminates the need for local film processing; indeed, the digital X-ray unit can be seen as an electronic extension of the radiology department, with important practical (and political) implications.

X-ray procedure rooms. These are larger than routine rooms and are usually about 36 m² (350 ft²). Correct siting of the table is essential. It is convenient for the radiologist (or radiographer/technologist) and the endoscopist to work at the same side of the table. The table can then be fixed nearer to one side of the

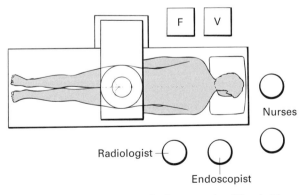

Fig. 2.2 ERCP room layout. Set up the fluoromonitor (F) and video monitor (V) side by side across the X-ray table from the endoscopist.

room, leaving plenty of space for the additional equipment and assistants.

It is essential to mount the video and fluoroscopy monitors side by side across from the endoscopist and radiology staff (Fig. 2.2), for convenient and efficient use. Rooms containing X-ray equipment need to be lead-lined with standard safety features (e.g. a light at the doorways indicating when the machine is activated). Some institutions require a trip switch so that the fluoroscopy is turned off when a door is opened. X-ray rooms using hard copy films (non-digital equipment) need rapid film-processing facilities nearby. Some lasers are bulky, and may need special plumbing arrangements. Rooms in which lasers are used must meet appropriate local safety standards for venting, eye protection and security.

Peri-procedure areas—preparation and recovery

Procedure rooms are the heart of an endoscopy unit, but patients (and their relatives) spend more time elsewhere — in waiting, preparation and recovery areas. The quality of the facilities for these activities and the good attitudes of the staff involved provide the main impressions for the clients. Preparation consists of the preliminary interview, teaching and consent process, undressing and setting up an intravenous line (best done with the patient lying down). After a sedated examination, the patient lies on the trolley (stretcher) on which the procedure was performed, for a period of 20–60 min, depending on the degree of sedation, health, etc. After dressing, the patient should be joined by relatives for consultation prior to discharge, preferably in a private area.

Physical arrangements vary considerably. Most units work on a *'production line' system* (Fig. 2.3). The patient is received into an interview room for discussion and consent, and then moves to an undressing/preparation room or bay. Clothes and valuables are placed in a fixed locker (or carried in a basket which can be

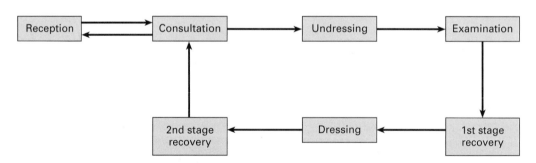

Fig. 2.3 'Production line' system of patient management for endoscopy.

stored underneath the examination stretcher). Intravenous access is established, and the patient is then wheeled (or walks) into the endoscopy room. After examination he is taken on the same stretcher into a recovery bay. When able to stand, he gets dressed again, and sits in a chair or recliner in that bay or a second stage recovery lounge, with a relative or friend who has been waiting outside. Finally he is seen again in the interview room by the doctor and nurse prior to discharge. The number of 'slots' needed for preparation and recovery depends on many factors, including the volume of out-patients, the efficiency of any transportation service for in-patients and local sedation practices.

Busy units require three 'slots' per (sedated) procedure room. The number can be reduced somewhat if there is a second stage recovery lounge. It is useful to have two types of 'slot'. Approximately half (for first stage recovery) are separated only by curtains. The remainder should have sound-proof walls and accordion doors.

Some units have sufficient resources to operate a *'personal room' system* (Fig. 2.4). The patient (and relative) is allocated a single preparation/recovery room, in which all of the periprocedural activities can take place. Privacy and comfort are maximized, but more staff are required to manage the recovery phase.

It is convenient to have a small kitchen area to provide drinks for (recovered) patients and staff.

Storage and cleaning space

Appropriate care of instruments and accessories is essential for their well-being, and to the patient; large areas are required for cleaning, disinfection, packaging and storage. Because toxic chemicals are used (e.g. glutaraldehyde), instrument disinfection should be restricted to one closed area with strong ventilation. A 'sequential' design is practical (Fig. 2.5). Used instruments are brought in through one door into a 'dirty' zone. They pass through a series of cleaning/disinfection processes, to end up hanging in the final 'clean' zone, accessible through a

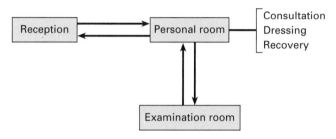

Fig. 2.4 'Personal room' system of patient management for endoscopy.

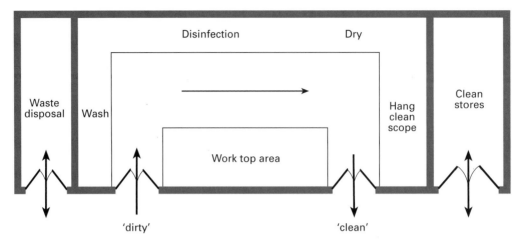

Fig. 2.5 Cleaning area: 'sequential' plan.

second door. A large work top is needed for packaging accessories (e.g. biopsy forceps, catheters) for central sterile processing. Storage needs are always underestimated in plans for endoscopy units. There are day-to-day supplies (linen, syringes, etc.) and many larger items, such as backup light sources and monitors. It is also helpful to have a small workshop where electronic equipment can be inspected and repaired.

Central work station

Larger units (say more than three procedure rooms) must have a central organizing work station—like the bridge of a ship. The captain, or 'triage officer', is usually a senior nurse. If possible, this organizing focus should be adjacent to the nurse station for patient preparation and recovery, to promote good communications and to provide cross-cover. Equally, it is helpful if the work station is close to the area for scheduling/secretarial activities. Figure 2.6 illustrates these relationships.

Reporting and archives

Reports are written, dictated or entered into computers immediately after procedures. Although this can be done within each endoscopy room, it may be more efficient to have a central reporting area with several work stations. Filing arrangements, image management and video-editing functions can also be centralized.

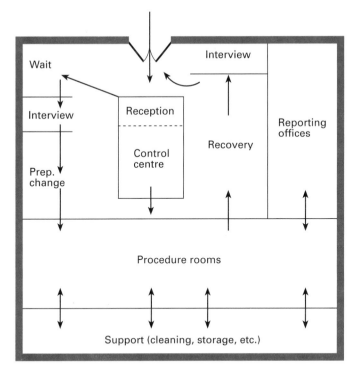

Fig. 2.6 A stylized endoscopy unit, emphasizing a central 'control area', a logical patient flow and separation of the patient from the support areas.

Teaching facilities

Most endoscopy teaching is done 'one on one' in the procedure rooms, greatly facilitated by modern video-endoscope systems. Most units should have a small conference room/library for teaching materials and seminars. Training centres need larger conference areas, including video and sound transmission from the procedure rooms.

Further reading

DiMagno EP. Setting up an endoscopy unit. In: Axon A, ed. *Infection in Endoscopy*. Gastrointestinal Endoscopy Clinics of North America, Vol. 3(3) (series ed. Sivak MV). Philadelphia: WB Saunders, 1993:507–71.

Overholt BF, Chobanian SJ. *Office Endoscopy*. Baltimore: Williams and Wilkins, 1990.

Waye JD, Rich ME. *Planning an Endoscopy Suite for Office and Hospital*. New York: Igaku-Shoin, 1990.

3

Preparation and Safety
Assessment, Consent, Medication, Disinfection and Complications

Many patients have benefitted greatly from gastrointestinal (GI) endoscopy. Unfortunately, some others have suffered severe (even fatal) complications. There are also some hazards for the staff. Our goal must be to maximize the benefits and minimize the risks. We need to be experts, working for good indications with patients who are fully prepared and protected, with skilled assistants, using optimum equipment. The basic principles are similar for all areas of GI endoscopy, recognizing that there are specific circumstances where the risks are greater, e.g. endoscopic retrograde cholangiopancreatography (ERCP), therapeutic procedures and emergency situations.

Emergency endoscopy is needed with increasing frequency because of its recognized value. Patients and equipment need as much care (if not more) as they do in elective situations. Procedures should be done by fully trained doctors, with on-call GI nurse assistants. Where they are done depends upon the circumstances; some patients are stable enough to be transported to the endoscopy unit, but many must be examined in other places, such as intensive care units, emergency rooms or even the operating suite. 'Travelling' endoscopy requires a safe and efficient method for transporting all the necessary equipment and ancillaries.

Regulation of endoscopic practice varies considerably between countries. Many have strict laws on occupational hazards and safety; most have stringent requirements for hospital settings, especially those receiving government funds. However, outpatient endoscopy facilities are often regulated less rigorously. Professional societies have developed practice guidelines. These are available from, amongst others, the American Society for Gastrointestinal Endoscopy (ASGE), the British Society of Gastroenterology (BSG) and the American Society of Gastroenterology Nurses and Associates (SGNA). Endoscopists and assistants must be familiar with the rules and guidelines promulgated within their own countries and working environments.

Assessment before procedure

Patient safety

This is the responsibility of the doctor performing the endoscopy. He must be satisfied that the examination is indicated, that there are no major contraindications, and that the patient understands and consents to it. The patient's records and relevant radiographs should be available at the time of examination. The extent to which the endoscopist should *personally* review the patient's fitness depends upon the circumstances. Many relevant details will be obtained during the nurse's initial assessment (Fig. 3.1). The endoscopist must be prepared to deny or delay examination, if necessary, pending further discussion or preparation.

Risk factors

Some procedures are clearly more dangerous than others. Complex endoscopies (e.g. ERCP) carry more risks than simple ones (e.g. flexible sigmoidoscopy); therapeutic manoeuvres increase the risk of any procedure. Sick in-patients are more likely to do badly than 'walk-ins'. It would be helpful to be able to measure these factors, and thereby come up with some form of aggregate 'risk score', which could be used for comparing different patient cohorts and predicting outcomes. It is not difficult to develop a list of *patient factors* which may increase the risk of endoscopic procedures; obvious examples include anticoagulation, immunosuppression and cardiorespiratory problems. The pre-procedure checklist should cover all of these possibilities. However, we do not yet have the data to calculate relative risks. The American Society for Anesthesiology (ASA) score can be used to give a crude measure of overall fitness or illness (Table 3.1). Risk factors related only to specific procedures (e.g. iodine allergy and ERCP) are covered in the relevant chapters.

1 = Healthy
2 = Minor problem, no systemic effects or continuous medication
3 = Significant illness, currently controlled by medication
4 = Major systemic illness, poorly controlled or uncontrolled
5 = Moribund

Table 3.1 ASA health status definitions (grades).

Explanation and consent

Explanation is crucial to success and safety. Many patients are fearful of endoscopy. Natural anxiety may be aggravated by horror stories from 'friends' or inappropriate remarks by endoscopy staff. Good technique is essential (and some medication is usually given) but the acceptability of endoscopy is also

GI ENDOSCOPY FLOW CHART

Name:

History number:

Pre-procedure assessment

Birth date:

Request by:

Doctor:

Procedure: Date:

Appointment:

Procedure to be done by:

Phone number (H) :
                                                                   (W) :

Problem:

Clinic/Ward:

Patient/Floor informed: Yes/No

Request approved by:

Prep given:

Previous GI procedures/Surgery (dates):

Risks

Allergies? Iodine/Opiates/Antibiotics/Local anaesthetics

Other:

Cardiac: Surgery/Valves/Endocarditis: Needs antibiotics: Yes/No   Given: Yes/No

Chest/Renal/Diabetes/Infection/Glaucoma/Pregnant/Immunosuppressed/Other?

Details

Medications: Anticoagulants/Antidepressants/Sedatives/Aspirin

Current:

Taken today:

Pre-procedure interview/Phone call: Date:

Comments: Signature/Title:

Weight: BP: Pulse: Resp: Temp:

Reviewed educational material:

Prep for procedure: Prep results:

Dentures/Loose teeth/Caps: PT: Hgb:

Travel arrangements: APTT: Hct:

Abd assessment: Consent signed: Yes/No

Comments: Special equipment anticipated:

Signature/Title:

Fig. 3.1 Nurses' pre-procedure form.

crucially dependent upon careful, empathetic explanation and a reassuring friendly atmosphere at the time of reception as well as during the examination. Endoscopy can become such a routine to the doctors and nurses concerned that patients' natural anxieties may be ignored and thereby increased. Patient education starts when the need for endoscopy is established. This is simple if the indication arises during consultation with the gastroenterologist who will himself perform the examination. However, patients are often referred to endoscopy units from other clinics or in-patient areas. Some doctors wish to see patients personally in a formal consultation before agreeing to perform endoscopy; others are prepared to offer an 'open' service. The first alternative is not always practical and some compromise must be reached which will be expressed in the design of any request/assessment form. If the patient is sent from another clinic direct to the unit for endoscopy, the referring doctor must give the patient some idea of what is involved. The instruction document given or sent to the patient with the appointment should also include a written explanation of the proposed procedure (Figs 3.2–3.4), which will contribute to the process of obtaining 'informed consent'. Patients who are already in the hospital should be seen beforehand by a member of the unit staff, to assess the indication for the procedure and its urgency, and to provide some explanation. Wherever the patient comes from, and whatever discussion has gone before, there should always be an opportunity for the patient to discuss the procedure with the doctor and nurse involved.

Informed consent should be obtained in writing before all endoscopic procedures. The extent of the explanation and the type of form used will vary according to the custom of the institution and the laws of the country. All patients (before being relieved of their spectacles) should be asked to sign a form stating that they understand the nature and purpose of the procedure, the possible risks and the alternatives. The doctor should countersign that he has given the patient the necessary information with which to make a judgement.

Sedation, analgesia and monitoring

Endoscopy procedures can be painful, and cause considerable anxiety. Most patients in most countries are given some form of sedation and/or analgesia, often termed 'conscious sedation' to distinguish it from anaesthesia. Since medication-induced respiratory depression is probably the most common cause of endoscopy-related deaths, it is evident that stringent policies should be established and enforced. Anaesthesiologists and their professional bodies are paying increased attention to this area; their advice should be welcomed.

UPPER GI ENDOSCOPY EXPLANATION SHEET

Upper GI endoscopy (OGD)

Upper GI endoscopy — or oesophagogastroduodenoscopy (OGD) — is a visual examination of the lining of your oesophagus, stomach and the first part of your intestine. This is performed by passing a small, long flexible tube through your mouth, under sedation. The doctor will be able to look for any abnormalities which may be present. If necessary, small tissue samples (biopsies) can be taken during the examination (painlessly) for detailed laboratory analysis.

Some treatments can also be done through the endoscope. These include stretching (dilating) narrowed areas of the oesophagus, stomach or duodenum, removing polyps and swallowed objects, and treatment of bleeding vessels and ulcers by internal injection or application of heat (using electrical diathermy, laser or heat probes).

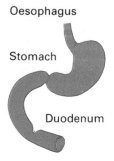

Oesophagus

Stomach

Duodenum

Preparation

Your stomach must be empty, so do not eat or drink anything after midnight. If you must take prescription medication, use only small sips of water. Do not take antacids.

What will happen

The doctor and/or nurse will explain the procedure and answer your questions. Please tell them if you have had any other endoscopic examinations, or any allergies or bad reactions to medications. You will be asked to sign a consent form, giving your permission for the examination. You will need to put on a hospital gown, and to remove your eyeglasses, contact lenses and dentures.

A local anaesthetic will be sprayed onto your throat, to make it numb. You may be given medication by injection through a vein to make you sleepy and relaxed. While in a comfortable position on your left side, the doctor will pass the endoscope through your mouth, and down your throat. A guard will be placed to protect your teeth. The instrument will not interfere with your breathing, nor cause any pain. The examination takes 5–30 minutes.

Afterwards

You will remain in the clinic area for up to 1 hour, until the main effects of any medication wear off. Your throat may feel numb and slightly sore. You should not attempt to eat or drink until your swallowing reflex is normal. After this you may return to your regular diet unless otherwise instructed. You may feel slightly bloated, due to the air which has been introduced through the endoscope; this will quickly pass.

If you have had a sedative injection, a companion *must* be available to drive you home. For the remainder of the day you should not drive a car, operate machinery, or make important decisions, as the sedation impairs your reflexes and judgement.

Risks?

Endoscopy can result in complications such as reactions to medication, perforation (tear) of the intestine, and bleeding. These complications are very rare (less than one in 1000 examinations), but may require urgent treatment, and even an operation. The possibility of complication is greater when the endoscope is used to apply treatment. Be sure to inform us if you have any pain, black tarry stools, or troublesome vomiting in the hours or days after endoscopy.

Questions or problems?

Contact the nurse in charge, Endoscopy Unit (Tel: ....) 8 a.m. to 4.30 p.m. Monday to Friday. At other times, in case of emergency, call the Hospital/Clinic Operator to contact the gastroenterologist on duty.

Fig. 3.2 Explanation sheet for upper endoscopy.

COLONOSCOPY EXPLANATION SHEET

Colonoscopy

Colonoscopy is a visual examination of the lining of your colon (large intestine). A long flexible tube (colonoscope) is passed through the rectum, and around the colon. Through this tube the doctor will be able to look for any abnormalities that may be present. If necessary, small tissue samples (biopsies) can be taken during the examination (painlessly) for laboratory analysis. Polyps (abnormal growths of tissue) can also be removed, using an electric snare wire and areas of bleeding can be treated.

Colon

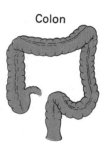

Preparation

To allow a clear view, the colon must be completely free of waste material. You will be given a laxative solution to drink the day before examination, and instructions to remain on clear fluids. Do not eat or drink anything after midnight. If you must take prescription medication, use only small sips of water. Avoid taking aspirin products or any iron preparations for 7 days before the examination.

What will happen

The doctor and/or nurse will explain the procedure and answer your questions. Please tell them if you have had any other endoscopic examinations, or any allergies or bad reactions to medications. You will be asked to sign a consent form, giving your permission to have the procedure performed. You will be asked to put on a hospital gown, and to remove your eyeglasses, contact lenses and dentures.

You will be placed in a comfortable position on your left side, and may be given medication by injection through a vein to make you sleepy and relaxed. The doctor will pass the colonoscope through your anus into the rectum, and advance it through the colon. You may experience some abdominal cramping and pressure from the air which is introduced into your colon. This is normal, and will pass quickly. You may be asked to change your position during the examination, and will be assisted by a nurse. The examination takes 15–60 minutes.

Afterwards

You will remain in the clinic area for up to 1 hour, until the main effects of any medication wear off. A companion *must* be available to drive you home as the sedation impairs your reflexes and judgement. For the remainder of the day you should not drive a car, operate machinery, or make important decisions. We suggest that you rest quietly.

Risks?

Colonoscopy can result in complications, such as reactions to medication, perforation (tear) of the intestine, and bleeding. These complications are very rare (less than one in 1000 examinations), but may require urgent treatment, and even an operation. The risks are slightly higher when the colonoscope is used to apply treatment, such as the removal of polyps. Be sure to inform us if you have any severe pain, bloody stools or troublesome vomiting in the hours or days after colonoscopy.

Questions or problems?

Contact the nurse in charge, Endoscopy Unit (Tel: ....) 8 a.m. to 4.30 p.m. Monday to Friday. At other times, in case of emergency, call the Hospital/Clinic Operator to contact the gastroenterologist on duty.

Fig. 3.3 Explanation sheet for colonoscopy.

ERCP EXPLANATION SHEET

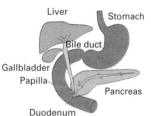

ERCP

ERCP (endoscopic retrograde cholangiopancreatography) is used in the diagnosis of disorders of the pancreas, bile duct, liver and gallbladder. The doctor passes an endoscope (a thin, flexible tube) through your mouth, to inspect your stomach and duodenum. The doctor then injects dye into the drainage hole (papilla) and takes detailed X-rays of the bile ducts and pancreas.

Preparation

To allow a clear view, you should not eat or drink anything after midnight. If you must take prescription medicines, use only small sips of water. Do not take antacids. Since X-rays are taken, you should inform us if there is any possibility of pregnancy.

What will happen

The doctor and/or nurse will explain the procedure and answer your questions. Please tell them if you have had any other endoscopy examinations, or any allergies or bad reactions to medications or dye. You will need to put on a hospital gown, and to remove your eyeglasses, contact lenses and dentures.

The examination is performed on an X-ray table. Local anaesthetic will be sprayed to numb your throat, and you will be given medication by injection through a vein to make you sleepy and relaxed. A guard will be placed to protect your teeth. You will be asked to lie on your left side with your left arm behind you so we can roll you onto your stomach once the procedure starts. While in this position, the doctor will pass the endoscope through your mouth and down your throat. The endoscope will not interfere with your breathing and will not cause any pain. The examination takes 30–90 minutes.

Afterwards

Your throat may feel numb and slightly sore. Because of the local anaesthetic and sedation you should not attempt to take anything by mouth for at least 1 hour. It is wise to keep to clear liquids for the remainder of the day. If you are an out-patient, you will remain in the clinic area for at least 1 hour. A companion *must* be available to drive you home as the sedation impairs your reflexes and judgements. For the remainder of the day you should not drive a car, operate machinery, or make important decisions. We suggest that you rest quietly.

Risks?

Endoscopy can result in complications, such as reactions to medication, perforation (tear) of the intestine, and bleeding. Injection of dye through the endoscope can cause allergic reactions, inflammation of the pancreas (pancreatitis) and of the bile duct (cholangitis). These complications are rare, but may require urgent treatment, and even an operation. Be sure to inform us if you have any pain, fever or vomiting in the 24 hours after ERCP.

Questions or problems?

Contact the nurse in charge, Endoscopy Unit (Tel: ....) 8 a.m. to 4.30 p.m. Monday to Friday. At other times, in case of emergency, call the Hospital/Clinic Operator to contact the gastroenterologist on duty.

ERCP treatments

Sphincterotomy. If the X-rays show a gallstone, or other blockage, the doctor can enlarge the opening of the bile duct at the papilla. This is called 'sphincterotomy', and is done with an electrically heated wire, which you will not feel. Any stones will be removed with a basket or balloon and left to pass through the intestine.

Stenting. A stent is a small plastic tube which is pushed through the endoscope and into a narrowed area in the bile duct. This relieves the obstruction (and any jaundice), by allowing the bile to drain freely into the intestine. Stents are also sometimes placed in the pancreatic duct when it is narrow or blocked.

Nasobiliary tube. Sometimes a small plastic tube is left in the bile duct, and brought out through the nose for a few days. This helps drainage of bile, and allows for further X-rays to be taken to check if the duct is clear. The presence of the tube may be slightly uncomfortable at first, but does not interfere with eating or drinking.

Risks. These treatments for stones and blockage have been developed and are recommended to you because they are simpler and safer than standard surgical operations. However, you should realize that they are not always successful, and problems can arise. Potential complications include perforation of the intestine, bleeding, inflammation of the pancreas (pancreatitis) and infection of the bile duct (cholangitis). These complications are rare, but may be serious enough to require urgent treatment, and even an operation. The risks of your discharge from hospital being delayed for several days by a complication is about 5%; complications may necessitate surgery in about 2% of patients; the risk of death resulting is less than 1%.

Late problems. It is very unusual for biliary problems to recur in the months or years after sphincterotomy, but jaundice, fevers, and even new stones can rarely occur. Usually these can be dealt with by another endoscopic procedure.

Stents can become blocked with debris after many months. This will result in recurrence of jaundice, usually associated with fevers and chills. If this happens, you should inform us or your local doctor within 1 or 2 days. You will need antibiotics, and consideration of a stent change.

Fig. 3.4 Explanation sheet for ERCP.

A few well-motivated and informed patients tolerate (simple) endoscopy procedures without any sedation or analgesia. Most endoscopists use local pharyngeal anaesthesia and a benzodiazepine (intravenously), often supplemented with an opiate analgesic. Our practice for particular procedures and circumstances is discussed in the relevant chapters.

Sedation

Pharyngeal anaesthesia

Pharyngeal anaesthesia (by spray or lozenge) is helpful when using little or no sedation. It is not necessary when using heavy sedation, and may increase the risk of pulmonary aspiration. Spray application is preferred since it can be directed to the posterior pharyngeal wall to suppress the gag reflex. Do not ask the patient to say 'aaah', since this exposes the larynx to anaesthesia, and may suppress the cough reflex.

Benzodiazepines

Diazepam (Valium) is the most popular sedative worldwide. Thrombophlebitis is a problem, particularly in small veins. This is avoided if it is presented in lipid emulsion (Diazemuls, Kabi-Vitrum). Diazepam is given by slow intravenous injection (over 1–2 min). The drug is titrated until the patient has reached an appropriate level of sedation as judged by continuous observation and conversation with the patient. Elderly patients and patients with coexisting pulmonary and hepatic disease are more sensitive than young, healthy patients to the sedative effects of diazepam and its active metabolite, desmethyldiazepam. Therefore, smaller doses should be titrated initially. Conversely, large doses of diazepam may have little effect in patients who have developed a tolerance to benzodiazepines or alcohol. The elimination half-time of diazepam is about 24h even in healthy patients. Large doses of diazepam may produce amnesia beyond the point where the patient appears to be awake and intelligent. Consultations even 2h after the procedure may be forgotten. Motor and cerebral dysfunction may occur for several days post-procedure. Recurrence of sedation 6–8h after diazepam administration may occur secondary to enterohepatic recirculation and the slow metabolism of the active metabolite desmethyldiazepam.

Midazolam (Versed, Dormicum) is a water-soluble benzodiazepine with negligible risk of producing thrombophlebitis. It is two to three times more potent than diazepam and, therefore, smaller doses are given. The amnesia induced by midazolam is more pronounced than after diazepam, which can be a problem, as well as a virtue. Significant hypoxia has occurred when mida-zolam is titrated too quickly, especially in the elderly and patients with coexisting pulmonary and hepatic disease. The elimination half-time of midazolam is 1–4 h in healthy patients. Though elderly patients experience an increased elimination half-time for midazolam and diazepam, the clearance of mida-zolam is more rapid. Central nervous system functions should return to normal more rapidly when midazolam is used com-pared to diazepam.

Analgesia

Opiates

Opioids are used to produce analgesia during endoscopic proce-dures, often in combination with benzodiazepines. Because of the synergism that exists between these classes of drugs, smaller doses of each are titrated to produce the desired end-point of analgesia and sedation. Elderly patients and patients with coex-isting pulmonary disease are sensitive to respiratory depression which may occur when opioids and benzodiazepines are used alone and, particularly, when they are used in combination. Intravenous *pethidine* (Demerol) (25–50 mg), followed by a smaller dose of diazepam (2–10 mg) or midazolam (1–3 mg) is a combination favoured by the authors, especially for younger patients and alcohol abusers. Meperidine is one-tenth as potent as morphine analgesia but is particularly effective in suppress-ing the gag reflex. It also produces useful euphoria in the very anxious without producing disinhibition which can result when high doses of benzodiazepines are used alone.

Fentanyl (Sublimaze) is a potent opioid. It is about 100 times more potent than morphine analgesia, with a rapid onset of action and rapid recovery. However, respiratory depression can be more marked than with pethidine. The use of fentanyl should be reserved for those practitioners experienced in its pharmaco-logical properties.

Naloxone (Narcan) is an opioid antagonist which may shorten the recovery time after examination by reversing the action of opioids. Intravenous administration of 0.2–0.4 mg has a rapid but short-lived effect (30–45 min) and it is therefore usually wise also to give the same dose intramuscularly. In painful pro-cedures, judicious use of naloxone may be warranted as acute reversal of opioid-induced analgesia may produce pain, hyper-tension, tachycardia and even pulmonary oedema.

Alternative medications

Droperidol, a neuroleptic agent, can be useful in sedating patients who are agitated, and appears particularly helpful in alcoholics.

Droperidol is given in increments of 0.5 mg up to 3.0 mg (occasionally 5.0 mg) in total. The blood pressure should be monitored carefully since hypotension can occur. Several centres use self-administered *nitrous oxide gas*, with good reported effects; recovery is almost instantaneous. It is sometimes necessary to suppress intestinal peristalsis, particularly during ERCP. Suitable agents include *Buscopan* (hyoscine N-butylbromide, 20–40 mg) and *glucagon* (0.1–0.5 mg i.v.).

General anaesthesia

General anaesthesia may be required in special circumstances, such as complex procedures in young children and for uncontrollable patients in whom normal sedative regimens are ineffective (alcoholics, drug addicts, etc.); it is safer than excessive doses of intravenous 'conscious' sedation. *Propofol* (Diprivan) has become a popular agent among anaesthetists.

Patient monitoring

The status of the patient during and after the procedure should be monitored by a trained nurse and the results documented (Fig. 3.5). The doctor (and other assistants) are often preoccupied with the technical complexities of the procedure. The nurse ensures that the airway and respiration are maintained and monitors vital signs (pulse, blood pressure, respiration and level of consciousness). A case is being made by some experts for giving oxygen continuously during all endoscopic procedures. Certainly oxygen should be readily available, along with resuscitation equipment and antidotes to sedatives.

The degree to which electronic monitoring is used varies considerably between countries. Although not mandatory, pulse oximeter monitoring is now standard practice in the USA. Continuous electrocardiographic monitoring is used selectively in patients with cardiac problems.

Discharge

Patients are observed in a recovery area after the procedure. The duration and intensity depends on the complexity of the procedure, the state of the patient and the degree of sedation. The patient and accompanying person should receive *written* discharge instructions (Fig. 3.6).

GI ENDOSCOPY NURSE REPORT

Patient name:

Procedure:

Date:

Performed by:

Scope number:

Time: Start: End:

i.v. started by unit/   Site: With: Fluids:

Assessment/Consent completed: Yes/No   Monitor attached: Yes/No

TIME	BP	PULSE	RESP	O$_2$SAT	LOC	MEDICATIONS (dose in mg) Local anaesthetic spray	COMMENTS Yes/No

Biopsies taken: Yes/No   Number of containers: Cytology: Yes/No

Diathermy used: Yes/No   Ground plate location: Settings:

Photos: Yes/No   35 mm/Videoprint/Videotape

Comments:

Signature/Title:

POST-PROCEDURE

TIME	BP	PULSE	RESP	LOC*	COMMENTS

*LOC = Level of consciousness

6 = Fully awake

5 = Easily aroused

4 = Arousable, may be confused

3 = Aroused only by vigorous stimuli, cannot communicate

2 = Responds only to pain

1 = Unresponsive

Discharged to: Time: With:

Discharge instruction sheet given:

Comments:

Signature/Title:

Fig. 3.5 Nursing flowsheet and report.

DISCHARGE INSTRUCTIONS

You have undergone a procedure called: Upper GI endoscopy (OGD)/Colonoscopy/ERCP/
Sigmoidoscopy with: ....

This procedure has been performed by Dr ....

1 It is essential that someone accompany you home if you received sedation. If so you
should not: drive a car, operate machinery, or drink any alcohol. The effects of the test
and medications should wear off by the next day and you will be able to resume
normal activities.

2 You may resume your normal diet unless otherwise instructed by your doctor.

3 You may resume your normal prescription medicines.

4 There may be some slight soreness where the instruments have been, but this will
wear off in a day or so.

5 Some bloating may be experienced if air has remained in your gastrointestinal tract
(stomach and/or bowel) and will resolve within a few hours.

6 Things to report to your doctor:
   – severe pain or vomiting
   – passage or vomiting of blood
   – temperature greater than 101°F/38°C
   – redness, tenderness and swelling at site of i.v. that persists for more than 48

7 Further advice about your condition and treatment will be given at your next clinic
appointment.

8 If specimens have been taken for analysis, the results may take several days.

9 If you have any questions or concerns, call the Endoscopy Unit (Tel: ....)
8 a.m. to 4.30 p.m. Monday to Friday, or at any other times call the Hospital/Clinic
Operator and ask for the gastroenterologist on call.

Fig. 3.6 Written discharge instructions.

Infection, endocarditis and antibiotic prophylaxis

Endocarditis

Bacteraemia occurs after many GI procedures (even after digital
rectal examination). The possible risk of provoking endocarditis,
and the value of antibiotic prophylaxis, has been much discussed. The overall risk is vanishingly small, and some argue
that the costs and risks of antibiotic prophylaxis are not justified.
Professional organizations have provided guidelines, based on
thoughtful consensus rather than scientific data. All support a

selective approach, emphasizing the need for prophylaxis in patients with 'high-risk' lesions (e.g. prosthetic heart valves and prior endocarditis) undergoing 'high-risk' procedures (in terms of bacteraemia), particularly variceal sclerotherapy and oesophageal dilatation. Most authorities also mention other cardiac lesions such as congenital cardiac malformations, rheumatic and acquired valve disease, hypertrophic cardiac myopathy and surgically constructed systemic pulmonary shunts. The importance of mitral valve prolapse is controversial.

The latest guidlines of the ASGE (published May 1995), which were developed in conjunction with the American Heart Association, actually *reduced* the recommended indications for antibiotics. Our guidelines for prophylaxis against endocarditis reflect this 'minimalist' strategy, which has the merit of simplicity.

We recommend that antibiotics should be given to all patients with:

1 prosthetic heart valves;
2 surgically constructed systemic pulmonary shunts;
3 a prior history of endocarditis;
4 a synthetic vascular graft less than 1 year old.

This applies to all flexible endoscopic procedures.

The usual regimen is parenteral ampicillin 1–2 g and gentamicin 1.5 mg/kg 30 min prior to the procedure. The same combination is repeated at 8 h (or a single oral dose of 1.5 g of amoxycillin). Patients who are allergic to penicillin are given vancomycin instead (1 g by slow i.v. infusion over 1 h).

The data are not sufficient to recommend routine prophylaxis in patients with other cardiac lesions, even in patients undergoing procedures with a higher risk of bacteraemia (e.g. variceal sclerosis, oesophageal dilatation).

Infection risks other than endocarditis

The special risks resulting from ERCP are discussed in the relevant chapters. Prophylactic antibiotics appear to reduce the risk of skin infection after percutaneous endoscopic gastrostomy or jejunostomy. Bacteraemia is common in patients with cirrhosis and ascites; prophylaxis with a broad spectrum cephalosporin or oral amoxycillin seems appropriate.

There is no evidence to support the routine use of antibiotics in patients with orthopaedic prostheses or prostheses in other non-cardiac and non-vascular sites.

Most authorities recommend antibiotics before interventional procedures in patients who are neutropenic or heavily immunocompromised (e.g. after bone marrow or solid organ transplantation).

It is important to emphasize that the decision for and against antibiotic prophylaxis belongs to the endoscopist, who is responsible for any adverse result. He should be mindful of the guidelines of his unit and national, professional organizations, and also of opinions expressed by the patient which usually reflect the advice of relevant specialists (e.g. cardiologists).

Instrument cleaning and disinfection

The infectious hazards of endoscopy received regrettably little interest in earlier years. Nowadays, there can be few endoscopists who are unaware of the need for proper cleaning and disinfection of endoscopes and accessories—and all endoscopy units worthy of the name have adopted rigorous standards. The need to face up to laborious and time-consuming cleaning routines was forced by a combination of awareness of the acquired immune deficiency syndrome (AIDS), individual case reports of *Salmonella* transmission and the realization that ERCP can provoke life-threatening sepsis unless the highest standards are applied. The risk of transmitting *Helicobacter pylori* is also pertinent. Even if the endoscope itself has been properly disinfected, catastrophe can originate from bacterial colonization of the water bottle or from inside the spiral wire of the biopsy forceps; even when instruments and accessories have been scrupulously managed, the results are useless if the mains water supply or a reprocessor (washing machine) proves to be contaminated with *Pseudomonas*.

Whereas certain procedures (e.g. ERCP), and certain patients (e.g. the immunocompromised) are obviously at a higher risk, in practice the correct attitude is *one standard for all*, since it is impossible to identify either carriers of pathogenic organisms or those who may be at an increased susceptibility to them. This is the principle of '*universal precautions*', in which continuously high standards throughout are the routine so that everyone, staff and patients alike, knows that they are protected. There are different interpretations of this irrevocable rule in different countries, and the degree of regulation varies. What follows is a synthesis of the recommendations of UK and US professional associations and represents a reasonable viewpoint in the mid 1990s.

A recent draft report of a multisociety American Ad Hoc Committee on Disinfection is reproduced in full (Fig. 3.7).

We realize that changes of materials, disinfectants and working practices may outdate these current views. For more detailed accounts the reader should consult other local sources and manufacturers' representatives. Infection control experts should also be welcomed as partners in this important exercise; they should be invited to participate in defining unit policies, and in monitoring their effectiveness.

AD HOC COMMITTEE ON DISINFECTION

The Ad Hoc Committee on Disinfection has developed recommendations for the disinfection of gastrointestinal endoscopes. This important 2-year project employed a thorough review of existing guidelines and the scientific literature and collaboration with representatives from the Food and Drug Administration (FDA), the Society of Gastrointestinal Nurses and Associates (SGNA), the Communicable Disease Center (CDC), and the American Practitioners of Infection Control (APIC). The Committee's recommendations, which have been approved, in concept, by the Governing Boards of both the ASGE and SGNA, are printed below in their entirety.

Recommendations of the ASGE Ad Hoc Committee on Disinfection

The following report represents a 2-year study of the appropriate reprocessing of gastrointestinal endoscopes. Inherent to these recommendations was a major emphasis on the importance of manual pre-cleaning prior to either manual or automated reprocessing with a disinfectant/sterilant solution. High-level disinfection was considered the appropriate standard of care for reprocessing gastrointestinal endoscopes. Specific recommendations include the following:

1 Each individual gastrointestinal endoscopy unit should have an effective quality assurance program with special emphasis on cleaning and disinfecting fiberoptic and video gastrointestinal endoscopes.

2 Each individual endoscopy unit must draft or adopt a clearly written, detailed cleaning and disinfection protocol. This should include structures and processes which:
   (a) Emphasize the manual pre-soaking and cleaning of gastrointestinal endoscopes as the first and most important step in removing the organic and microbial burden from an endoscope.
   (b) Permit only those individuals who have the ability to read and understand and implement instructions on the proper cleaning and disinfecting of endoscopes to reprocess such instruments.
   (c) Only individuals who have met written endoscopic processing competency standards should reprocess endoscopes. Temporary personnel should, under no circumstances, be allowed to manually pre-clean or disinfect instruments in a manual or automated endoscopic reprocessor.
   (d) Infection control education is a critical part of the orientation and continued education in the gastrointestinal endoscopic setting. It is to be emphasized that no endoscopic reprocessors replace manual pre-cleaning of the entire endoscope.

3 Certain endoscopes, especially ERCP/duodenoscopes, may require special reprocessing techniques. The elevator channel of the ERCP scopes will require additional manual cleaning and disinfection.

4 Special attention should be paid to prevent cross contamination in the endoscopic procedure room.

5 Endoscopic reprocessing should occur in a room separate from the performance of the gastrointestinal endoscopic procedure.

6 In the context of a strict quality assurance program for the manual pre-cleaning and disinfecting of gastrointestinal endoscopes, a 20-minute exposure time at 20°C to a verified active 2.4% glutaraldehyde solution is adequate for disinfection of gastrointestinal endoscopes after effective manual cleaning.

7 OSHA guidelines clearly impact on gastrointestinal nurses, assistants, technicians, and gastroenterologists. It is important that each gastrointestinal endoscopic unit be familiar with and adhere to OSHA guidelines.

8 The Ad Hoc Committee recommended that the American Practitioners of Infection Control (APIC) guidelines be followed with regard to the reporting of infections identified in individual gastrointestinal units. This notification should include:
   (a) Those responsible for institutional control.
   (b) The FDA.
   (c) The State Health Department.
   (d) The Centers for Disease Control and Prevention.
   (e) The manufacturer (manufacturers).

9 Manufacturers' recommendations to achieve high-level disinfection would be appropriate for solutions other than the 2.4% glutaraldehyde disinfectant/sterilant. It is important that a test strip, specific for the concentration of the glutaraldehyde solution, be used to monitor the potency of such solutions. This should be done each day of use of the gastrointestinal reprocessing or more frequently in units with high-volume use.

10 Because it is impossible to sufficiently clean and disinfect endoscopes that cannot be completely immersed in liquid, the use of nonimmersable endoscopes is now unacceptable in gastroenterology.

11 The ASTM/FDA Committee report, 'Standard Practice for Cleaning and Disinfection of Flexible Fiberoptic and Video Endoscopes Used in the Examination of Hollow Viscera', with the modifications or emphasis described above, is considered an appropriate document as a guideline for gastrointestinal reprocessing. A narrative, more user-friendly document for use at endoscopy centers by technicians, nurses, or physicians is in the process of being completed and will be made available to the ASGE and SGNA memberships and other individuals interested in the reprocessing of gastrointestinal endoscopes.

12 The ASGE and SGNA Governing Boards support increased research for the important area of endoscopic reprocessing and strongly encourage manufacturers to develop future gastrointestinal endoscopes that can be more easily disassembled for greater ease and verification of the cleaning and disinfection process.

Fig. 3.7 Draft report of the American Ad Hoc Committee on Disinfection (1995).

Disinfection or sterilization?

Higher standards are needed in endoscopy than in a bar or restaurant because of the selective concentration of risky organisms and at-risk patients. However, there are different levels of risks, which define the disinfection needs. *Critical accessories* are those which enter body cavities and the vasculature or penetrate mucous membranes; examples include biopsy forceps, sclerotherapy needles and sphincterotomes. These require formal sterilization. *Semicritical accessories* are those which come into contact with mucous membranes, e.g. endoscopes and oesophageal dilators. These require high-level disinfection. *Noncritical accessories* come into contact with intact skin, and require only low-level disinfection; examples include cameras and endoscopic furniture. The important distinction in practice is between endoscopes and their accessories—at least those which may breach the mucosa or enter sterile duct systems (e.g. biopsy forceps and catheters). Most accessories can be sterilized (see below).

Flexible endoscopes cannot be formally sterilized. High-level disinfection kills bacteria and viruses (and *Mycobacterium tuberculosis*), but not necessarily spores. Disinfectants are assessed on their 'log kill' capability on the basis that, for a given concentration, perhaps 99.9% of test organisms may be rapidly inactivated by the disinfectant whereas the remaining few may be more resistant. As a generalization, much of the effect of a disinfectant is in the first few seconds, with full clinical efficacy after a minute or two of exposure. 'Exposure' presumes chemical contact, which may be achieved in the test system but not in working practice if mucus, blood and other organic matter acts as a physical barrier, reacts chemically to neutralize the disinfectant or, as is often the case, a combination of both. Glutaraldehyde, for instance, reacts with organic matter, denaturing it into a hard impenetrable layer which protects underlying infective agents— hence the need for excellent preliminary mechanical and detergent cleaning.

'Infectivity' is an important parallel concept. For most infections such as hepatitis B or salmonellosis, a substantial dose of the infective agent is needed to penetrate body defences and cause clinical illness. On the other hand, introducing a single *Pseudomonas* organism into the perfect culture medium of a stagnant biliary system could theoretically achieve colonization and cholangitis. Infectivity is also the experimental gold standard for assessing the success or failure of a disinfection regimen. Since this requires a suitable animal model, it is not surprising that data are scarce. The recommendations for disinfection exposure are therefore based on a body of expert clinical, bacteriological and virological experience, with an extra 'safety factor' deliberately built in. Most infective agents, with the notable exception of mycobacterial spores, are rather easily inactivated; reassuringly, the AIDS virus is extremely sensitive to disinfectants and even hepatitis B virus (contrary to early reports) is no more resistant than representative bacteria.

The choice of disinfectant is inevitably constrained by the materials used in endoscope construction, particularly the delicate silicone rubber covering of the bending section, the bonding agents used in the lens mounting and elsewhere, and the waterproofing rubber seals in the control head. Even in this respect there is some latitude; for instance short (3–4 min) repeated exposure of the bending section to 70% ethyl alcohol is reported to have no damaging effect during thousands of test immersions, whereas long continued exposure is damaging. Ask the manufacturers before you consider using a new cleaning or disinfection agent.

Mechanical cleaning

Thorough cleaning to remove all blood, mucus, other body secretions or organic debris is the first and main essential in the disinfection process, so that the chemical agent(s) subsequently employed can penetrate for effective bacterial or viral inactivation. Detergents of any kind, but especially enzyme detergents, are useful in removing organic matter and blood, both in areas which can be reached for brushing, swabbing or other methods of physical cleaning and for perfusing the inaccessible parts such as the air and water channels of an endoscope. Non-foaming domestic enzyme detergents can be used in endoscope washing machines. Accessories, which include the air/water and suction buttons, toothguard, water bottles and the cleaning brushes, must all be cleaned equally scrupulously (see below).

Leak testing

Instruments should be inspected carefully and leak tested to avoid subsequent inward leakage of fluids resulting in damage and expensive repairs. Leak testing is done by inflating the endoscope shaft under pressure, paying particular attention to the rubber of the bending section.

Water supply

Excellence of the water supply should not be assumed. Surprisingly large particles can be present with potential for blockage of the smaller endoscope channels and clogging of the filters of a reprocessor. The water supply or its pipework can become the source of *Pseudomonas* contamination, rendering useless during the final rinse of an instrument all the careful disinfection which has gone before. We recommend installation of an in-line bacterial filter which effectively produces a sterile water supply.

Disinfectants

Glutaraldehyde

Glutaraldehyde (2% alkaline solution) and closely related products constitute the only disinfectants which can be globally recommended for endoscopic use at the present time. It destroys all viruses and bacteria within 4 min, is non-corrosive and has a low surface tension which helps penetration. Glutaraldehyde is related chemically to formaldehyde, and has similar toxic effects on human skin and mucous membranes, with the capability of causing severe dermatitis, sinusitis or asthma. Unless closed-system washing machines and excellent ventilation/extraction systems are used, there is a serious risk of sensitization of endoscopy staff, the risk increasing with increasing levels and time of exposure. Heavy domestic-grade rubber gloves should be worn when using glutaraldehyde since normal thin medical glove material is permeable to it, and goggles and/or a face mask can protect against splashes. Alternatives to glutaraldehyde are being investigated. Peracetic acid and some quaternary ammonium compounds have been proposed.

Ethyl alcohol

Ethyl alcohol (70%) soaking for 4 min may be acceptable after 2 min in a bactericidal detergent. Alcohol constitutes a fire hazard; handling and disposal must be carefully regulated.

Rinsing and drying

The disinfectant must be removed from the instrument completely by flushing all the channels. Bacteria multiply in a moist environment; the importance of drying instruments after disinfection cannot be overemphasized. The drying properties of alcohol are useful in this regard. The air, water and suction channels should be perfused with 70% alcohol and dried with forced air before storage: This removes any residual water, which otherwise leads to a risk of bacterial regrowth when the endoscope is stored overnight. Instruments should be hung vertically in a well-ventilated cupboard; the transportation suitcase should not be used for storage between examinations because its absorbent lining cannot be disinfected and the closed, potentially moist, atmosphere inside can encourage growth of micro-organisms. If vertical storage is impractical (long enteroscopes, travel, etc.), the risks of colonization must be addressed by assiduous disinfection *before* each examination.

Cleaning facilities

Although initial endoscope flushing should be done immediately in the endoscopy room, formal cleaning and disinfection procedures should take place in a purpose-designed area. There should be clearly defined and separated clean and dirty areas, multiple worktops, double sinks and a separate hand wash-basin, endoscopic reprocessors (washing machines) and an ultrasound cleaner. Suction and compressed air should be available. Good ventilation/extraction facilities are essential. The room should have at least 10 air exchanges per hour. An appropriately placed fume hood is also desirable.

Reprocessors (washing machines)

A variety of endoscope reprocessors, manual, semiautomatic and automatic, are available. Most take only a single scope, some take two or more at a time. Some require special three-phase electricity supply and high-pressure water input; others are mobile with tanks that must be filled or emptied by hand before and after the session. Some include the control head of the instrument and its accessories in the wash/rinse/disinfect/rinse/dry cycles; others do not. In deciding which machine to purchase an on-site trial is strongly advised, to ensure that the staff concerned are satisfied, that all routine scopes can be handled by it and that the machine is suitable for the space available. Take advice from expert centres.

Remember that reprocessors *do not* remove the need for scrupulous mechanical cleaning. They do reduce exposure to glutaraldehyde, ensure properly timed perfusion cycles and release staff for other more productive activities during the disinfection period. Care is needed for periodic disinfection of the reprocessor itself, especially any reservoirs, and attention must be paid to the tendency for gradual dilution of the disinfectant. The concentration can be assayed directly with test strips, and replaced as necessary.

Routine endoscope cleaning and disinfection

All endoscopes marketed now are fully immersible and have been designed to facilitate cleaning and disinfection. Their major advantage over earlier equipment lies not just in their immersibility, but in the ability to irrigate all channels with positive pressure. Most endoscopes have three channels; suction/biopsy, air and water. Side-viewers fitted with a bridge/elevator have a fourth smaller channel which carries the bridge elevator cable and others may have a separate injection channel. All channels must be included in the cleaning and disinfection process, as all are potential reservoirs for transmissible infection.

External cleaning

If the instrument has just been removed from a patient, flush the air/water channel for 10–15 s to eject any refluxed blood or mucus (a special cleaning air/water channel adaptor is available for some endoscopes to force flush these channels selectively). Aspirate detergent through the biopsy/suction channel for about 10–15 s to remove gross debris.

Totally immerse the instrument in warm water and neutral detergent. Wash the outside of the instrument thoroughly with gauze swabs. Brush the distal end with a soft toothbrush, paying particular attention to the air/water outlet jet and bridge/elevator where fitted. All valves are removed (air/water, suction and biopsy valves) and are cleaned and disinfected as described separately. Additional valves should be available for busy lists. Clean the biopsy channel opening and suction port using a cotton bud.

Brushing through the suction/biopsy channel

Use a clean brush suitable for the instrument and channel size, and brush through the suction channel several times until clean, in the steps described below, and clean the cleaning brush itself in detergent with a soft toothbrush each time it emerges.
1 Introduce the cleaning brush via the biopsy port, through the shaft, until it emerges from the distal end at least three times.
2 Pass the cleaning brush through the suction channel opening (having removed the suction button) and down the shaft until it emerges from the distal end at least three times.
3 Pass the cleaning brush from the suction channel opening in the other direction, through the umbilical, until it emerges from the suction connector at least three times.

After the channel has been thoroughly brushed, either put the endoscope into a reprocessor to complete cleaning and disinfection, or alternatively follow the manual method described below.

Flushing the internal channels

Flush each internal channel with detergent fluid. This should be done independently for each separate channel. Alternatively, an all-channel irrigator supplied by the manufacturer may be used, but, if so, ensure that detergent is seen to emerge through the air/water nozzle at the distal end of the insertion tube and out of the water and suction (and, on colonoscopes, carbon dioxide) connectors on the light guide. It is essential to confirm that all air is expelled from the channels.

On scopes with a bridge/elevator, attach the bridge channel adaptor and flush this additional channel using a 2 ml syringe.

Some endoscopes also incorporate an auxiliary washing channel which should be flushed similarly. Flush all channels as above using clean water followed by air to expel as much water as possible prior to disinfection.

Disinfection

If a closed system is not available, disinfection should be carried out under a fume canopy, wearing gloves and an eye shield. Totally immerse the instrument in 2% glutaraldehyde (or an approved alternative disinfectant). Fill each internal channel with disinfectant and leave the instrument for the recommended contact time. A clock timer should be used for accuracy.

Rinsing

Following disinfection, rinse the instruments internally and externally to remove all traces of disinfectant, using the all-channel irrigator.

Drying

Dry the endoscope externally, paying particular attention to the light guide connector and eye piece. Flush air through each channel, preferably using a compressed air source, or reconnect the endoscope to the light source (or the special pump supplied by the manufacturers) and fit the disinfected valves. Switch on the pump and expel the fluid from the air/water channel by simultaneously occluding the water bottle connector on the endoscope and depressing the air/water valve. Connect the instrument to the suction system and dry the suction channel by depressing the suction valve several times.

Practical decisions — disinfectant and timing

Most authorities agree on the general principles of cleaning and disinfection as described above. Endoscopy unit directors have to make several very practical decisions. The important questions include:

1 Which disinfectant?
2 How long to soak?
3 Disinfect *before* sessions?

Sources of advice include the instrument manufacturers, professional organizations dealing with endoscopy, nursing and infection control, and safety regulations. These vary between countries and institutions. Manufacturers of disinfectants and machines also offer advice.

Glutaraldehyde is still the most popular disinfectant, but recommended soak times vary between 4, 10, 20 and 45 min. The longer times are particularly recommended when a scope may have been exposed to *Mycobacterium tuberculosis*, and *before* use in immunocompromised patients and before ERCP. Even longer soak periods (90–120 min) have been recommended in patients with known infection with *M. avium intracellulare* or other highly resistant mycobacteria. The American Ad Hoc Committee on Disinfection recommends a 20 min soak time for standard situations, assuming adequate pre-cleaning (see Fig. 3.7).

Should all endoscopes be re-disinfected *before* starting an endoscopy list? The answer is yes for high-risk patients and procedures (e.g. immunocompromised patients and ERCP), but there may be some latitude for other routine procedures. It clearly depends on how long instruments remain disinfected. Simple tests after proper cleaning and disinfecting (and drying) show no significant contamination after overnight storage. Thus, many busy units do not re-disinfect routine upper scopes and colonoscopes every morning if they have been used on the previous work day. This is certainly simpler for the staff, but the purist may be unhappy. If pre-disinfection is not the routine, there must be some way of knowing when the instrument was last disinfected.

Documentation and validation

The disinfection policy should be written down and understood by all staff. Ensuring and documenting adherence to the policy is a crucial responsibility of the unit director and head nurse. A record should be made after each endoscope is cleaned and disinfected, at the simplest a tag should be left on it with the date and time of the procedure, but better still the endoscope should be left with a completed and initialled proforma (which can be kept for medicolegal purposes). Routine bacteriological test cultures are not essential once a disinfection routine has been established and initially validated, but should be done whenever there is any change of routine and may be undertaken on an occasional basis, especially for ERCP instruments. A bile culture taken during ERCP, looking for *Pseudomonas*, is probably the most critical test as well as the most clinically relevant.

Endoscopic accessories

Endoscopic accessories should be sterilized by standard techniques (i.e. autoclave or ethylene oxide gas). Complex instruments (e.g. spiral guidewires and sphincterotomes) are increasingly supplied for one-time use. Disposability solves the sterility problem, but also increases the cost substantially.

Reusable accessories (including water bottles) must be cleaned and sterilized between procedures.

1 Wash immediately after use in fresh detergent solution.

2 Dismantle as far as possible; remove the handles and withdraw the inner parts where these exist — for example, remove snare wires from sheaths and inner tubes from injection needles.

3 Brush away adherent debris with a cleaning brush or toothbrush.

4 Flush the detergent solution through the lumens of all the hollow components using the syringe attachments where these are available.

5 Place in an ultrasonic cleaner. It is almost impossible to clean complex metal items (e.g. biopsy forceps) without this facility.

6 Rinse thoroughly, flushing the lumens of hollow items well, blow dry and place in a pack for sterilization.

7 Sterilize by the method most appropriate to the local environment:

(a) steam autoclaving (where recommended by the manufacturer, since some plastics melt);

(b) ethylene oxide gas; or

(c) low-temperature steam and formaldehyde.

A portable electric autoclave on site is practical and inexpensive.

Logistical consequences of disinfection

Following the above recommendations for proper cleaning and using even the shortest disinfection exposure times (whether manually or by machine) means that endoscopes cannot be 'turned around' in less than about 30 min. It follows that at least two endoscopes are required for a busy list (as well as others for backup purposes in case of breakage), and that a nurse or assistant will be kept busy full-time in managing the cleaning routines. Disassembly, cleaning, disinfection and re-assembly of accessories, and their packing and transmission for sterilization, is time-consuming and requires an appropriate number of extra accessories. These are conveniently stored in see-through sealed bags for immediate use when required.

Endoscopy environmental hazards

Patients and staff may be exposed to hazards other than those directly due to the procedures (and sedation).

Electrical hazards

The combinations of various fluids and electric cables constitute an obvious potential risk. Commonsense precautions should be taken. Electric cables should be suspended if possible and electric devices should not be used carelessly (e.g. using the light source as a worktop). Inappropriate use of electrosurgical apparatus (e.g. inadequate grounding) has caused injuries. There has been concern about the use of electrocautery in patients with implanted cardiac devices (e.g. pacemakers). However, there is probably no hazard with low-power units, abdominal procedures and a distant patient plate (e.g. on the thigh). The ASGE Technology Assessment Committee recommends deactivating any implantable cardioverter defibillator during endoscopic electrosurgery.

Radiation

Staff working in procedure rooms with X-rays should wear protective aprons and exposure badges. Thyroid shields and special glasses may be appropriate for those with more frequent exposure. All staff and practices should be supervised by a radiation safety officer.

Lasers

Some lasers use high-power electrical sources which can constitute an electrical and fire hazard. Laser beams can cause immediate and irreversible eye damage. Appropriate room design, security and protective eyewear are mandatory. The smoke and laser plume is a hazard, especially during tumour ablation treatments. Viable cells and viral particles have been recovered from the plume. Focal venting and special laser goggles and masks should be available.

Toxic agents

The need for staff to be protected from the hazards of glutaraldehyde and alcohol have been mentioned. Other toxic substances (e.g. solid carbon dioxide) are sometimes employed in endoscopy units, and should be managed appropriately. All drugs must be managed professionally and safely.

Infection risks for staff

Endoscopists and assistants are at risk of cross-infection from patient fluids. All staff should wear gloves and water-resistant gowns. Video-endoscopes have somewhat reduced the risk of splashing to the eyes, but there is a strong case for using a face shield, particularly when working close to the patient (or the endoscope biopsy valve) in high-risk situations such as bleeding. Frequent hand washing, rigorous use of paper towels or gauzes when handling soiled accessories, putting soiled items directly into a sink or designated area (not on clean surfaces), covering sores or skin wounds with a waterproof dressing and general maintenance of good hygienic practice throughout the unit is more logical and safe than dressing up as for outer space and then being unthinkingly messy.

Needle-stab injuries are a particular worry. Safety can be enhanced by a rigid attitude towards the immediate disposal of sharps, and avoiding re-sheathing of needles. Use a toothpick rather than a needle for handling small biopsy specimens. A needle-free environment is feasible and desirable (using a stop cock for injections). Spiked biopsy forceps are also a potential problem. The literature suggests that even when a needle-stick injury has occurred, human immunodeficiency virus (HIV) sero-conversion is fortunately almost unknown. Hepatitis B is a greater risk; immunization should be routine for all endoscopy staff, with their antibody status checked.

Complications

We all hope and plan for our procedures to be successful, pain-less and uncomplicated—but must recognize that some adverse outcomes are unavoidable. Positive outcomes are discussed in Chapter 12 and specific complications are discussed in relevant sections.

The word complication carries an unfortunate connotation; it suggests blame or malpractice. Some complications certainly arise from negligence, but the vast majority do not. This is the essence and importance of truly informed consent; the patient signs regarding potential benefits *and* risks.

We cannot measure bad outcomes or complications without agreed definitions. The first difficulty is to define the threshold. Many undesired events occur during and after complex procedures; at what level do they become sufficiently im-portant to be called complications? Few endoscopists would count a transient drop in oxygen saturation, or minor self-limited oozing after sphincterotomy, or local phlebitis after an injection of diazepam. We suggest defining a complication as an undesired event which needs management by a doctor after the procedure is completed, and which requires in-patient hos-pital care — either unplanned admission or prolongation of planned stay.

Other undesired events not reaching this threshold need a dif-ferent descriptor — maybe *incidents*. They should be mentioned in the procedure report, but not counted in the complication statistics.

Complications are categorized by *nature* (type) and whether they are *focal* or *non-specific*. Focal complications are those which occur at the point of endoscopic contact (e.g. perforation, bleed-ing, pancreatitis). Non-specific complications are problems which occur in organs which have not been traversed or touched (e.g. cardiopulmonary or renal problems).

Timing categories are also important.

1 *Immediate complications* are evident during or shortly after completion of the procedure.

2 *Early complications* present within the immediate recovery period (i.e. within a few hours); examples include pancreatitis after ERCP, and bleeding after polypectomy.

3 *Delayed complications* occur after the patient leaves initial supervision, up to an arbitrary time limit. A 30-day cut-off seems reasonable for direct focal complications, but may be much too long for non-specific adverse events. Most of us would probably not wish to count a myocardial event if it occurred 29 days after a routine endoscopy procedure. However, we might well accept an aetiological connection if the same event occurred within a few days (especially if we had changed the medications, such as anticoagulants or non-steroidal anti-inflammatory drugs). We therefore suggest a time limit of 3 days for delayed non-specific complications.

4 *Late complications* are adverse events which are obviously connected with the procedure, but which may not present for many months or years; examples include oesophageal stricturing after sclerotherapy or stenosis after sphincterotomy.

Another category of complication has been introduced in the surgical literature — that of adverse sequelae. This indicates an undesirable but inevitable result of the procedure (e.g. loss of the leg when amputating for cancer of the toe). Examples in the endoscopic field include the loss of sphincter activity inherent in balloon dilatation for achalasia and sphincterotomy for stones; both may have adverse consequences (e.g. oesophageal reflux and bacterobilia).

Adverse events also vary widely in severity — from trivial to fatal. Complication rates cannot be assessed or compared unless they include a measure of severity. Most experts considering this problem have devised stratifications based on the discomfort or inconvenience which they cause to the patient. Indices which might be used include loss of work, repeated medical consultations, hospitalization, intensive care and unexpected additional interventions (e.g. interventional radiology or surgery).

We have published a simple scale for grading the severity of complications.

1 *Grade 1 (mild):* requires hospitalization for 1–3 days.

2 *Grade 2 (moderate):* requires hospitalization for 4–10 days.

3 *Grade 3 (severe):* requires hospitalization for more than 10 days or intensive care or surgery.

4 *Grade 4 (fatal):* death due to an immediate, early or delayed complication (as defined above).

It is important also to decide what constitutes an 'endoscopic procedure'. This is not just the period of intubation; it should include preparation and early recovery, say the whole period of sedation or anaesthesia. For completeness, we should also count adverse reactions to the preparation (e.g. prophylactic antibiotics or problems during bowel preparation), even if the endoscopy never takes place.

Managing complications and medicolegal issues

All active endoscopists will encounter complications. It is essential to understand the basic principles of management, and the types of behaviour which will provide most protection for the patient, and for yourself in the event of legal action. Most complications do not lead to lawsuits, even in litigious countries. Lack of communication is the main cause of trouble. The doctor who takes time to go through the informed consent process thoroughly with the patient and relatives, and establishes a caring relationship, will be in a good position to help them through any complications and to avoid medicolegal problems. It is essential to recognize an adverse event quickly (or to consider the possibility), to communicate your thoughts appropriately with the patient and others involved and to act decisively. For medical endoscopists, this often means obtaining a surgical consultation early (although the indications for surgical intervention are limited). It is necessary to be professional, attentive and sympathetic, without becoming obsequious or apparently wracked with guilt. We may feel very bad about the complications, but profuse apologies are usually misinterpreted. Make sure you continue to visit the patient, and talk with the relatives, if a patient is transferred to another service (intensive care or surgery). It can be tough to do, but failure will look like abandonment and disinterest.

The best defence against a claim for malpractice (apart from being properly trained and doing procedures only for accepted indications), is to document everything compulsively. The cliche states 'if it is not written down, it was not done'. This applies to the process of informed consent, the procedure report and the chart records of early recognition and appropriate, prompt management (including consultation requests). The worst errors are to downplay a patient's complaint, to delay investigation and management, and to fail to get appropriate help when necessary. Never be tempted to alter chart records; this can be detected and is surely an admission of guilt.

Resuscitation equipment and training

It is self-evident, but important to emphasize, that endoscopy staff must be ready to deal with any emergency. Endoscopists and assistants should be trained in resuscitation methods, and a fully stocked emergency cart must be available close by. Policies and equipment should be checked and tested on a regular basis and documented.

Further reading

Sedation and monitoring

American Society for Gastrointestinal Endoscopy. *Monitoring Equipment for Endoscopy*. ASGE Technology Assessment Status Evaluation. Manchester: American Society for Gastrointestinal Endoscopy, 1994.

American Society for Gastrointestinal Endoscopy. *Sedation and Monitoring of Patients Undergoing Gastrointestinal Procedures*. ASGE Publication 1022. Manchester: American Society for Gastrointestinal Endoscopy, 1989 (revised 1995).

British Society of Gastroenterology. Recommendations for standards of sedation and patient monitoring during gastrointestinal endoscopy. *Gut* 1991;**32**:823–7.

Freeman ML. Sedation and monitoring for gastrointestinal endoscopy. In: Blade EW, Chak A, eds. *Upper Gastrointestinal Endoscopy*. Gastrointestinal Endoscopy Clinics of North America, Vol. 4 (series ed. Sivak M). Philadelphia: WB Saunders, 1994:475–99.

Infection/disinfection and antibiotics

American Ad Hoc Committee of Disinfection. *ASGE News* 1995;**3**:13.

American Society for Gastrointestinal Endoscopy. *Antibiotic Prophylaxis for Gastrointestinal Endoscopy*. ASGE Publication 1027. Manchester: American Society for Gastrointestinal Endoscopy, 1995.

Axon ATR, ed. *Infection in Endoscopy*. Gastrointestinal Endoscopy Clinics of North America, Vol. 3(3) (series ed. Sivak MV). Philadelphia: WB Saunders, 1993.

Axon ATR, Bond W, Bottrill PM *et al.* Endoscopic disinfection: Working Party Report to the World Congress of Gastroenterology. *J Gastroenterol Hepatol* 1991;**6**:23.

British Society of Gastroenterology. Cleaning and disinfection of equipment for gastrointestinal flexible endoscopy: interim recommendations of a working party. *Gut* 1988;**29**:1134.

British Society of Gastroenterology. Aldehyde disinfection and health in endoscopy units. *Gut* 1993;**34**:164–5.

Cowen A. Infection and endoscopy; patient to patient transmission. In: Axon ATR, ed. *Infection in Endoscopy*. Gastrointestinal Endoscopy Clinics of North America, Vol. 3(3) (series ed. Sivak MV). Philadelphia: WB Saunders, 1993:483–96.

Dajani AS, Bison AL, Chung KL *et al.* Prevention of bacterial endocarditis: recommendations by the American Heart Association. *J Am Med Assoc* 1990;**264**:2919.

Endocarditis Working Party of the British Society for Antimicrobial Chemotherapy. Antibiotic prophylaxis of infective endocarditis. *Lancet* 1990;**335**:88.

Gruber M *et al.* Electrocautery and patients with implanted cardiac devices. *Gastroenterol Nurs* 1995;**38**:49–53.

Meyer GW. Antibiotic prophylaxis for gastrointestinal procedures: who needs it? *Gastrointest Endosc* 1994;**40**:645–6.

O'Connor HJ. Risk of sepsis in endoscopic procedures. In: Axon ATR, ed. *Infection in Endoscopy*. Gastrointestinal Endoscopy Clinics of North America, Vol. 3(3) (series ed. Sivak MV). Philadelphia: WB Saunders, 1993:459–68.

Rutala WA. APIC guidelines for selection and use of disinfectants. *Am J Infect Control* 1990;**18**:99.

Zeroske J. Practical disinfection technique. In: Axon ATR, ed. *Infection in Endoscopy*. Gastrointestinal Endoscopy Clinics of North America, Vol. 3(3) (series ed. Sivak MV). Philadelphia: WB Saunders, 1993.

Other risks — ASGE guidelines

Electrocautery use in patients with implanted cardiac devices. *Gastrointest Endosc* 1994;**40**(6):794–5.
Quality safeguards for ambulatory gastrointestinal endoscopy. *Gastrointest Endosc* 1994;**40**(6):799–800.
Radiation safety during endoscopy. *Gastrointest Endosc* 1994;**40**(6):801–4.
The recommended use of laboratory studies before endoscopic procedures. *Gastrointest Endosc* 1993;**39**:892–4.

Risk stratification

Cotton PB. Outcomes of endoscopic procedures: struggling towards definitions. *Gastrointest Endosc* 1994;**40**:514–18.
Fleischer DE. Better definition of endoscopic complications and other negative outcomes. *Gastrointest Endosc* 1994;**40**:511–14.

Risk management

American Society for Gastrointestinal Endoscopy. *Risk Management. An Information Resource Manual.* Manchester: American Society for Gastrointestinal Endoscopy, 1990.
Plumeri PA. Risk management for gastrointestinal endoscopists. In: Cotton PB, Tytgat GNJ, Williams CB, eds. *Annual of Gastrointestinal Endoscopy*. London: Current Science, 1992:1–4.

Diagnostic Upper Endoscopy

4

Indications

Full assessment of the clinical role of upper gastrointestinal (GI) endoscopy is outside the scope of this book. It varies with local circumstances, and with the available radiological and endoscopic expertise. Endoscopy is appropriate when a patient's symptoms are persistent and unresponsive to simple conservative management, since a precise diagnosis is needed to apply cost-effective focused therapy—whether medical, endoscopic or surgical.

Endoscopy was used initially to examine patients who had undergone barium X-ray studies which had not completely answered the clinical question, or had raised other questions. The endoscopic task was then straightforward, for the precise target and question were defined. Barium studies are now used only for investigation of motility and outlet problems, and to provide roadmaps of strictures or gross morphology prior to complex surgery. Endoscopy has taken over the primary role in most clinical situations, which makes the task more difficult and the endoscopist's responsibility greater in achieving both accuracy and a high level of safety and patient acceptability. The examiner must be capable of doing a complete and reliable survey of the oesophagus, stomach and proximal duodenum. It is relatively easy to see, describe and sample a lesion, but much more experience and skill are needed to say with certainty that no lesion is present.

The need for cancer screening, and repeated endoscopic surveillance in patients with pre-malignant conditions (e.g. Barrett's oesophagus and the operated stomach) remains controversial.

Although endoscopy appears to be an example of expensive Western high tech medicine, the technique is cost-effective and has become popular in developing countries—where X-ray facilities are more expensive and radiologists are rare.

Patient preparation, position and medication

Details of explanation, consent and safety issues are discussed in Chapter 3. Patients are instructed not to eat or drink for 4–6h before endoscopy (although small sips of water are permissible for comfort). It is kinder to perform examinations during the morning so that most patients need only fast overnight. Patients with oesophageal or gastric outlet obstruction should be fasted

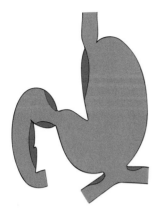

Fig. 4.1 Some areas (grey shading) are more difficult to see with a forward-viewing endoscope.

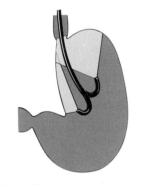

Fig. 4.2 Tip retroversion visualizes the gastric fundus.

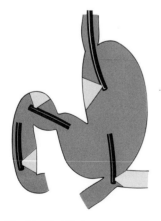

Fig. 4.3 The blind areas are well seen with a side-viewer.

for longer periods; aspiration of the oesophagus or formal gastric lavage may be necessary in these circumstances. The patient should partly undress and put on a gown or protective bib. Dentures and spectacles (including contact lenses) should normally be removed and stored safely.

The patient lies on the examination trolley/stretcher on the *left* side with the intravenous access line in the *right* arm. The head is supported on a small but firm pillow, with a disposable towel to collect secretions. Monitoring sensors are applied as appropriate (see Chapter 3), and a mouthguard is inserted. We prefer a type which can be strapped into place, and which also includes an oxygen feed.

Medication practices vary widely between different centres and cultures. Pharyngeal anaesthesia is used almost universally, and most units give sedation. We use a combination of pethidine (Demerol) and diazepam (Valium), or midazolam (Versed, Dormicum) in the majority of patients. Details of these and other drugs (e.g. antibiotics) are given in Chapter 3. Selected patients are managed without sedation, relying on good technique, rapport and speed. This is tolerated better by older patients than by younger ones and in procedures using small endoscopes (and lateral-viewing instruments which have a rounded tip); it may be safer in patients with pulmonary problems. Endoscopy is also easier to organize when sedation is avoided; there is no need for formal recovery, and fit patients can drive or return immediately to work or play.

Choice of endoscope

Routine upper endoscopy is done with a long forward-viewing instrument. With the modern degree of tip deflection and wide-angle lenses available, it is usually possible to perform a complete survey of the stomach and duodenum. Some areas are slightly more difficult to see face-on (Fig. 4.1), as is necessary for optimal tissue sampling (e.g. high lesser curve gastric ulcers), although a skilled endoscopist can usually achieve this by suitable manoeuvres, including tip retroversion (Fig. 4.2). These areas are well seen with side-viewing instruments (Fig. 4.3), which are essential for examination (and cannulation) of the papilla of Vater. Only very rarely is it necessary nowadays to withdraw a forward-viewing instrument and replace it with a side-viewing endoscope. There is a trend towards smaller 'paediatric' endoscopes. These are essential for small children and are useful in patients with strictures. Surprisingly, very small endoscopes (5–6mm diameter) can be more difficult to pass than standard instruments, as the bending section is more floppy; it is easy to get lost in the pharynx unless insertion is done under direct vision.

The proliferation of therapeutic techniques has lead to the

development of larger 'therapeutic' endoscopes, with bigger channels (4 mm or greater, compared with the standard 2.8 mm). These channels allow the passage of larger and more robust probes and more effective suction (e.g. of blood clots).

A unit offering a comprehensive service for upper endoscopy should have a variety of different instrument types, and a sufficient total number to allow for rapid patient turnover with complete disinfection schedules. A single procedure room unit would need four endoscopes (two standard, one paediatric and one therapeutic). Busy rooms will alternate three endoscopes in a session of upper GI endoscopy. The more specialized instruments can be shared when there are several procedure rooms. Backup instruments are necessary to cover breakages. Each room must have appropriate light sources and sufficient accessories (water bottles, biopsy forceps, etc.) to ensure that sterile replacements are always available.

When video-endoscopes are used (or a video convertor onto a fibrescope), it is important to site the monitor in a place convenient for the endoscopist and main assistant — which means across the patient (Fig. 4.4). The patient and other assistants may appreciate a second monitor at a site convenient for them. If television systems are not in use, a side-arm 'teaching attachment' should be available.

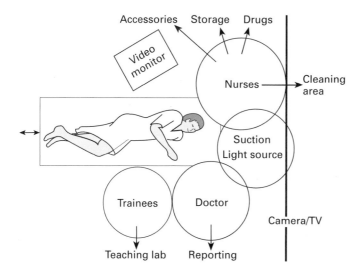

Fig. 4.4 Functional planning is important in the endoscopy room.

Stance and instrument handling

The endoscopist should stand comfortably and hold the instrument in such a way that it runs in a gentle curve directly to the patient's mouth (rather than drooping below the examination table, which reduces torque control). Inexperienced endoscopists often stand too close to the patient in a cramped and uncomfortable position (Fig. 4.5). Video-endoscopes, not requiring the endoscopist to hold the control body to the eye, are particularly easy to handle in this respect (Fig. 4.6).

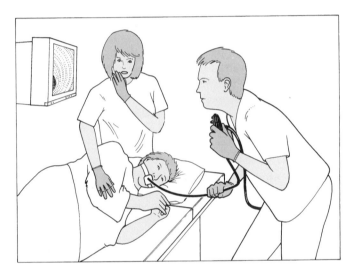

Fig. 4.5 Wrong: an obviously incompetent endoscopist with clumsy stance and handling.

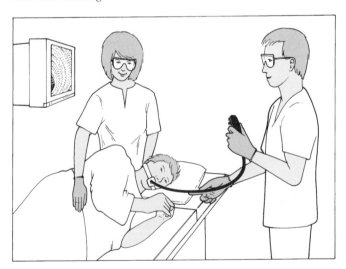

Fig. 4.6 Right: confident and balanced stance with a straight instrument, gently handled.

The endoscope should be held delicately in the fingers, avoiding sudden or aggressive shaft movements which tend to provoke gagging. Twisting (torqueing) movements of the control body and a straightened shaft can add to the fluency of the examination.

The grip. Like a golf club or violin, the endoscope has to be held correctly to produce good results. Its head should be placed in the palm of the left hand, and gripped between the fourth and little fingers and the base of the thumb, with the tip of the thumb resting on the up/down control (Fig. 4.7). This grip leaves the first finger (forefinger) free to activate the air/water and suction buttons. The second (middle) finger assists the thumb as a 'ratchet' during major movements of the up/down control. With practice, the left/right control can also be managed with the left thumb (Fig. 4.8). The left thumb is used to control the lever for the forceps elevator, where present. The right hand thus remains free to push, pull and torque the instrument and also to control accessories such as the biopsy forceps and cameras. The right hand may be used intermittently to manage the left/right tip control and the brakes, but for fluent 'single-handed' endoscopy this is avoided as much as possible.

The basic left-hand grip should be maintained throughout the examination. Acute rotation of the instrument should be effected by rotating the hand, not by rotating the instrument in the hand. Some endoscopists find it convenient to ask the nurse to push and pull the instrument, leaving both hands free to manage the controls. This method may be easier for beginners, but is not generally recommended.

Orientation conventions. When referring to tip deflection, it is convenient to use 'up/down' and 'left/right' in relation to the instrument view and the neutral position of the instrument head (i.e. buttons up), rather than to the ceiling or floor. Thus, turning the up/down control anticlockwise as seen from the right (pushing the bottom of the wheel away from the endoscopist with the thumb) always moves the tip 'up' relative to the field of view (Fig. 4.9). This applies whatever the shaft rotation; if the hand and the (straight) scope are rotated so that the buttons face the floor, 'up' deflection of the tip now points it towards the floor (Fig. 4.10). Fibreoptic instruments have a small mark at 12 o'clock in the field of view (Fig. 4.11) to facilitate orientation for photography (and the endoscopist viewing down a teaching side-arm), and 'up' deflection always deviates the tip towards that mark; video-endoscopes do not need this facility since the monitor does not rotate. Remember that tip movements cause the view to move in the opposite direction (Fig. 4.12). The lens in side-viewing instruments always faces upwards towards the buttons, and the same conventions apply.

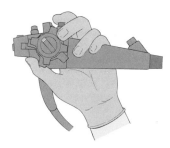

Fig. 4.7 The thumb rests on the up/down control wheel, the forefinger on the air/water button and the middle finger can also assist.

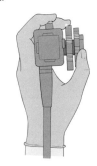

Fig. 4.8 The thumb can reach across to the left/right control.

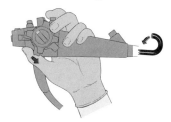

Fig. 4.9 The thumb pushes away from the endoscopist to angle the tip 'up'.

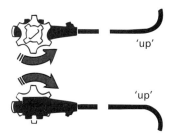

Fig. 4.10 Inversion of the endoscope and the 'up/down' convention.

12 o'clock marker

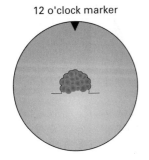

Fig. 4.11 Fibrescopes have a marker for photography.

12 o'clock marker

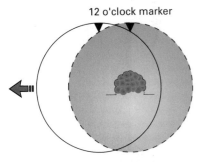

Fig. 4.12 Tip movements move the view in the opposite direction.

Passing the instrument

Pre-check the endoscope for proper functioning and lubricate the distal 20 cm of the shaft (lightly) with jelly. Avoid waving the instrument around in front of a nervous patient; a little subtlety, sleight of hand and smooth talking are appropriate at this moment. Just before inserting the endoscope through the tooth-guard, pre-rehearse up/down movements of the controls to ensure that the tip moves in the correct longitudinal axis to follow the pharynx (Fig. 4.13). If necessary, adjust the lateral knob or twist the shaft appropriately so that it does so, and will track automatically down the midline, rather than impacting laterally into a piriform fossa.

There are three basic methods for passing an endoscope.

Method 1 Steering down under direct vision

This is the safest, most exact and (with a little practice) the quickest method of inserting a forward-viewing instrument. With the mouthguard in position, hold the endoscope shaft at the 30 cm mark (so that changes of hand position are not needed during insertion), pre-rehearse up-angling to check the axis and then pass the tip into the mouthguard. Look for a rough, pale surface of the tongue horizontally in the upper (anterior) part of the view (Fig. 4.14a) and keep the interface between it and the red

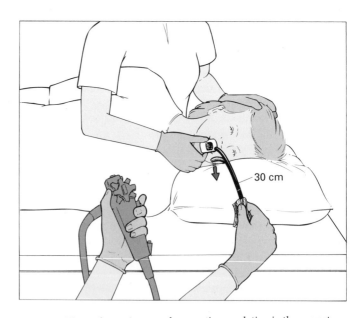

Fig. 4.13 The endoscopist pre-rehearses tip angulation in the correct axis before insertion.

surface of the palate in the centre of view by angling up appropriately, whilst advancing inwards over the curve of the tongue. Simultaneously, take care to stay in the midline by watching for the linear 'median raphe' of the tongue or the convexity of its midpart, correcting if necessary by twisting the shaft; if the view is lost, or the teeth are seen, withdraw and start again. The uvula is often seen transiently, projected upwards in the lower part of the view (Fig. 4.14b). Then, as the tip advances, the epiglottis and, finally, the cricoarytenoid cartilage with the 'false' vocal cords above it are visible in the upper part of the view (Fig. 4.14c; Plate 4.1). In a few patients with forcefully bulging tongues the view may be poor; in others gagging movements can be reduced by asking for deep breathing which automatically reduces retching. The normal tonic contraction of the cricopharyngeal sphincter means that the entrance to the first, or pharyngeal, part of the oesophagus is poorly seen except transiently during swallowing. To reach it, angle down (posteriorly) so that the tip passes inferior to the curve of the cricoarytenoid cartilage, preferably passing to one or other side of the midline since the midline bulge of the cartilage against the cervical spine makes central passage difficult (Fig. 4.14d). At this point there will often be a 'red-out' as the tip impacts into the cricopharyngeal sphincter; insufflate air, maintain *gentle* inward pressure, and the instrument should slip into the oesophagus within a few seconds. If necessary, ask the patient to swallow, and push in quickly as the sphincter opens. Keep watching carefully to ensure smooth mucosal 'slide-by' as the instrument passes semiblind into the upper oesophagus, for it is here that there is the occasional danger of entering a diverticulum.

After insertion to the cricopharyngeal region under direct vision the instrument will be in the midline, with no possibility of impaction into one of the piriform fossae. The endoscopist can therefore have confidence that the instrument will pass correctly, safely and rapidly into the oesophagus, even when a less than perfect view is obtained. The adequate views of the region normally obtained, including the vocal cords, are a bonus denied to those using the old-fashioned 'blind' insertion technique.

Method 2 Blind tip manipulation

This is an alternative insertion method. Standing facing the patient, the operator holds the instrument control head and tip close to each other. The nurse places the mouthguard, and holds the patient's head slightly flexed (see Fig. 4.13). With the right hand, the endoscopist passes the instrument tip through the mouthguard and over the tongue to the back of the mouth; using the left thumb on the control knob, the tip is then actively deflected upwards so that it curls in the midline over the back of the tongue and into the midline of the pharynx. The tip is

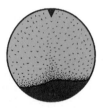

Fig. 4.14 (a) Follow the centre of the tongue . . .

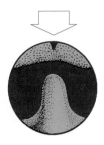

(b) . . . past the uvula . . .

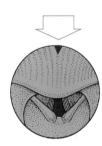

(c) . . . and the epiglottis . . .

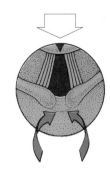

(d) . . . to pass below the cricoarytenoid on either side.

advanced slightly and the thumb is removed from the tip control. While slight forward pressure is maintained, the patient is asked to swallow when the 20 cm mark on the endoscope shaft is just visible outside the mouthguard. This relaxs the cricopharyngeal sphincter, which lies at 15–18 cm from the incisor teeth. As in the direct insertion method, constant reassurance and encouragement should accompany this phase ('swallow please, this is the worst part, you've nearly done it, swallow please, well done, almost finished', etc.).

Passage of the tip through the cricopharyngeal sphincter is easily felt by the right hand as resistance is lost. If the tip does not pass after two or three good swallows, it is probably not in the midline. This can be checked by view or finger (see method 3 below), but it is often better to remove the instrument and to reinsert it after re-orientation and further reassurance.

Method 3 Finger guidance

Finger insertion is not recommended as a routine. The head of the instrument is held by an assistant (avoiding contact with the control knobs) or can be draped over the endoscopist's shoulder. The mouthguard is fitted over the shaft. The endoscopist puts the second and third fingers of his gloved left hand over the back of the tongue. With the right hand he then passes the tip of the instrument over the tongue and uses the inserted fingers of the left hand to guide it into the midline of the pharynx (Fig. 4.15).

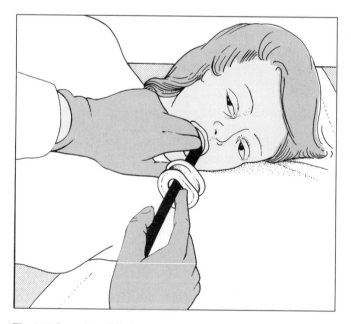

Fig. 4.15 Sometimes 'blind' insertion is helped by guiding the instrument between two fingers.

The patient is asked to swallow after the fingers are withdrawn and the mouthguard is slid into place. If swallowing is not effective, the tip of the instrument has probably fallen into the left pyriform fossa; it may be necessary to reinsert a finger to lift the tip back into the midline.

We strongly recommend passing the instrument under direct vision (method 1). Method 2 is applicable for lateral-viewing endoscopes which have smooth rounded tips. Method 3 may be necessary on occasions, but is risky. Bites to the fingers and the instrument can be dangerous and expensive.

Passage of an endoscope is a co-operative venture between patient and endoscopist; rapport and safety should never be compromised by persisting when the patient is distressed. If in doubt, remove the instrument, and only try again when the patient is ready. The addition of pethidine (Demerol) 20–50 mg i.v. is helpful if anxiety or retching are problematic.

Endotracheal tubes present no problem for the endoscopist inserting under direct vision. Deflating the balloon of the tube may be necessary occasionally to allow easier passage, especially with larger instruments.

Nasogastric tube position can be maintained during endoscope insertion by the simple means of inserting a stiff guidewire down the tube beforehand.

The routine survey

Whatever the precise indication, it is usually appropriate to examine the entire oesophagus, stomach and proximal duodenum. A complete survey may sometimes be prevented by stricturing from disease or previous surgery, or can be curtailed for other reasons. It is important to develop a systematic routine to reduce the possibility of missing any area. The instrument is always advanced under direct vision, using air insufflation and suction as required, and delaying occasionally during active peristalsis (if antispasmotics have not been used). Mucosal views are often better during instrument withdrawal, when the organs are fully distended with air, but inspection during insertion is also important since minor trauma by the instrument tip (or excessive suction) may produce small mucosal lesions with consequent diagnostic confusion. Lesions noted during insertion are best examined in detail (and sampled for histology or cytology) following a complete routine survey of other areas. As well as being systematic in survey, be precise in movements and decisive in making a 'mental map' of what is being seen. A careful, unhurried gastroscopy can be achieved in less than 5 min by avoiding unnecessary movements and repeated examinations of the same area.

Remember two golden rules for endoscopic safety:

1 do not push if you cannot see;
2 if in doubt, inflate and pull back.

Oesophagus

After the cricopharyngeal sphincter, other landmarks seen during oesophagoscopy may include indentation from the left main bronchus, and pulsation of the left atrium and aorta. The oesophagogastric mucosal junction is clearly seen (at 38–40 cm from the incisor teeth in adults) where pale pink squamous oesophageal mucosa abuts darker red gastric mucosa; this junction is often irregular and therefore called the 'Z-line'. The diaphragm normally clasps at or just below the oesophagogastric mucosal junction. The position of the diaphragmatic hiatus can be highlighted by asking the patient to sniff or to take deep breaths, and is recorded as the distance from the incisors. In any patient, the precise relationship of the Z-line to the diaphragmatic hiatus varies during an endoscopy (depending on the patient position, respiration, gastric distension, etc.). In normal patients, the gastric mucosa is often seen at least 1 cm above the diaphragm; hiatus herniation is diagnosed if the Z-line remains more than 2 cm above the hiatus. From the clinical point of view, however, the presence or degree of herniation may be less important than any resulting oesophageal lesions (e.g. oesophagitis or columnar transformation).

Stomach

Endoscopes are easy to pass through the cardia unless there is stenosis; the tip is simply advanced gently under direct vision. The distal oesophagus usually angles to the patient's left as it passes through the diaphragm, so it may be necessary to turn the instrument tip slightly to remain in the correct axis (Fig. 4.16). Unless the cardia is unduly lax, the mucosal view is lost momentarily as the tip passes through, passage being felt by the advancing hand as a slight 'give'. If the tip is further advanced in the same plane, it will abut on the posterior wall of the lesser curvature of the stomach so that pushing in blindly risks retroflexing towards the cardia. Thus, as soon as the tip has passed through the cardia, the instrument should be rotated somewhat to the 'left' (counterclockwise), further air inflated and the tip withdrawn slightly to disimpact from the wall of the fundus or the pool of gastric juice on the greater curve.

With the patient in the left lateral position and the instrument held correctly (buttons up), the disimpacted endoscopic view is predictable (Figs 4.17 & 4.18). The smooth lesser curvature is on the endoscopist's right with the angulus distally, the longitudinal folds of the greater curve are to the left and its posterior aspect is below (Plate 4.2). The pool of gastric juice should be

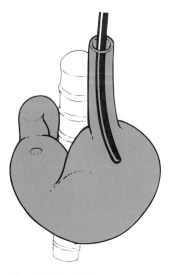

Fig. 4.16 The distal oesophagus angles the scope into the posterior wall of the lesser curve.

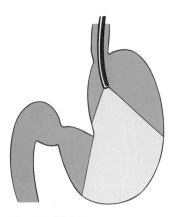

Fig. 4.17 With the gastroscope high on the lesser curve . . .

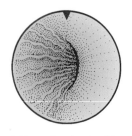

Fig. 4.18 . . . the view is of the angulus in the distance, with the greater curve longitudinal folds on the left.

aspirated to avoid reflux or aspiration during the procedure and the stomach then inflated sufficiently to obtain a reasonable view during insertion. When the mucosal view is obscured by foaming or bubbles, it is helpful to inject a suspension of silicone (simethicone) down the biopsy channel. The four walls of the stomach are examined sequentially by a combination of tip deflection, instrument rotation and advance/withdrawal. The field of view during the advance of a four-way angling endoscope can be represented as a cylinder angulated over the vertebral bodies; the distended stomach takes up an exaggerated J-shape with the axis of the advancing instrument corkscrewing clockwise up and over the spine, following the greater curvature (Fig. 4.19). Thus, the endoscopist, after first turning the tip to his left and somewhat down on entering the stomach, must increasingly angle it up, and rotate the shaft clockwise, following the longitudinal folds as the instrument is advanced down over the vertebral column and into the antrum (Fig. 4.19).

This clockwise corkscrew rotation through approximately 90° during insertion brings the angulus and antrum into end-on view (Fig. 4.20); downward deflection of the tip brings it into the axis of the antrum (Fig. 4.21). The antrum and pylorus should first be examined from a distance, waiting as necessary for any peristaltic waves to pass.

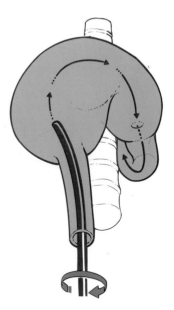

Fig. 4.19 The route to the pylorus and down the duodenum is a clockwise spiral around the vertebral column.

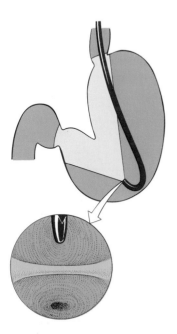

Fig. 4.20 The angulus and antrum come into view . . .

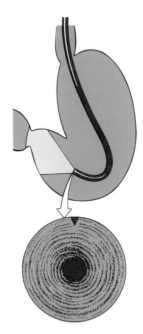

Fig. 4.21 . . . then angle down to see the pylorus in the axis of the antrum.

The tip is then again advanced past the angulus into the antrum (Fig. 4.22). The motor activity of the antrum, pyloric canal and pyloric ring should be carefully observed. Any asymmetry during a peristaltic wave is a useful indicator of present or previous disease.

Through the pylorus into the duodenum

The pyloric ring is approached directly for passage into the duodenum. During the manoeuvre it is particularly convenient to use only the left hand to maintain the instrument tip in the correct axis. When the pyloric ring fills the field of view, the tip is advanced and is seen or felt to pass into the duodenal cap (Figs 4.23 & 4.24) which is recognized by its more granular and paler surface. Some patience may be needed to pass the pylorus, especially if there is spasm or deformity; downward angulation of the tip or deflation may help its passage.

As the instrument tip passes the resistance of the pylorus, the loop which has inevitably developed in the stomach straightens out and accelerates the tip to the distal bulb (Fig. 4.24). This makes it necessary to withdraw the shaft considerably to disimpact the tip (and insufflate some air) before a view is obtained (Fig. 4.25). Like the stomach, the bulb is scanned by circumferential manipulation of the tip during advance and withdrawal. The area immediately beyond the pyloric ring, especially the inferior part of the bulb, may be missed by the inexperienced, who fail to withdraw sufficiently for fear of falling back into the stomach. Buscopan (or Glucagon) can be given intravenously if visualization is impaired by duodenal motility — but avoid excessive air insufflation, which will leave the patient uncomfortably distended.

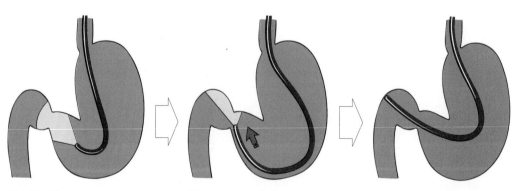

Fig. 4.22 The scope passes from the antrum . . .

Fig. 4.23 . . . to the pylorus and duodenal cap . . .

Fig. 4.24 . . . and tends to impact in the duodenum.

Passage into the descending duodenum

This must be effected with care. The superior duodenal angle is the important landmark (Fig. 4.25). The instrument is advanced into the angle, so that the tip lies at the junction of the first and second parts of the duodenum. The shaft is rotated about 90° to the right, and the tip is then angled to the right and acutely up to corkscrew round the bend (Fig. 4.26), and provide a tunnel view of the descending duodenum. Paradoxically, the tip is best advanced beyond the flexure by *withdrawing* the shaft, since straightening the loop in the stomach presses the tip inwards, and the straightening shaft also corkscrews more efficiently round the superior duodenal angle (Figs 4.27 & 4.28). Inexperienced endoscopists mistakenly push to attempt passage into the descending duodenum. Using the correct 'pull and twist' method, the tip slides in to reach the ampullary region with only 55–60 cm of instrument inserted. Duodenoscopy with more than 70 cm of shaft inserted is inelegant and uncomfortable.

A forward-viewing instrument gives tangential and often restricted views of the convex medial wall of the descending duodenum and the papilla of Vater. With small acute-angling instruments, it is sometimes possible to view this area more directly in a partly retroflexed manner (Fig. 4.29), but care should be taken.

Be gentle when trying to pass standard instruments further into the third part of the duodenum. Attempts at pushing may simply form a loop in the stomach (Fig. 4.30). Further pressure may advance the tip but often at the cost of considerable discom-

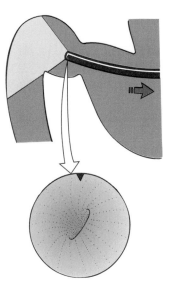

Fig. 4.25 Withdraw the scope to disimpact the tip and see the superior duodenal angle — an important landmark.

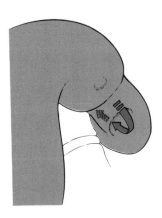

Fig. 4.26 Corkscrew the tip clockwise around the superior duodenal angle, using twist, right- and up-angulation simultaneously.

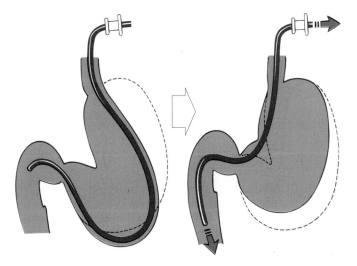

Fig. 4.27 Because of the loop in the greater curve . . .

Fig. 4.28 . . . withdrawal helps to advance the scope into the second part of the duodenum.

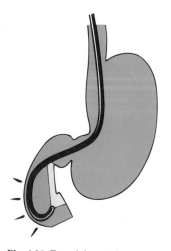

Fig. 4.29 Forceful partial retroflexion may give a view of the papilla, but take care.

fort to the patient; pulling back, deflating or even applying pressure on the patient's upper abdomen may be more effective.

Retroflexion

Retroflexion of the tip of the instrument is achieved by complete 180° upward angulation (combining both angling controls) with simultaneous inward pressure if the tip of the instrument is in the antrum, and the stomach distended. This manoeuvre should demonstrate the angulus, the entire lesser curve and the fundus as the instrument is withdrawn (Fig. 4.31). The retroversion (or 'J') manoeuvre is probably best performed after examining the duodenum so as to avoid overinflation on the way in. Some patients (particularly those with a lax cardia) find it difficult to hold enough air to permit an adequate view. If retroversion proves difficult, it may be made easier by rotating the patient slightly onto the back to give the stomach more room to expand. Having examined the lesser curvature from below, the retroflexed shaft is rotated through 180° in either direction to swing the tip around and provide views of the greater curvature and fundus (Fig. 4.32). Close-up cardia views are obtained by withdrawing further still, again rotating the retroverted instrument as necessary.

During all of these manoeuvres, it is particularly important to keep the shaft of the instrument relatively straight from the patient's teeth to your hands. This reduces the strain on the endoscope, helps orientation and ensures that rotatory movements are precisely transmitted to the tip.

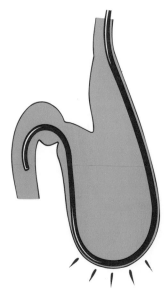

Fig. 4.30 Trying to reach the third part by force simply forms a loop in the stomach.

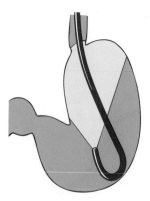

Fig. 4.31 Angulation of 180° retroflexes the tip to see the lesser curve . . .

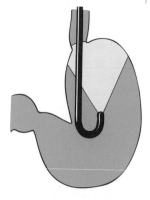

Fig. 4.32 . . . and swinging the retroflexed tip around gives a view of the fundus and cardia.

Having examined the proximal stomach and cardia, the instrument tip is straightened back to the neutral position by de-angling the controls and pulling back.

Removing the instrument

The duodenum, stomach and oesophagus should be surveyed carefully once again during withdrawal. Under the different motility conditions and organ shapes produced by distension and instrument position, areas previously seen only tangentially on insertion may be brought into direct view on the way out. Remember to aspirate air (and fluid) from the stomach completely on withdrawal, and to take the brakes off from the control knobs.

The instrument should be wiped and its channel flushed immediately after it is removed from the patient, before proteinaceous secretions and blood can dry in the channels. The endoscopist or assistant should place the tip of the instrument into water and press down on both control buttons; this flushes both the suction/biopsy and the air/water channels. Details of formal cleaning and disinfection methods are given in Chapter 3.

Problems during endoscopy

Patient distress

Endoscopy should be terminated quickly if any patient shows distress, the cause of which is not immediately obvious and remediable. Many patients have an understandable anxiety about choking. The airway should be checked and any residual oral sections aspirated. If reassurance does not calm the patient, remove the instrument and consider giving additional sedation or analgesia (especially pethidine). Inadvertent bronchoscopy is not rare if insertion is done by the 'blind' method. It is obvious from the unusual view and impressive coughing. Discomfort may arise from inappropriate pressure during intubation, or from distension due to excessive air insufflation. Most sedated patients are able to belch; when performing endoscopy under general anaesthesia, it may be wise to keep the abdomen exposed so that overinflation can be detected, especially in children. Remember to keep inflation to a minimum, and to aspirate all the air at the end of the procedure. Severe pain during endoscopy is very rare, and indicates a complication such as perforation or a cardiac incident. It is extremely dangerous to ignore warning signs.

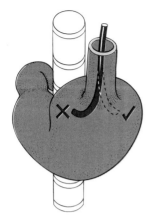

Fig. 4.33 Angling right (rather than left) on entering the fundus can cause retroflexion and can result in getting lost.

Getting lost

The endoscopist may become disorientated, and the instrument looped, in patients with congenital malrotations, major pathology (e.g. achalasia, large diverticula and hernias, 'cup and spill' deformities) and after complex surgery. Careful study of any available radiographs should help. The commonest reason for disorientation in patients with normal anatomy is inadequate air insufflation due to a defect in the instrument or air pump (which should have been detected before starting the examination). Inexperienced endoscopists often get lost in the fundus, especially when the stomach is angled acutely over the vertebral column. Having passed the cardia, the instrument tip should be deflected to the endoscopist's *left* and slightly downwards (Fig. 4.33). A wrong turn to the right will bring the tip back up into the fundus. When in doubt, withdraw, insufflate and turn sharply left to find the true lumen.

A curious endoscopic view may indicate perforation (which is not always immediately painful). If in any doubt, abandon the examination and obtain radiological studies.

Inadequate mucosal view

Lack of a clear view means that the lens is lying against the mucosa or is obscured by fluid or food debris. Withdraw slightly and insufflate air; double check that the air pump is working and that all connections are firm. Try washing the lens with the normal finger-controlled water jet. This may not be effective if the instrument lens is covered by debris (or mucosa which has been sucked onto the orifice of the biopsy channel). Pressure can be released by brief removal of the rubber cap of the biopsy port, but it may be necessary to flush the channel with water or air, using a syringe. Small quantities of food or mucus obscuring an area of interest can be washed away with a jet of water. Foaming can be suppressed by adding a few drops of silicone suspension. Since most patients obey instructions to fast beforehand, the presence of excessive residue is an important sign of outlet obstruction. Standard endoscope channels are too small for aspiration of food; prolonged attempts simply result in blocked channels. The instrument can usually be guided along the lesser curvature over the top of the food to allow a search for a distal obstructing lesion. The greater curvature can also be examined if necessary by rotating the patient into the right lateral position. However, any examination in the presence of excess fluid or food carries a significant risk of regurgitation and pulmonary aspiration. The endoscopist should only persist if the immediate benefits are thought to justify the risk. It is usually wiser to stop and to repeat the examination only after proper lavage.

Recognition of lesions

This book is concerned mainly with techniques rather than lesions. We recommend that beginners should study several of the excellent atlases which are now available. Certain points, however, are worth emphasizing here.

Oesophagus

Oesophagitis normally follows acid reflux and is most apparent distally, close to the mucosal junction. There is no clear macroscopic dividing line from normality; the earliest visible changes consist of mucosal congestion and oedema, which obscure the normal fine vascular pattern. At a more advanced stage, the mucosa becomes friable and bleeds easily on touching; there are patches of exudate and areas of reddening or ulceration, usually in the long axis of the oesophagus. The process culminates in a symmetrical stricture above which the mucosa (now protected from reflux) may appear almost normal. Columnar lining of the oesophagus (Barrett's oesophagus) is easily recognized (Plates 4.3 and 4.4). Red gastric-type mucosa extends more than 2 cm above the diaphragmatic hiatus; initially in longitudinal stripes or plaques, it can coalesce to involve the entire circumference. Monilial oesphagitis is characterized by white spots or plaques (Plate 4.5).

Oesophageal carcinoma usually causes asymmetrical stenosis, with areas of exuberant abnormal mucosa, and sometimes an irregular ulcer with raised edges. Carcinoma of the gastric fundus may also infiltrate upwards submucosally to involve the oesophagus. The correct diagnosis is then easily made if the endoscope can be passed through the stricture to allow retroverted views of the cardia.

Diverticula in the mid- or distal oesophagus are easily recognized, but the instrument may enter a pulsion diverticulum or pouch in the upper oesophagus without the true lumen being seen at all. Lack of view and resistance to inward movement are (as always) an indication to pull back and reassess. Webs or rings (Plate 4.6), such as the Schatski ring at or just proximal to the oesophagogastric junction, may not be obvious to the endoscopist due to a combination of 'flat' bright endoscope illumination and distortion from the wide-angled lens view. If in doubt, skilled radiology (with video taping) should be used to define the situation before therapeutic endoscopy.

Varices lie in the long axis of the oesophagus as tortuous bluish mounds covered with relatively normal mucosa. They resemble varicose veins elsewhere in the body.

Mallory–Weiss tears are 5–20 mm longitudinal mucosal splits lying either side of or across the oesophagogastric mucosal junction. In the acute phase the tear is covered with exudate or clot and may sometimes be seen best in a retroverted view.

Motility disturbances of the oesophagus should be diagnosed by radiology and manometry, but their consequences — such as dilatation, pseudodiverticula, food retention and oesophagitis — are well seen at endoscopy, which is always needed to rule out obstructing pathology. Hypermotility is probable when recurrent oesophageal contractions are seen in spite of antispasmodics and sedation; the inco-ordinate non-propulsive contractions of oesophageal dysfunction being known as 'tertiary' contractions.

Achalasia allows the endoscope to pass easily through the cardia, in contrast to the fixed narrowing of pathological strictures due to reflux oesophagitis or malignancy (Plates 4.7 and 4.8).

Stomach

The appearance of the normal gastric mucosa varies considerably. Reddening (hyperaemia) may be generalized (e.g. with bile reflux into the operated stomach) or localized; sometimes it occurs in long streaks along the ridges of mucosal folds. Localized (traumatic) reddening with or without petechiae or oedematous changes is often seen on the posterior upper lesser curve in patients who habitually retch. Macroscopic congestion does not correlate well with underlying histological gastritis, and care should be taken when considering clinical relevance. Biopsy samples should be taken from any odd-looking mucosa.

Gastric folds vary in size, but the endoscopic assessment also depends upon the degree of gastric distension (Plate 4.2). Very prominent fleshy folds are seen in Ménétrièr's disease and are best diagnosed by a snare-loop biopsy. Patients with aggressive duodenal ulceration often have large gastric folds with spotty areas of congestion within the areae gastricae and excess quantities of clear resting juice. With gastric atrophy, there are no mucosal folds (when the stomach is distended) and blood vessels are easily seen through the pale atrophic mucosa. Atrophy is often associated with intestinal metaplasia which appears as small grey-white plaques.

Erosions and ulcers are the most common localized gastric lesions. A lesion is usually called an erosion if it is small (<5 mm diameter) and shallow with no sign of scarring. Acute ulcers and erosions are often seen in the antrum and may be capped with, and partially obscured by, clots. Oedematous erosions appear as small, smooth umbilicated raised areas, often in chains along the folds of the gastric body. When these are multiple, the condition has been called 'chronic erosive gastritis'. However, gastritis is a term best reserved for histological use.

The classic chronic benign gastric ulcer is usually single and is most frequently seen on the lesser curvature at, or above, the angulus. It is typically symmetrical with smooth margins and a clean base (unless eroding adjacent structures). Multiple and punched-out ulcers (sometimes odd-shaped and very large), occur in patients on non-steroidal anti-inflammatory drug (NSAID) therapy.

Malignancy may be suspected if an ulcer has raised irregular margins (or different heights around the circumference), a lumpy haemorrhagic base or a mucosal abnormality surrounding the ulcer. Mucosal folds around a benign ulcer usually radiate towards it and reach the margin. Inexperienced endoscopists cannot hope to separate benign from malignant ulcers on macroscopic appearance alone; tissue specimens must always be taken. Unfortunately, gastric cancer is usually diagnosed at an advanced stage in Western countries, when it is all too obvious at endoscopy. Diffusely infiltrating carcinoma (linitis plastica) may be missed unless motility is carefully studied. Early gastric cancer may mimic a small benign ulcer, chronic erosion or flat polyp. Polypoid lesions under 1 cm in diameter are usually inflammatory in origin. However, since all malignant lesions start small and are curable if detected at an early stage, odd mucosal lumps and bumps should not be ignored; a tissue diagnosis must be made. Submucosal tumours are characterized by normal overlying mucosa and bridging folds; leiomyomas and plaques of aberrant pancreatic tissue (characteristically found in the floor of the antrum) usually have a central dimple or crater (Plate 4.9).

Duodenum

Duodenal ulcers, either current or previous, often cause persistent deformity of the pyloric ring. The ulcers occur most commonly on the anterior and posterior walls of the bulb and are frequently multiple. When active they are surrounded by oedema and acute congestion. Scarring often results in a characteristic shelf-like deformity which partially divides the bulb and may produce a pseudodiverticulum; a small linear ulcer or scar is seen running along the apex of this fold. The mucosa of the bulb often reveals small mucosal changes of dubious clinical significance. Areas of mucosal congestion with spotty white exudate ('pepper and salt' ulceration) merge into even less definite macroscopic appearances labelled as 'duodenitis'. Small mucosal lumps in the proximal duodenum usually reflect underlying Brunner's gland hyperplasia or gastric metaplasia (ectopic islands of gastric mucosa). Primary duodenal tumours are rare; papillary lesions are described in Chapter 6.

Ulceration and duodenitis in the second part of the duodenum suggests Zollinger–Ellison syndrome or underlying pancreatic disease. Crohn's disease may be suspected by the presence of small aphthous ulcers in the second part; there are typical granulomas on histology.

Coeliac disease can be recognized microscopically (in the second part of the duodenum and beyond), especially when viewed close up. The fine villus pattern is lost and the mucosa appears knobbly and oedematous.

Dye-enhancement techniques

These may assist the recognition of inconspicuous lesions—such as coeliac disease. Dye coating is best achieved by spraying with a tube and fine nozzle applied close to the mucosa. The dye fills the interstices, highlighting irregularities in architecture. Indigo carmine is used most frequently, but simple pen ink (1:5 dilution of washable blue) is also effective. Intravital staining is an alternative approach to lesion enhancement. Dyes such as methylene blue, Lugol's solution and toluidine blue may be taken up preferentially in diseased mucosa (such as intestinal metaplasia). Fluorescent stains (given intravenously) may highlight lesions under special conditions such as ultraviolet illumination.

Specimen collection

It is important to emphasize the need for close collaboration between endoscopy and laboratory staff. The diagnostic yield from endoscopic specimens will be maximized if laboratory staff are involved in defining the policy for specimen handling and transmission. Specimens should reach the laboratory with precise details of their origin, and the specific clinical question which needs to be answered. Pathologists who routinely receive a copy of the endoscopy findings (and later follow-up) are more likely to give timely and relevant reports. Regular review sessions should be part of the quality improvement process.

Biopsy specimens

Biopsy specimens are taken with cupped forceps. The lesion should be approached face-on, so that firm and direct pressure can be applied to it with the widely opened cups; the forceps are then gently closed by an assistant and withdrawn. At least six good specimens should be taken from any lesion—perfectionists would ask for many more. Forceps with a central spike make it easier to take specimens from lesions which have to be approached tangentially (e.g. in the oesophagus). Some experts prefer not to use spiked forceps because of the risk of accidental skin puncture.

Ulcer biopsies should include samples from the base and from the ulcer rim in all four quadrants; basal specimens are sometimes diagnostic, but usually yield only slough. When sampling proliferative tumours, it is wise to take several specimens from the same place to penetrate the outer necrotic layer. A larger final tumour biopsy may be obtained by grabbing a protuberant area and deliberately *not* pulling the forceps through the channel; the instrument is withdrawn with the specimen still outside the tip.

The methods for handling and fixing specimens should be established after discussion with the relevant pathologist; some prefer samples to be gently flattened on paper or other surfaces such as cellulose filter (Millipore, etc.). The cellulose filter method of biopsy mounting has considerable advantages for the management of multiple small endoscopic biopsies. They adhere well to the filter and are rarely lost, they are mounted in sequence so that errors of location are impossible, and they allow the histopathologist to view serial sections of six to eight biopsies at a time in a row across a single microscope slide. A 15 mm strip of cellulose filter (just less than the width of a glass slide) has a pencil-ruled or printed central line and a notch or mark made at one end (Fig. 4.34a). Each biopsy is eased out of the forceps cup with the tip of a micropipette or toothpick (Fig. 4.34b) (to avoid needle-stick injuries), placed exactly onto the line and patted flat (Fig. 4.34c). The strip with its line of biopsies is placed into fixative (Fig. 4.34d). In the laboratory it is processed, wax-mounted in the correct orientation (Fig. 4.34e),

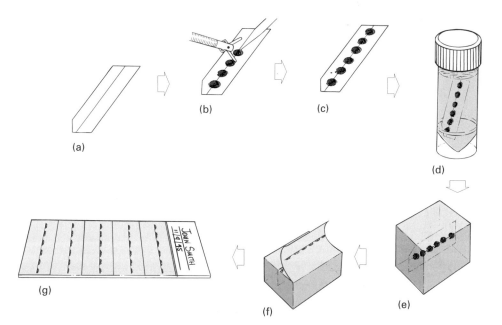

Fig. 4.34 (a–g) Stages in placing biopsies onto the filter, then fixing, sectioning and mounting the specimens.

sectioned through the line of biopsies on the filter (Fig. 4.34f), positioned on the microscope slide (Fig. 4.34g), and then stained and examined without handling the biopsies individually at any stage.

A dissecting microscope or hand lens can be used to orientate mucosal specimens before fixation if information is required about the mucosal architecture (e.g. duodenal biopsies in malabsorption).

Detection of *Helicobacter pylori* infection has become important recently. A biopsy specimen should be taken from the gastric antrum and placed in a rapid urease test; a formalin-fixed specimen is sent to the laboratory only if the urease test is negative.

Biopsy sites often bleed trivially, but sometimes sufficiently to obscure the lesion before adequate samples have been taken; if so, the area should be washed with a jet of water or adrenaline (epinephrine) solution (1:100 000). Bleeding of clinical significance is exceptionally rare.

Cytology specimens

Cytology specimens are taken under direct vision with a sleeved brush (Fig. 4.35) which is passed through the instrument channel. The head of the brush is advanced out of its sleeve and rubbed and rolled repeatedly across the surface of the lesion; a circumferential sweep of the margin and base of an ulcer is desirable. The brush is then pulled back into the sleeve, and both are withdrawn together. The brush is protruded, wiped over two to three glass slides and then rapidly fixed before drying damages the cells. The precise method of preparation (in the unit or laboratory) is determined by the cytologist. Brushes should not be re-used. Bleeding of clinical significance is exceptionally rare. A trap (Fig. 4.36) can be used to collect cytology specimens. Suction through the channel after a biopsy procedure also produces useful cellular material ('salvage cytology').

The value of brush cytology depends largely on the skill and enthusiasm of the cytopathologist. Many studies indicate that the combination of brush cytology and biopsy provides a higher yield than biopsy alone. In practice, most endoscopists reserve cytology for lesions from which good biopsy specimens are difficult to obtain (e.g. tight oesophageal strictures) and when resampling a suspicious lesion.

Sampling submucosal lesions

Histology reports are usually normal in patients with submucosal lesions (such as benign tumours), since standard biopsy forceps do not traverse the muscularis mucosa. Larger and deeper specimens can be taken with a diathermy snare loop; the technique is described with polypectomy in Chapter 10. Larger

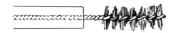

Fig. 4.35 Cytology brush with outer sleeve.

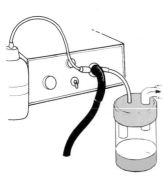

Fig. 4.36 A suction trap to collect fluid specimens.

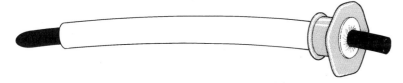

Fig. 4.37 An overtube with toothguard over a rubber lavage tube.

specimens can also be taken with 'jumbo' forceps or even larger experimental forceps which have to be 'muzzle loaded', i.e. the forceps are threaded backwards up the biopsy channel before the instrument is passed into the patient — with an overtube (Fig. 4.37) to protect the pharynx and oesophagus during intubation. An alternative method for obtaining deeper tissue samples is to use a needle to obtain aspiration samples for cytology. Good results have been reported for this technique, but it has not become popular.

Patient recovery and discharge

With standard sedation regimens, most patients rest after the procedure for about 15–30 min on a trolley (stretcher) or in a reclining chair in view of the nursing staff. The accompanying relative or friend can sit with the patient if space permits. Drinking is usually delayed for 20 min if pharyngeal anaesthesia has been used. However, the effect of pharyngeal anaesthesia can be displaced in a few seconds if the patient is able to gargle (and spit out) two mouthfulls of water. Most patients who have been sedated are fit to leave in the care of a relative or friend 30–60 min after a routine examination. They are again instructed to go home, and not to drive or take any responsible action on the same day; these instructions should also be given in writing.

Every patient should leave the unit with an idea of what has been discovered and what should happen next. Consultation should take place in the presence of an accompanying relative because of the potential for significant amnesia after sedation. Staff must ensure that the patient has further appropriate appointments. All of this process is simpler if patients are managed without sedation.

Diagnostic endoscopy under special circumstances

Operated patients

Unless prevented by postoperative stenosis, endoscopy is the best method for diagnosis and exclusion of mucosal inflammation, recurrent ulcers and tumours after upper GI surgery. The endoscopist can document the size and arrangement of any outlet or anastomosis, but standard barium radiology and nuclear medicine techniques may be needed to give more information about motility and emptying disorders.

Experience is needed to appreciate the wide range of 'normal' endoscopic appearance in the operated patient. Partial gastrectomy, gastroenterostomy and pyloroplasty result in reflux of bile and intestinal juice; resultant foaming in the stomach may obscure the endoscopic view and should be suppressed by flushing with a silicone suspension. Gastric distension is difficult to maintain in patients with a large gastric outlet; avoid pumping too much air and overdistending the intestine. Most patients who have undergone partial gastrectomy or gastroenterostomy have impressively hyperaemic mucosae. Initially this is most marked close to the stoma, but atrophic gastritis is progressive and plaques of greyish-white intestinal metaplasia may been seen. There is an increased risk of cancer in the gastric remnant, particularly close to the stoma. Many cancers in this site are not recognized endoscopically, so during endoscopy of an operated stomach the opportunity should be taken to obtain multiple biopsy (and cytology) specimens from within 3 cm of the stoma — in every case, whatever the level of suspicion.

Ulcers following partial gastrectomy or gastroenterostomy usually occur at, or just beyond, the anastomosis. Endoscopic diagnosis is usually simple, but the area just beneath the stoma may sometimes be difficult to survey completely using a forward-viewing instrument. A lateral-viewing endoscope may also sometimes allow a more complete survey in a scarred and tortuous pyloroplasty. Many surgeons use non-absorbable sutures when performing an intestinal anastomosis; these can ulcerate through the mucosa and appear as black or green threads and loops. Their clinical significance remains controversial; when sutures are associated with ulcers, it is justifiable to attempt their removal with biopsy forceps or with a diathermy snare loop. Endoscopy is occasionally performed (for bleeding or stomal obstruction) within a few days of upper GI tract surgery; if so, air insufflation should be kept to a minimum.

Acute upper gastrointestinal bleeding

Bleeding provides special challenges for the endoscopist and details are given in Chapter 5.

Endoscopy in children

Paediatric endoscopy is simple with appropriate instruments and preparation; examination techniques are similar to those used in adults. The standard adult forward- and lateral-viewing instruments (10–12 mm diameter) can be used down to the age of about 2 years. Smaller paediatric instruments (5 mm diameter) may be needed in infants.

Endoscopy can be performed with little or no sedation in the first year of life. Fasted babies usually swallow the instrument avidly. A few endoscopists prefer to use general anaesthesia beyond this age and into the mid-teens (especially for complex procedures) but most are satisfied with heavy sedation alone. This usually consists of a small dose of a benzodiazepine and generous doses of pethidine (Demerol). Even an apparently calm or well-sedated child may suddenly become briefly uncontrollable during intubation and it is essential to swaddle the upper body and arms completely within a blanket before beginning, and to have an experienced nurse in charge of the mouthguard (and suction). There is a risk of excessive air insufflation when using heavy sedation or anaesthesia; it is wise to keep the abdomen exposed during examination and to palpate it regularly. Careful monitoring of oxygenation and the pulse is essential. Impending shock in a neonate is indicated by the baby suddenly becoming still and floppy; this is an indication to abort the procedure rapidly.

Complications

Upper GI endoscopy should be very safe, but there are many potential hazards. Large surveys suggest that simple diagnostic endoscopy carries a risk of significant complications in about one in 1000 procedures, and of death in about one in 10 000. Problems are more likely to be encountered in the elderly and acutely ill, and during emergency and therapeutic procedures. Definitions, risk factors and general precautions are discussed in Chapter 3. The most important factors are inexperience, incompetence, overconfidence and oversedation.

Medication reactions

Medication reactions may result from idiosyncrasy or overdosage. Allergy to local anaesthetics is not unusual and should always be checked prior to examination. Small doses of sedatives may produce coma in patients with respiratory or hepatic insufficiency. Medication problems may occur after patients leave the unit. Prolonged effects of various sedatives may affect co-ordination and judgement, and patients must not drive or operate machinery on the same day. Anticholinergics will not affect treated glaucoma but may precipitate an acute painful attack in occult chronic glaucoma, which is a good thing since it leads to diagnosis and appropriate treatment; there is therefore no ocular contraindication to the use of anticholinergics. Superficial thrombosis occasionally occurs at injection sites; the glycol carrier medium used for diazepam is particularly irritating and should not be given into small veins. The risk is reduced with diazepam in lipid emulsion form (Diazemuls) or water-soluble midazolam (Versed).

Pulmonary problems

These are not unusual, and hypoxia has been shown to be a common event with standard medication regimens. Significant hypoxia is best prevented by careful oximeter monitoring with appropriate responses to any drop in saturation (stimulation, oxygen or antidotes to narcotics). Aspiration pneumonia can also occur, especially in patients with oesophagogastric retention (e.g. achalasia, pyloric stenosis) or in those with active bleeding. Aspiration is more likely to occur in elderly patients, and when the gag reflex has been suppressed by pharyngeal anaesthesia and excessive sedation.

Cardiac dysrhythmias

Cardiac dysrhythmias can be induced by endoscopy, especially in the presence of hypoxia. Electrocardiographic monitoring, used routinely in many units, is certainly advisable when endoscopy is performed in patients with cardiac problems. Full resuscitation equipment must always be available.

Perforation

Peroration can occur at all levels of the upper gut. It is more common in the pharynx and cervical oesophagus where the endoscope is passed blindly, but can occur also at the cardia and superior duodenal angle, especially when these areas are distorted or diseased. Perforation is more likely to occur during therapeutic dilatations, either when passing a stiff guidewire blindly or during the dilatation itself. Imprudent force is usually responsible, but excessive air insufflation alone may occasionally result in perforation of an existing lesion. Perforation is immediately painful in the neck and mediastinum, but more distal perforation may not be apparent for some hours. Perforation may be obvious (by the bizarre view), or recognized only later by subsequent development of subcutaneous emphysema, and by the characteristic appearances on abdominal radiographs. The management of evident or suspected perforation is discussed in Chapter 5.

Instrument impaction

This can occur in a hiatus hernia or the distal oesophagus during the retroversion manoeuvre. Blind and forceful withdrawal should not be attempted if impaction has occurred. Disimpaction is best achieved by *advancing* the instrument, preferably under fluoroscopic guidance. Rarely, a mechanical failure in a diagnostic device (cytology brush, biopsy forceps or snare loop) may prevent its withdrawal through the instrument tip; the instrument and device must be carefully withdrawn together.

Bleeding

Bleeding can be induced by forceps biopsy, especially in patients with impaired coagulation and portal hypertension. Aggravation of bleeding during urgent endoscopy is difficult to detect or disprove. Bleeding is more common after therapeutic procedures.

Transmission of infection

This is discussed in Chapter 3.

Further reading

See further reading list in Chapter 5.

5 Therapeutic Upper Endoscopy

Over the last two decades, gastroenterologists have taken an increasing role in the interventional treatment of many upper gastrointestinal problems. This chapter discusses the techniques and applications in dysphagia, benign and malignant oesophageal stenoses, achalasia, gastric polyps, gastric and duodenal stenoses, instrument perforation, foreign bodies, acute bleeding and nutritional support.

Dysphagia

There are specific techniques used in managing different causes of dysphagia, but some important common principles. The nature, site and extent of the causative lesion must be evaluated carefully before a management strategy is determined (Plates 4.7 and 4.8). Many endoscopists rely almost exclusively on endoscopy, but a radiological roadmap is helpful with tight and tortuous strictures, and functional data (e.g. manometry and 24-h pH monitoring) may be needed. It is essential to have 'control' of the stricture, i.e. with a guidewire. Hurrying is dangerous and invites perforation. Objective outcome measures should be used (e.g. swallowing scores and quality of life indices). Good dietary advice and appropriate medications may be as important as aggressive therapeutic interventions.

Benign oesophageal stenosis

Most benign strictures are due to longstanding gastro-oesophageal acid reflux. Dilatation is used only as part of an overall treatment plan, with due attention to diet, medication and the possible need for surgical intervention. The patient must understand the treatment plan and recognize the risks and alternatives. Instrumental dilatation can provoke bacteraemia; antibiotic prophylaxis against endocarditis should be given to patients with significant cardiac lesions (see Chapter 3).

Dilatation techniques

Many techniques and variations of equipment are available. Mild strictures can be treated simply with mercury-weighted dilators (such as Maloney's bougie) without sedation. Other techniques are necessary when the stenosis is tight or tortuous, along with endoscopic and/or fluoroscopic control (over a guidewire), to ensure correct placement.

When the narrowing is not suitable for Maloney dilatation, the main question is whether to use dilating balloons or tapered bougies. Both methods are effective and their relative merits are debated. It has been suggested that the *radial* force applied by distending a balloon is likely to be more effective and safer than the tangential *shearing* force of a bougie, but these claims have not been proven. Bougie techniques give a better 'feel' of the stricture, which may be an important safety factor.

Through the scope (TTS) balloon dilatation. Balloons designed to be passed via the endoscope channel are 3–8 cm in length and of various diameters. We use 10, 15 and 18 mm diameter balloons, and usually prefer the 5 cm length (Fig. 5.1). These are easier to pass than longer balloons, but less likely to 'pop out' of the stricture than shorter ones. Passage is easier if the balloons are well maintained and 'furled' in the same direction on each occasion. Lubrication should be applied, either directly to the balloon with a silicone spray or by injecting 1–2 ml of silicone oil down the endoscope channel followed by 10 ml of air. Suction should be maintained on the balloon whilst it is passed through the channel. The stricture is examined endoscopically, and the soft tip of an appropriately sized balloon is passed gently through the stricture under direct vision. The balloons are fairly translucent, so that it is usually possible to observe the 'waist' of the balloon endoscopically during the procedure and to note the extent of dilatation. Most manufacturers recommend inflation to a fixed pressure, but, in the oesophagus, many experts dilate by feel. It is helpful to use a smaller syringe (15–20 ml) for easy inflation, changing to a larger one (50 ml) for more rapid evacuation. For tight strictures or maximal dilatation, the efficiency of balloon inflation is improved by using water (or contrast medium) rather than air, since fluids cannot be compressed. To do this, the balloon must be fluid-filled and all air extracted before insertion down the endoscope.

TTS balloon dilatation has become popular for several reasons. It can be performed as part of the initial endoscopy, and does not normally require fluoroscopic monitoring. The results of dilatation should be obvious immediately; the endoscope can be passed through the stricture (if this was not possible previously) to complete the endoscopic examination, including a retroverted view of the cardia in low lesions. However, balloons must be handled with care and are relatively expensive.

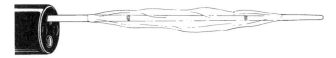

Fig. 5.1 A deflated TTS balloon dilator.

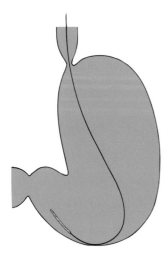

Fig. 5.2 A dilator guidewire positioned in the gastric antrum.

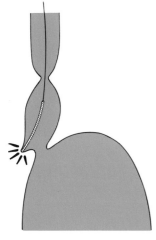

Fig. 5.3 Take care not to impact the guidewire.

Wire-guided bougie dilatation. This depends on endoscopic passage of a guidewire through the stricture into the stomach (Fig. 5.2) Standard guidewires are rigid 'piano' wires with floppy tips. Biliary-type guidewires, which are more flexible (see Chapter 6), may help find the lumen in tight and tortuous strictures. Endoscopic injection of contrast may also be instructive. The presence of the guidewire provides the security of knowing that the dilator will pass correctly through the stricture (and not into a diverticulum or necrotic tumour, or through the wall of a hiatus hernia) (Fig. 5.3). This security exists only if fluoroscopy is being used during the dilatation process — which can be a problem since many endoscopists do not have immediate X-ray access. However this is essential when tight and complex strictures are being treated.

Savary–Guilliard bougies are popular throughout the world. These are simple plastic wands with a long taper (Fig. 5.4), a distal metal marker and a radio-opaque band at the 'neck'. Variants of this design are available from other manufacturers. Diameters range from 3 to 20 mm. Eder–Puestow bougies were initially more popular in Europe; these are a series of metal olives (21–53 French gauge) which attach to a shaft and leader (Fig. 5.5). They give good 'feel', but the dilatation is relatively abrupt.

The following steps should be performed when dilating.

1 Choose a bougie which will pass relatively easily through the stricture and slide it over the guidewire down close to the mouth; lubricate the tip of the bougie.

2 Hold the bougie shaft in the left hand and push in, simultaneously applying countertraction on the guidewire with the right hand. Keep the left elbow extended (Fig. 5.6) so that the dilator cannot travel too far when resistance 'gives' (with the potential for distal perforation or a punch in the face for the patient).

3 Increase the size of the bougies progressively, but do not use more than three sizes above that at which significant resistance is felt.

4 Check the guidewire position repeatedly by fluoroscopy or by placing its end against a fixed external object.

5 After dilatation check the effect endoscopically; take biopsy and cytology samples if necessary.

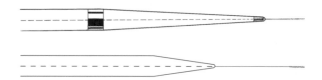

Fig. 5.4 Tips of Savary–Guilliard (above) and American Endoscopy (below) dilators for use over a guidewire.

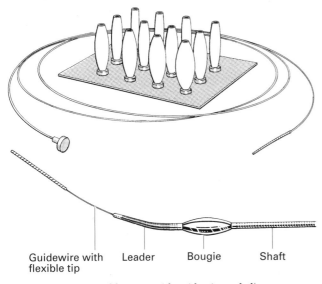

Guidewire with   Leader   Bougie   Shaft
flexible tip

Fig. 5.5 Eder–Puestow dilator set with guidewire and olives.

Certain strictures, particularly those due to irradiation or corrosive ingestion are particularly difficult to dilate. The process may take many procedures (which should start early after corrosive ingestion) and too rapid an increase in dilator size will result in perforation.

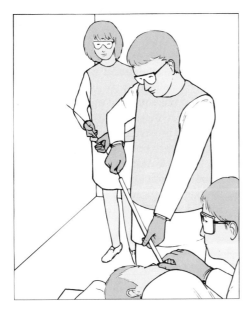

Fig. 5.6 Advance the dilator with the left hand and the elbow extended to avoid sudden overinsertion. Keep traction on the wire with the right hand.

Post-dilatation management

The patient should be kept under observation for at least 1 h, and considerably longer if the stricture is complex and the dilatation has been difficult. Patients are kept 'nil by mouth' during this first period and observed in the recovery area for any sign of perforation. The patient should always be reviewed by the endoscopist concerned (or his designated deputy), who should personally give the patient a trial drink of water if progress has been satisfactory. The patient is then discharged with instructions to keep to a soft diet overnight, plus appropriate medication and a follow-up plan. Dilatation can be repeated within a few days in severe cases, and then subsequently every few weeks until swallowing has been restored fully.

Achalasia

Manometry provides the gold standard for the diagnosis of achalasia, but endoscopy is also important, to demonstrate the absence of any local lesions such as a submucosal malignancy (Plates 4.7 and 4.8). The optimal treatment for achalasia is currently under review. To the longstanding techniques of 'brusque' balloon dilatation and open surgery, have recently been added two new methods of considerable promise — laparoscopic myotomy and endoscopic injection of botulinus toxin.

Balloon dilatation techniques are still widely used. The patient should be on a clear liquid diet for several days before the procedure. When, despite this, the endoscopist finds significant residue, he should remove the endoscope and perform lavage with a large-bore tube. Many different techniques and balloons have been used for achalasia dilatation. The position can be checked radiologically, or under direct vision with the endoscope alongside the balloon shaft, or even by a retroversion manoeuvre with the balloon fitted on the endoscope shaft. We prefer to place a guidewire endoscopically, and then dilate with a balloon under fluoroscopic control (Fig. 5.7). Achalasia balloons are available with diameters of 30, 35 and 40 mm. We start with the smallest balloon, warning the patient that repeat treatments may be necessary if symptoms persist or recur quickly. Inflation is maintained at the recommended pressure for 1–2 min if tolerated. There is usually some blood on the balloon after the procedure.

Close observation is mandatory for at least 4 h to detect any sign of perforation. Overnight admission is usually not necessary, but may be appropriate in selected cases. A chest X-ray and water-soluble contrast swallow should be done once the patient has recovered from sedation. Nothing should be given by mouth until the patient and the X-rays have been examined by the endoscopist personally. A trial drink of water is given under

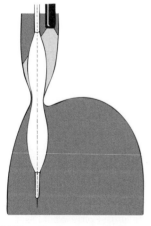

Fig. 5.7 Achalasia dilating balloons (before full inflation). (a) Checked fluoroscopically.

(b) Visualized endoscopically.

supervision. The uncomplicated patient can return to a normal diet on the next day. A formal follow-up review is arranged.

Malignant oesophageal stenosis

Barium studies and endoscopy have complementary roles in assessing the site and nature of oesophageal neoplasms. Endoscopic ultrasonography is the most accurate staging tool. Endoscopic management can help to improve swallowing in the majority of patients who are unsuitable for surgery because of intercurrent disease or tumour extent.

The abrupt onset of severe dysphagia may be due to the impaction of a food bolus which can be removed endoscopically (see below). The bulk of an exophytic tumour can be reduced by diathermy, lasers or an injection of toxic agents such as alcohol. Malignant strictures can be dilated using balloons or wire-guided bougies, but improvement is brief. Recurrence of dysphagia after dilatation can be prevented by inserting an oesophageal stent.

Oesophageal stents

The best candidates for stents are patients with mid-oesophageal tumours who are not expected to survive for more than a few months. Stents cannot be used when the tumour extends to within 2 cm of the cricopharyngeus, and stent function is less predictable with lesions at the cardia because of the angulation (Fig. 5.8). Appropriate stents provide good palliation for patients with malignant tracheo-oesophageal fistulae.

There are two main types of oesophageal stents: plastic and expandable metal mesh stents.

Plastic stents

Some experts make their own stents, since they wish to be able to tailor the length and shape precisely to the individual patient. However, a variety of stents are available commercially. Designs are broadly similar, with lumens of at least 10 mm, upper and lower flanges to prevent migration and radio-opaque markings (Fig. 5.9). They are flexible enough for ease of insertion and comfortable 'seating', but strong enough not to collapse. There are several lengths, and narrower tubes are available for special circumstances. A stent with a self-inflating cuff is available for use in patients with fistulae (Fig. 5.10).

Stent insertion

The lesion is assessed carefully by radiology and endoscopy, and the patient fully informed about the aims and risks of the proce-

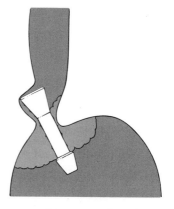

Fig. 5.8 Plastic stents through angulated tumours at the cardia may not function well.

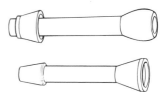

Fig. 5.9 Typical plastic oesophageal stents.

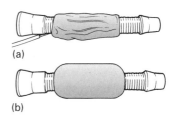

(a)

(b)

Fig. 5.10 Plastic-sleeved stent for fistulae. (a) Collapsed. (b) Sleeve expanded.

dure and the (usually few) available alternatives. Antibiotic prophylaxis should be considered. The stricture is then dilated by standard methods using wire-guided dilators, up to 50 French gauge (16 mm). The process must not be hurried since there is a significant risk of perforation by splitting the tumour; several sessions may be required. Dilatation may be more difficult and perhaps more hazardous after radiation therapy.

Placing a plastic stent is simple in principle. However, the procedure is technically demanding, and requires a fine blend of dexterity, caution and force; it is not for the inexperienced.

The Dumon–Guillard introducer consists of a long 10.5 mm diameter Savary bougie, a range of stents and a semirigid polyvinyl pusher tube (Fig. 5.11). The stiff guidewire is left in

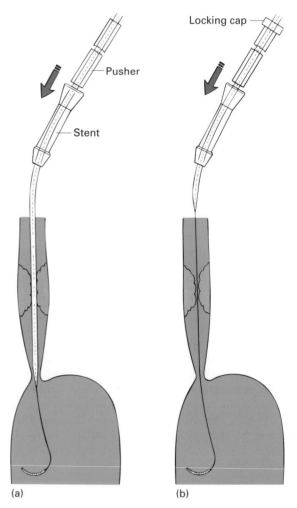

(a)   (b)

Fig. 5.11 'Over the dilator' methods for dilatation. (a) The stent is pushed over the static dilator. (b) The stent and pusher tube are locked onto the dilator and move in together over the guidewire.

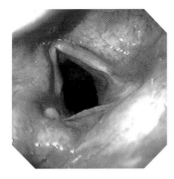

Plate 4.1 Ulcer close to the vocal cords in a patient with severe acid reflux presenting with nocturnal cough.

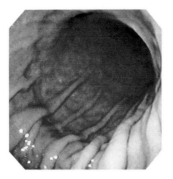

Plate 4.2 Normal gastric mucosa and folds in the body of the stomach, with the angulus in the distance.

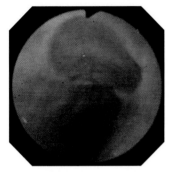

Plate 4.3 Gastric mucosa in the upper oesophagus – 'Inlet patch'.

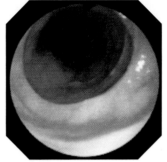

Plate 4.4 High squamo – columnar junction in the distal oesophagus – Barrett's oesophagus.

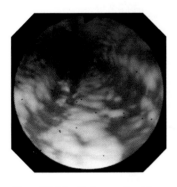

Plate 4.5 Monilial oesophagitis – typical adherent white plaques.

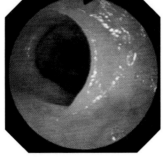

Plate 4.6 Oesophageal web – thin smooth membrane without inflammation.

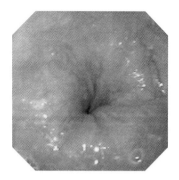

Plate 4.7 Pseudoachalasia – narrowing of the cardia, as viewed from the oesophagus.

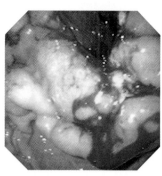

Plate 4.8 Pseudoachalasia – retroverted view of the fundal carcinoma.

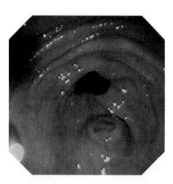

Plate 4.9 Ectopic pancreatic tissue in the floor of the gastric antrum – note characteristic central dimple.

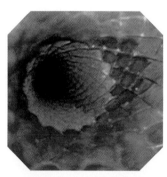

Plate 5.1 Covered expandable metal mesh stent in the mid oesophagus.

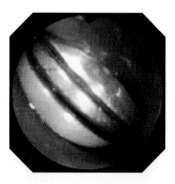

Plate 5.2 Three coins impacted in the mid oesophagus.

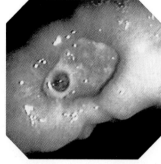

Plate 5.3 Visible vessel in a benign gastric ulcer.

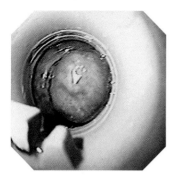

Plate 5.4 Endoscopic view after sucking a varix into the banding device, before firing.

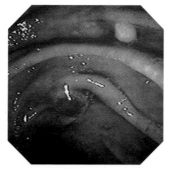

Plate 6.1 Normal major and minor papillas in the descending duodenum.

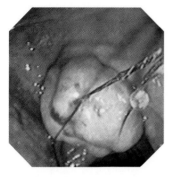

Plate 6.2 Villous adenoma of the papilla – placing an endoscopic snare for papillectomy.

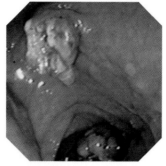

Plate 6.3 Villous adenoma of the papilla – appearance after papillectomy.

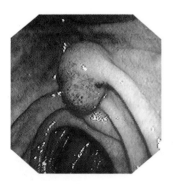

Plate 6.4 Swollen papilla due to an impacted stone – direct needle-knife puncture over the stone may be needed.

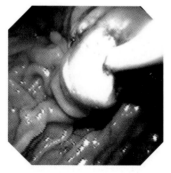

Plate 6.5 Catheter in the main papilla has exited through a biliary fistula, caused by a prior passage of a stone, or surgical dilator.

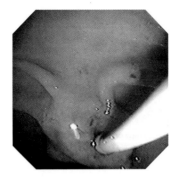

Plate 6.6 Cannulation of the papilla in a patient after Billroth II gastrectomy – the anatomy is 'upside down'.

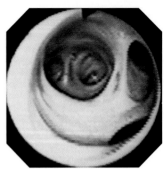

Plate 6.7 Peroral endoscopic choledochoscopy – views at the liver hilum.

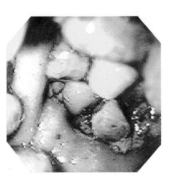

Plate 7.1 Multiple stones in the duodenum after sphincterotomy.

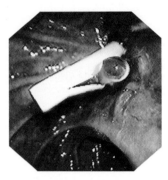

Plate 7.2 Stent draining bile – note short intraduodenal portion with flap well positioned.

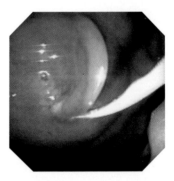

Plate 7.3 Turbid fluid draining after endoscopic transgastric diathermy puncture of a pseudocyst.

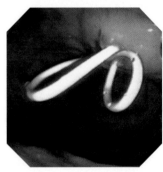

Plate 7.4 Two pigtail stents placed after endoscopic pseudocyst-gastrostomy.

place after bougie dilatation to 50 French gauge (16 mm) and its position checked fluoroscopically. A suitable stent of appropriate length is selected, and mounted on the long dilator with the pushing tube behind it. The assembly is lubricated and passed over the guidewire like a dilator—with backward traction of the guidewire. It is often necessary for the endoscopist to 'help' the stent around the pharynx using his fingers. Correct positioning is monitored fluoroscopically. Usually it is easy to feel when the stent enters the stricture and when the proximal funnel abuts its upper end. Rather than relying solely on feel, it is wise to place distance markers on the pusher tube shaft, having made the appropriate measurements (to the top and bottom of the tumour from the incisor teeth) during endoscopy after the final dilatation. Correct placement of the stent is also facilitated by prior endoscopic injection of contrast (lipiodol) at the upper and lower limits of the tumour, using a sclerotherapy needle.

When the stent appears to be correctly placed, the dilator and guidewire are removed, leaving the pusher tube in place. Endoscopy is then performed through the pusher, after it has been withdrawn 1–2 cm to separate it from the stent (Fig. 5.12). With the scope in place as a guide, the stent position can be adjusted forwards with the pusher or withdrawn somewhat if the tip is in the stomach, by pulling back with sharp retroversion (Fig. 5.13).

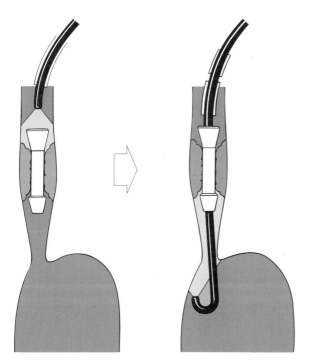

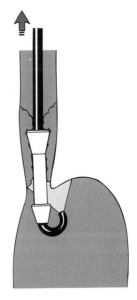

Fig. 5.12 Pass the scope through the pusher to check the final position of the stent.

Fig. 5.13 Use the hooked scope to pull back the stent—providing the tip is in the stomach.

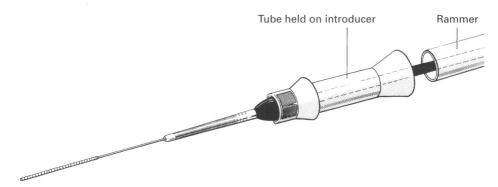

Fig. 5.14 The 'Nottingham introducer' system—the black expanding leader grips the stent tip firmly.

A variant method employs a flexible metal shaft with a device which can be expanded to grasp the inside of the stent (the Nottingham system) (Fig. 5.14). The system is passed over a standard guidewire after appropriate dilatation (Fig. 5.15). The stent is deposited by releasing the lock and removing the inserting assembly and guidewire. A pushing tube can also be used with this system, to hold the stent in place and to facilitate check endoscopy.

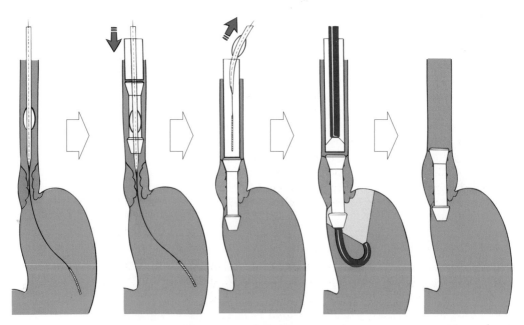

Fig. 5.15 The sequence of events for stent insertion using the 'Nottingham introducer' system.

Post-stent management

Patients with large tumours in the upper oesophagus may develop respiratory distress due to tracheal compression as the stent is placed. Always be prepared to remove a stent rapidly should this occur.

Stent insertion carries a perforation risk of 5–10%. Patients are kept in the hospital overnight under observation. Chest X-ray and water-soluble contrast swallow examinations are performed after about 2 h. Clear fluids can be given after 4 h if there have been no adverse developments.

Patients must understand the limitations of the stent, and the need to maintain a soft diet with plenty of fluids during and after meals. Written instruction should be provided and relatives counselled. Overambitious eating or inadequate chewing may result in obstruction. When this occurs, the food bolus can usually be removed or fragmented at endoscopy using snares or biopsy forceps. Sometimes the stent must be removed and replaced.

Stent dysfunction due to tumour overgrowth can be managed by endoscopic diathermy, laser photocoagulation or placement of another (smaller) stent inside the first. Gastro-oesophageal reflux can be a problem with stents crossing the cardia. Stents can deteriorate with time and may eventually disintegrate. Occasionally, a good result from chemotherapy or radiotherapy may make it possible to remove a stent entirely.

Stent extraction

Complete removal of a stent can be difficult, especially if there has been tumour overgrowth. Reversing the 'Nottingham introducer' technique (see Fig. 5.14) is effective. Alternatively, sufficient purchase can usually be provided with a large (unlubricated) TTS balloon inflated within the stent. When a stent has migrated downwards, removal is easier if it is first pushed into the stomach, rotated and withdrawn with the distal tip leading. If the stent cannot be gripped by inflating a large TTS balloon within its lumen, a polypectomy snare may be employed (Fig. 5.16). Fortunately, plastic stents which have migrated into the stomach rarely cause problems if left *in situ*.

Expandable metal mesh stents

There are several varieties of metal mesh stents and the technology is developing rapidly. The principle is simple. The nitinol (memory metal) or stainless steel device is compressed inside an introducing tube of 8–10 mm diameter (20–25 French gauge). This is inserted over a guidewire under fluoroscopic control after some initial dilatation (less than that required for a plastic

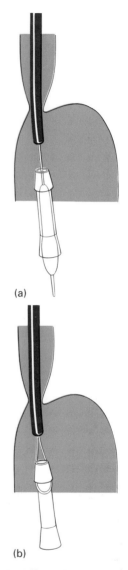

(a)

(b)

Fig. 5.16 Removing a stent, after rotation, using (a) a TTS balloon or (b) polypectomy snare.

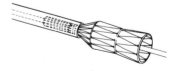

Fig. 5.17 Metal mesh oesophageal stent (partially expanded).

stent). The stent is released by gradual withdrawal of the covering sleeve (Fig. 5.17). The overall maximal luminal diameter of these stents is 15–18 mm. However, they vary considerably in expansile force. Most expand gradually over a period of days, and become fully incorporated in the oesophageal wall so that they cannot be removed. Less powerful stents—although easy to place and well tolerated—may not expand sufficiently to relieve the patient's symptoms, even with balloon dilatation.

The main problem with metal mesh stents (apart from their cost) is the tendency for tumour ingrowth through the mesh. This can be managed by endoscopic debulking (see below) or by placement of a second stent. The problem of ingrowth is being addressed by the development of metal mesh stents with plastic covering sleeves (Plate 5.1).

Tracheo-oesophageal fistulae are best managed with sleeved metal stents. A plastic stent with a self-expanding cuff is also available (see Fig. 5.10).

Tumour debulking

Obstructing tumour tissue can be destroyed endoscopically by several techniques. Scanning (especially endoscopic ultrasonography) may be helpful beforehand to assess the depth and size of tumours, and their relationships to important local structures (such as the aorta). It is pertinent to inform patients that dysphagia may worsen temporarily, for a few days, after some of these treatments, before the oedema subsides and the tumour sloughs.

Snare-loop diathermy. This is a simple method for debulking polypoid and exophytic tumours.

Local injection. Local injection of toxic agents will produce similar debulking results. Absolute alcohol is applied in aliquots of 0.2–0.5 ml using a sclerotherapy needle; it is rarely necessary or wise to exceed a total of 10 ml as extensive necrosis and mediastinitis have resulted. The effect is best judged after about 7 days and repeated as necessary. Other methods are preferred for longer and less exophytic lesions.

Laser photocoagulation. This vaporizes tumour tissue, so that the result can be assessed immediately if the smoke is aspirated continuously. The principle is simple, but the practice can be tedious and difficult for both endoscopist and patient. Repeated treatments are usually required. Lasers are expensive; safety goggles and venting systems are needed. The neodymium-yttrium aluminium garnet (YAG) laser has been used most commonly, at settings of 80–100 W, applied with a 300 µm fibre in a catheter with a coaxial gas jet. Laser energy can also be applied at low power using contact (sapphire tip) techniques, and the argon beam coagulator is becoming popular in this context.

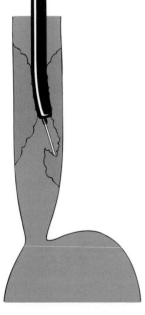
Fig. 5.18 Laser treatment is best performed from below upwards.

Laser treatments should be applied from below upwards (Fig. 5.18), since starting from the top may cause oedema, and obscure the view completely. Starting from below may require prior dilatation, which carries its own risks. It is preferable to use an endoscope with a large operating channel (or two channels) to be able to aspirate smoke and vent excessive insufflated gas; often there is not room for anything other than a small instrument. The probe should be activated about 1 cm away from the lesion. Treatment from a greater distance reduces the effect, whereas treating too close (which is often difficult to avoid) causes 'drilling' and splatter of charred debris onto the endoscope lens. The tip of the instrument itself can be damaged if the laser fibre is withdrawn inadvertently too far into the channel, or by reflected light energy.

The BICAP tumour probe. This is a cylindrical bipolar coagulator which can be passed over a guidewire (Fig. 5.19). Several sizes are available. Treatment is applied from below upwards after initial dilatation. The process is monitored fluoroscopically, and with an endoscope passed alongside the probe. This method is applicable only with circumferential tumours and has not been widely used.

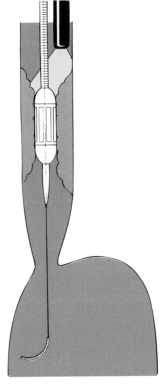

Fig. 5.19 The BICAP tumour probe over a guidewire—the procedure is monitored endoscopically.

Stents or tumour ablation?

Stenting is (theoretically) a once-only treatment performed after the initial dilatation. Stents are particularly useful in patients with straight mid-oesophageal lesions. The tumour probe is suited to long circumferential tumours. It is easiest to apply snare diathermy and injection to short exophytic lesions and to local recurrences after surgery or stenting. Laser therapy can be used in all of these contexts, but is becoming less popular because of its complexity and cost.

Endoscopists should be aware of their limitations, and be able to balance technological enthusiasm with full consideration of the patient's quality of life. These treatments are palliative, risky and only partially effective at best. They often need to be repeated. Even achieving a large lumen will not restore normal swallowing. The goal must be to restore 'adequate but not perfect' swallowing, at the lowest risk, cost and inconvenience to the patient.

Photodynamic therapy

Photodynamic therapy utilizes the fact that certain light-sensitive drugs (photosensitizers) concentrate selectively in malignant tissue when injected intravenously. Endoscopic laser light is used to produce toxic singlet oxygen from the photosensitizer, with destruction of the malignant tissue. The potential of this 'targeted' tumour therapy is considerable, and may have application in other conditions (e.g. Barrett's oesophagus). This treatment method is being studied actively in several centres using different photosensitizers and lasers. Its ultimate clinical role cannot be predicted.

Gastric and duodenal polyps

The principles and techniques of endoscopic polypectomy are described in Chapter 10 in relation to colonic polyps. Gastric and duodenal polyps are seen much less frequently; oesophageal polyps are rare. Endoscopic treatment of early oesophageal and gastric cancers (mucosectomy) is under investigation in Japan.

Upper GI polyps rarely have the long, thin stalks which make most colonoscopic polypectomies easy and safe. Many upper GI polyps are sessile, and some are largely submucosal. The possibility of a transmural lesion should be considered, in which case endoscopic ultrasonography may be helpful in making a treatment decision; surgical (or laparoscopic) resection may be safer. Because of the risk of bleeding, we usually inject the base of gastric and duodenal polyps with adrenaline (1 : 10 000) prior to snare diathermy; using saline (rather than aqueous) adrenaline solution slows the bleb dispersal.

Snare diathermy techniques can also be used to obtain large biopsy specimens when the gastric mucosa appears thickened, and standard biopsy techniques have failed to provide a diagnosis.

Gastric polypectomy and snare-loop biopsy techniques leave an ulcer; it is probably wise to prescribe appropriate medication for a few weeks.

Gastric and duodenal stenoses

Functionally significant stenoses may occur in the stomach or duodenum as a result of disease (tumours and ulcer healing) and following surgical intervention (e.g. hiatus hernia repair, gastroenterostomy, pyloroplasty, gastroplasty). Dilatation techniques as applied in the oesophagus (see above) can be used in these contexts, albeit often with less satisfactory results. Balloon dilatation of surgical stomas is usually effective (except in the case of banded gastroplasty with a rigid silicone ring). Pyloro-duodenal stenosis caused by ulceration can be relieved by balloon dilatation, but recurrence is common. Plastic and expandable metal mesh stents have been used to palliate malignant obstruction of the stomach and duodenum, with only marginal benefit.

Instrument perforation

Oesophageal dilatation is relatively safe using optimal techniques. However, perforations do occur, especially with complex and malignant strictures approached by inexperienced or overconfident endoscopists. The rate is approximately 0.1% in benign oesophageal strictures, 1% in achalasia dilatation and 5–10% in malignant lesions. Never try to dilate to the largest balloon or bougie simply because it is available. The risk is minimized by taking the process step by step — gradually and deliberately.

Early suspicion and recognition of perforation is the key to successful management, and no complaint should be ignored. The problem is usually obvious clinically; the patient is distressed and in pain. Signs of subcutaneous emphysema may not develop for several hours. Electrocardiograph (ECG), chest X-ray and water-soluble X-ray contrast swallow examinations should be performed. Surgical consultation is mandatory when perforation is seriously suspected or confirmed. Many confined perforations have been managed conservatively, with no oral intake, intravenous fluids or antibiotics—with or without placement of a sump tube across the perforation (with the suction holes above and below it). The choice between surgical and conservative management (and the timing of surgical intervention if conservative management appears to be failing) are difficult decisions; review of the literature shows varied and strong opinions. Conservative management is more likely to be appropriate when the perforation is in the neck; since the mediastinum is not contaminated, local surgical drainage can be performed simply when necessary. Perforation through a malignancy can be treated with a sleeved stent if the lumen can be found.

Foreign bodies

Foreign bodies are mainly found in children, in elderly patients with poor teeth and in the drunk and deranged. The problem is obvious if the patient is distressed and cannot swallow, and especially if a missing object is visible on a radiograph. However, many instances are less straightforward. Patients may not know that they have swallowed a bone or a drink-can pull and these items are not radio-opaque. It is therefore necessary to maintain a high index of suspicion.

Chest and abdominal radiographs (with lateral views) are appropriate. A water-soluble contrast swallow examination is helpful in patients with oesophageal symptoms, but is not necessary and potentially hazardous if dysphagia is complete.

Treatment should be initiated within hours in the following circumstances.

1 Patients who cannot swallow saliva.
2 Impacted sharp objects.
3 Ingestion of button batteries (which can disintegrate and cause local damage).

Other situations are usually less urgent. Indeed many foreign bodies should be managed conservatively, at least initially; food

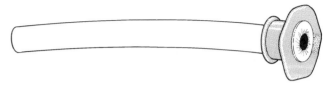

Fig. 5.20 An overtube with toothguard.

boluses and coins often pass spontaneously. An intravenous injection of Glucagon (0.5–1 mg) may help release oesophageal impactions.

Extraction techniques

Objects impacted at, or above, the cricopharyngeus, are usually removed by surgeons with rigid instruments. Foreign bodies in the oesophagus have also been approached traditionally with a rigid oesophagoscope. This allows good suction and the use of large grasping tools; however, general anaesthesia is required and the technique carries risks. Flexible endoscopy now takes precedence in most (but not all) situations. This procedure is easier for patients and does not usually require general anaesthesia. The use of an overtube increases the therapeutic options (Fig. 5.20).

Food impaction

If endoscopy is performed soon after the food has been ingested, meat can be removed as a single piece using a polypectomy snare, triprong grasper or retrieval basket. An increasingly popular approach is to use strong suction on the end of an overtube or a banding sleeve (Fig. 5.21). The biggest risk is losing the bolus in the region of the larynx. Food that has been impacted for several hours can usually be broken up (e.g. with a snare), and the pieces pushed into the stomach. This must be done carefully, especially if there is any question of a bone being present. Sometimes it is possible to manoeuvre a small endoscope past the food bolus and to use the tip to dilate the distal structure; the food can then be pushed through the narrowed area.

Most patients with impacted food have some oesophageal narrowing (benign reflux stricture or Schatski's ring). The endoscopist's task is not complete until this has been checked and treated. Usually, dilatation can be performed at the time of food extraction, but should be delayed if there is substantial oedema or ulceration.

Enzyme preparations (meat tenderizer) should not be used since severe pulmonary complications have been reported.

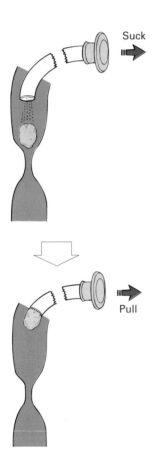

Fig. 5.21 Use an endoscopic overtube (after removing the scope) with suction to remove a food bolus.

True foreign bodies

Foreign bodies should always be removed if they are trapped in the oesophagus (Plate 5.2). Sharp objects (such as open safety pins) should be withdrawn into the tip of an overtube (Fig. 5.22); sometimes it is safer to use a rigid oesophagoscope.

Most objects entering the stomach will pass spontaneously, but there are a few indications for early removal. Sharp and pointed objects have a 15–20% chance of causing perforation (usually at the ileocaecal valve), and should be extracted whilst still in the stomach or proximal duodenum. Foreign bodies wider than 2 cm and longer than 5 cm are unlikely to pass from the stomach spontaneously and should be removed if possible. Once they have reached the stomach, button batteries usually pass spontaneously; a purgative should be given to accelerate the process. Endoscopists should resist the temptation to attempt removal of condoms containing cocaine or other hard drugs since rupturing the containers can lead to a massive overdose; surgical removal is the safest option.

The golden rules for foreign body removal are:
1 be sure that your extraction procedure is really necessary;
2 think before you start, and rehearse outside the patient;
3 do not make the situation worse;
4 do not be slow to get surgical or anaesthesia assistance;
5 protect the oesophagus, pharynx and bronchial tree during withdrawal with an overtube or endotracheal anaesthesia.

The endoscopist should have several specialized tools available, in addition to the overtube. There are forceps with claws or flat blades designed to grasp coins (Fig. 5.23), and a triprong extractor is useful for meat (Fig. 5.24). Many objects can be grasped with a polypectomy snare or stone-retrieval basket. Any object with a hole (such as a key or ring) can be withdrawn by passing a thread through the hole. The endoscope is passed into the stomach with biopsy forceps or a snare closed within its tip, grasping a thread which passes down the outside of the instrument (Fig. 5.25). It is then simple to pass the thread through the hole in the object by advancing the forceps, dropping the end and picking it up on the other side.

Gastric bezoars

Gastric bezoars are aggregations of fibrous animal or vegetable material. They are usually found in association with delayed gastric emptying (e.g. postoperative stenosis or dysfunction). Most masses can be fragmented with biopsy forceps or a polypectomy snare, but more distal bolus obstruction may result if fragmentation is inadequate. Various enzyme preparations have been recommended to facilitate disruption, but these are rarely necessary or effective. Large gastric bezoars are best disrupted and removed by inserting a large-bore (36 French gauge,

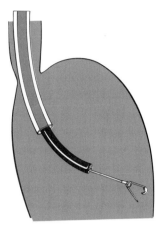

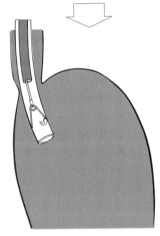

Fig. 5.22 Remove sharp foreign bodies with a protecting overtube.

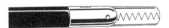

Fig. 5.23 Foreign-body extraction forceps.

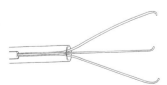

Fig. 5.24 A triprong grasping device.

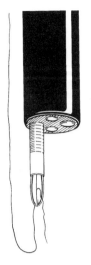

Fig. 5.25 Take a thread down with the forceps to pass through any object with a hole in it, e.g. a ring or key.

12 mm) lavage tube, and instilling and removing 2–3 litres of tap water with a large syringe. The cause of gastric-emptying dysfunction should be evaluated.

Upper gastrointestinal bleeding

Acute upper GI bleeding (haematemesis and/or melaena) is a common medical problem, for which endoscopy has become the primary diagnostic and therapeutic technique. Barium radiology is obsolete in this context and surgical intervention has been markedly reduced in recent years.

The timing of endoscopy is important and somewhat controversial. Examination can be delayed to a convenient time (e.g. the next morning) in most patients who appear to be stable, but the endoscopic team must be prepared to go into action within hours (after immediate resuscitation) in certain circumstances.

Emergency endoscopy

Indications for emergency endoscopy include the following:
1 Continued active bleeding requiring intervention.
2 Suspicion of variceal bleeding.
3 When the patient has an aortic graft.
4 To check the upper tract before severe rectal bleeding is attributed to a colonic source.

Emergency endoscopy is a challenging task. There is considerable potential for benefit — but there are also risks. These techniques require experience, nerve and judgement. The endoscopist should be expert, must know the equipment and should be assisted by an experienced GI nurse. Unstable patients should be under supervision in an intensive care environment. Safety considerations are paramount. Sedation should be given cautiously in unstable patients, and every precaution must be taken to minimize the risk of pulmonary aspiration. Patients with massive bleeding are often best examined under general anaesthesia, with the airway protected by a cuffed endotracheal tube. Even in less acute situations, blood clots may obscure the view in the stomach and duodenum. Standard gastric lavage is rarely effective, even when performed personally with a large-bore tube. Endoscopes with a large channel (or two channels) allow better flushing and suction. An alternative approach is to start the procedure with an overtube over the endoscope (see Fig. 5.20). If blood is encountered, the endoscope can be removed; blood clots can be sucked directly through the overtube or after flushing with a lavage tube. A diagnosis can usually be made even if the stomach cannot be emptied completely. Lesions are rare on the greater curvature, where the blood pools in the standard left lateral position. Changing the patient's position some-what should improve the survey, but turning completely on the right side is hazardous unless the airway is protected.

Lesions which cause acute bleeding are well known. Endoscopy has highlighted the fact that many patients are found to have more than one mucosal lesion (e.g. oesophageal varices *and* acute gastric erosions). A complete examination of the oesophagus, stomach and duodenum should be performed in every bleeding patient, no matter what is seen *en route*. A lesion should be incriminated as the bleeding source only if it is actu-ally bleeding at the time of examination, or is covered with clot which cannot be washed off with a jet of water. An ulcer whose base is haemorrhagic, or contains a visible vessel, can be assumed to have bled recently (Plate 5.3). If the patient has pre-sented with haematemesis, and endoscopy shows only a single lesion (even without any of these features), it is likely to be the bleeding source. This is not necessarily the case if the presenta-tion has been with melaena, or if the examination takes place more than 48 h after bleeding since acute lesions such as mucosal tears and erosions may already have healed.

Treatment modalities

Many different endoscopic techniques have been developed. These include injection sclerosis, rubber banding, thermal probes (heat probe, bipolar or monopolar electrocoagulation and lasers), clipping and simple adrenaline (epinephrine) injec-tion. Many randomized trials have compared different tech-niques, but the experience of the endoscopist — and his familiarity with a particular technique — is probably the most important determinant of success. Laser photocoagulation initially became popular because it was assumed that it was safer not to *touch* the lesion. However, it has become clear that direct pressure with some probes (and injection treatment) pro-vides an additional important tamponade effect. Standard laser photocoagulation is now rarely used because of its complexity and cost, but the argon beam coagulator is useful for certain lesions.

Variceal treatments

Endoscopic treatment of oesophageal (and gastric) varices can be helpful in patients who are bleeding, or have recently bled. Prophylactic treatment is controversial. Techniques include injection sclerosis, banding and combination techniques. Clips and loops have also been used recently. Endoscopic management should be seen as only a part of a patient's overall care.

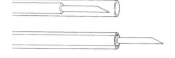

Fig. 5.26 A retractable sclerotherapy needle.

Injection sclerotherapy

This has been used for decades, originally with rigid oesophago-scopes; flexible instruments are now used routinely. Many adjuvant devices have been described, including overtubes with a lateral window and the use of balloons—either in the stomach to compress distal varices or on the scope itself to permit tamponade if bleeding occurs. However, most experts use a simple 'free-hand' method, with a standard large-channel endoscope and a flexible, retractable needle (Fig. 5.26). Injections are given directly into the varices, starting close to the cardia (and below any bleeding site) and working spirally upwards for about 5 cm. Each injection consists of 1–2 ml of sclerosant, to a total of 20–30 ml.

Precise placement of the needle within the varix (as guided by co-injection of a dye such as methylene blue or by simultaneous manometric or radiographic techniques) may improve the results and reduce the complications. However, some experts believe that paravariceal injections are also effective, and it is often difficult to tell which has been achieved. If bleeding occurs on removal of the needle, it is usually helpful to tamponade the area simply by passing the endoscope into the stomach.

Several sclerosants are available. Sodium morrhuate (5%) and sodium tetradecylsulphate (STD) (1–1.5%) are popular in the USA. Polidocanol (1%), ethanolamine oleate (5%) and STD are widely used in Europe. Various experts use mixed sclerosant 'cocktails' (some containing alcohol). Efficacy, ulcerogenicity and the risk of complications run together, since it is the process of damage and healing by fibrosis which eradicates or buries the communicating veins, but may equally result in stricture. In general, excessive volumes, especially if given paravariceally, increase the risk of ulceration or stricture, whereas higher concentration of stronger agents (e.g. 3% STD) increases the likelihood of perforation.

Endoscopic polymer injection is another alternative. The two agents most commonly used (*n*-butyl-2-cyanoacrylate and isobutyl-2-cyanoacrylate) are not available in the USA. These polymers solidify almost immediately on contact with proteinaceous material. The endoscopist and nurse must be very aware of how to use these polymers in order to provide an effective injection without gluing up the endoscope. Preliminary results appear to be excellent, especially in gastric varices (which do not respond well to standard sclerotherapy).

Variceal ligation (banding)

Variceal ligation is a method originally used for the treatment of haemorrhoids which has become popular for the management of oesophageal (and gastric) varices. The device consists of a friction-fit sleeve on the endoscope tip, an inner cylinder preloaded with an elastic band and a trip wire (passing up the endoscope channel) to move the inner cylinder and release the band (Fig. 5.27). The varix is sucked into the sleeve, and the band fired by pulling on the nylon trip wire (Plate 5.4). Early devices contained only one band which meant that the endoscope had to be passed repeatedly. This was facilitated by using an overtube, but there were concerns about safety. The need for repeated passage has been greatly reduced by the development recently of devices which contain five or more bands. Banding can also be applied to gastric varices and to small ulcers (e.g. Dieulafoy lesions).

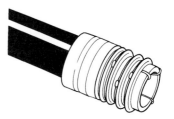

Fig. 5.27 An oesophageal banding device.

Repeated treatments are necessary (initially at 5–7 days, then every 2–3 weeks) until the varices are obliterated, whichever method is used.

Actively bleeding varices are more difficult to treat. It may be helpful to tilt the patient slightly head up, or to apply traction on a gastric balloon. Sometimes it is wiser to defer endoscopy for several hours and temporize with a pharmacological agent (vasopressin or somatostatin) or a Sengstaken–Blakemore tube. The TIPS (transvenous interventional porto-systemic shunt) procedure provides a useful alternative when these treatments fail.

Risks of variceal treatment include all of the complications of emergency endoscopy (especially pulmonary aspiration). Severe ulceration and stricturing are more common after sclerotherapy than after banding. Medications to lower gastric acid and/or protect the mucosa are given until the treatment sequence is complete.

Treatment of bleeding ulcers

Duodenal and gastric ulcers are the commonest cause of acute bleeding. About 80% will stop spontaneously, but it is now possible to predict those patients likely to rebleed and select them for endoscopic treatment. Certain clinical features (e.g. size of the bleed and type of presentation) give some predictive information. We pay most attention to the appearance of the lesion itself. Active 'spurters' continue to bleed (or rebleed soon) in 70–80% of cases. Ulcers with a 'visible vessel' have about a 50% chance of rebleeding. Clean ulcers do not rebleed. An important question is whether it is appropriate to wash clots off the base of an ulcer simply to check for these stigmas. Most endoscopists will do so in high-risk patients provided they are poised for treatment. Endoscopic Doppler devices can be used to 'listen' for feeding vessels.

The most popular haemostatic methods now are injection, heat probe and bipolar probe.

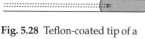

Fig. 5.28 Teflon-coated tip of a
heat probe with a water-jet
opening.

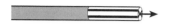

Fig. 5.29 The tip of a multipolar
BICAP probe with a central water
jet.

1 *Injection treatment.* Adrenaline (epinephrine) in 1:10000 to
1:20000 dilution, is applied with a standard sclerotherapy
needle in 0.5–1.0 ml aliquots around the base of the bleeding site,
up to a total of 10 ml; diluting it in saline solution (0.9–1.8%)
gives a more localized bleb. Some experts use absolute alcohol in
much smaller volumes (1–2 ml in 0.1 ml aliquots) or combinations of adrenaline with alcohol or with the sclerosants used for
the treatment of varices.
2 *The heat probe* (Fig. 5.28) provides a constant high temperature;
the setting (usually 30 J) reflects the duration of application.
3 *The bipolar probe* (Fig. 5.29) provides bipolar electrocoagulation, which is assumed to be safer than monopolar diathermy
(which produces an unpredictable depth of damage). Use the
larger 10 French gauge probe at 30–40 W for 10 s.

These treatment devices share some common principles. All
can be applied tangentially, but (apart from injection) are better
used face-on if possible. When the vessel is actively spurting,
direct probe pressure on the vessel or feeding vessel will reduce
the flow and increase the effectiveness of treatment. The bipolar
and heat probes incorporate a flushing water jet which helps
prevent sticking.

Know when to stop treatment and when not to start

Treatment attempts should not be protracted if major difficulties
are encountered; the risks rise as time passes. There are some
patients and lesions in which endoscopic intervention may be
foolhardy, and surgery is more appropriate, e.g. a large posterior
wall duodenal ulcer which may involve the gastroduodenal
artery.

Follow-through

A single endoscopic treatment is not an all-or-nothing event.
It is necessary to continue other medical measures, to maintain
close monitoring and to plan ahead for further intervention
(endoscopic, radiological or surgical) if bleeding continues or
recurs. The job is not complete until the lesion is fully healed.
Eradication of *Helicobacter pylori* reduces the risk of late
rebleeding.

Complications of ulcer haemostasis

The two most important hazards of ulcer haemostasis are pulmonary aspiration and provocation of further bleeding. It is difficult to know how often endoscopy causes rebleeding which
would not have occurred spontaneously, but major immediate
bleeding is unusual and can usually be stopped. The risk of pulmonary aspiration is minimized by protecting the airway using

pharyngeal suction and a head-down position, or a cuffed endo-tracheal tube. Perforation can be induced with any of the treatment methods if they are used too aggressively, especially in acute ulcers which have little protecting fibrosis.

Treatment of mucosal lesions

All of the modalities described above can be used to treat vascular malformations such as angiomas and telangiectasia. The risk of full-thickness damage and perforation is greater in organs with thinner walls (e.g. the oesophagus and small bowel) than in the stomach and duodenum. Lesions with a diameter of more than 1 cm should be approached with caution, and treated from the periphery inwards to avoid provoking haemorrhage. Laser photocoagulation and the argon beam coagulator provide the best control.

Nutrition

Feeding and decompression tubes

Tubes for short-term feeding (and gastric decompression) are normally placed blindly, but can also be passed under fluoroscopic guidance or after endoscopic placement of a guidewire. Two direct endoscopic methods can be used when necessary, for example to advance tubes through the pylorus or a surgical stoma.

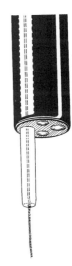

Through-the-channel method. The simplest technique is to advance a 7 French gauge plastic tube through a large-channel endoscope, over a standard (400 cm long) 0.035-inch diameter guidewire (Fig. 5.30). The tube and guidewire are advanced through the pylorus under direct vision, and subsequent passage is checked by fluoroscopy. When the tip is in the correct position, the endoscope is withdrawn whilst further advancing the tube (and guidewire) through it. Finally, the guidewire is removed and the tube is rerouted through the nose (see Chapter 7).

Fig. 5.30 The feeding tube and guidewire are passed through a large-channel scope.

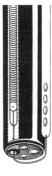

Alongside-the-scope method. This technique allows the placement of a tube larger than the endoscope channel, and is appropriate when a therapeutic instrument is not available—or when there is a need to pass a large decompression tube. A short length of suture material is attached to the end of the tube and is grasped within the instrument channel with a biopsy forceps or snare (Fig. 5.31). The endoscope is passed into the stomach and the tube is then pushed through the pylorus (or stoma) under direct vision. Once in position (checked by fluoroscopy), the thread is released and the endoscope is removed. It is helpful to make the

Fig. 5.31 A tube is carried alongside the scope by a thread grasped with a biopsy forceps.

tube stiffer with a large-gauge guidewire to avoid dislodgement while withdrawing the endoscope. The final position should be checked by fluoroscopy.

Percutaneous endoscopic gastrostomy (PEG)

Nasoenteric feeding can be used for several weeks but is inconvenient and unstable, and it is probably often responsible for pulmonary aspiration and pneumonia. PEG is now a popular method for long-term feeding, particularly to permit the transfer of patients with chronic neurological disability from acute care hospitals into nursing homes. The technique can be extended into a feeding jejunostomy by the use of appropriate tubes. Studies comparing PEG with operative gastrostomy have shown some advantages for the endoscopic method, but surgical (and laparoscopic) options should always be considered, especially in circumstances (e.g. ascites) where the endoscopic approach may be more difficult or hazardous.

Although many variants have been described, there are two major methods for PEG — the 'pull' and the 'push' methods. The risk of skin sepsis may be reduced by using antibiotics prophylactically; some experts also recommend disinfectant mouthwashes.

Methods of insertion

The 'pull' technique. A standard endoscope is passed into the stomach and the gastric outlet is checked. The patient is rotated onto the back, the stomach distended with air and the room darkened. Darkening is particularly important with video-endoscopes which provide less illumination.

1 The tip of the endoscope is directed towards the anterior wall of the stomach.

2 The abdominal wall is observed for transillumination and the assistant indents the site with a finger.

3 The endoscopist checks that the indentation can be seen and that it is in an appropriate part of the body of the stomach.

4 The assistant marks this spot on the anterior abdominal wall, applies disinfectant and infiltrates local anaesthetic into the skin, subcutaneous tissues and fascia.

5 A short (about 5 mm) skin incision is made with a pointed blade, extending into the subcutaneous fat.

6 An 18 gauge needle catheter is pushed through the anterior abdominal wall and its entrance into the stomach is observed by the endoscopist, who has meanwhile placed a polyp snare under the area of indentation and maintained gastric distension (Fig. 5.32a).

7 A guidewire (or silk suture) at least 150 cm long is passed

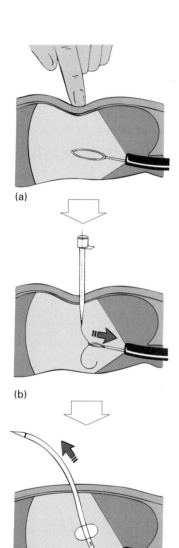

(a)

(b)

(c)

Fig. 5.32 (a–c) Stages in PEG tube placement—the 'pull' technique (see text).

through the needle and grasped with the snare (Fig. 5.32b).

8 The endoscope and snare are withdrawn through the mouth, carrying the guidewire, ensuring that the free end of the wire remains outside the abdominal wall.

9 The wire at the mouth is then tied to the PEG catheter, which is pulled down the oesophagus and through the anterior abdominal wall (Fig. 5.32c). It should not be pulled tight, since compression necrosis of the gastric wall has been described. This position is checked after the endoscope is replaced (Fig. 5.32c).

10 The tube is anchored at the skin by various disc devices.

11 Feeding can be commenced on the day after the procedure if there are no complications.

A simplified 'pull' technique. A variation of the 'pull' technique eliminates the necessity to pass the endoscope twice.

1 Pass the endoscope, pulling the guidewire or long suture down *alongside* it (holding the tip with forceps in the channel) (see Fig. 5.25).

2 Grasp the guidewire with a polyp snare (without the sheath) which has been passed by the assistant through the needle traversing the abdominal wall.

3 Withdraw the snare loop and guidewire.

4 Pull the PEG tube down through the mouth (alongside the endoscope) and into the correct position.

The 'push' technique. This method is inherently simpler. The feeding tube is pushed through the abdominal wall (rather than pulling it down from the mouth). The stomach is distended and an appropriate position chosen by transillumination and finger indentation, as with the other methods. The skin and subcutaneous tissues are infiltrated with local anaesthetic to allow a wider and deeper skin incision.

1 Insert a needle through this incision into the stomach, and pass a guidewire through it (Fig. 5.33a).

2 Withdraw the needle and pass a larger trochar with a plastic 'peel-away' catheter over the guidewire with pressure and rotation.

3 Withdraw the trochar once the catheter enters the stomach (Fig. 5.33b).

4 Pass the feeding tube through the catheter.

5 Remove the outer 'peel-away' catheter and fix the tube to the abdominal wall (Fig. 5.33c).

This 'push' method eliminates contamination of the feeding tube by passage through the mouth, and requires only one insertion of the endoscope. It can be performed under fluoroscopy without endoscopy. However, it is sometimes difficult to push the trochar and catheter through the abdominal and gastric walls.

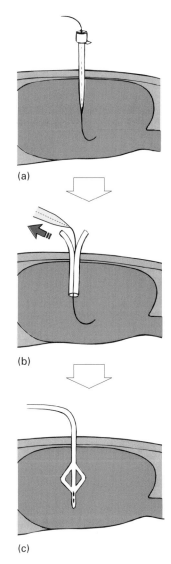

(a)

(b)

(c)

Fig. 5.33 (a–c) Stages in PEG tube placement—the 'push' technique (see text).

Problems and risks

PEG placement cannot be performed in patients with oesophageal strictures too tight to permit the passage of an endoscope. Technical difficulties and risks are higher in patients who have previously undergone abdominal surgery, particularly with partial gastric resection, and in patients with ascites or obesity. Local infection can occur (even spreading fasciitis), particularly if the skin incision is too small or if the tube has been pulled too tight against the gastric wall. A small pneumoperitoneum is not uncommon, and usually benign, but major and persisting leakage requires operative correction. Injury to the transverse colon may result in a gastrocolic fistula.

Tube dislodgement was distressingly frequent with original Foley catheter-type tubes, but should occur only rarely with other commercial devices unless the patient pulls on them. Early dislodgement usually results in peritonitis requiring surgical repair. A blocked or displaced tube can be replaced once a fibrous tract has formed (after a few weeks) by the simple insertion of a Malecot-type catheter, or one of the 'buttons' that are available commercially.

Percutaneous endoscopic jejunostomy (PEJ)

Jejunal feeding is often recommended in patients with gastro-oesophageal reflux to reduce the risk of pulmonary aspiration. Current evidence suggests that this hope may not always be realized. The jejunostomy tube may be inserted (under endoscopic guidance) through an established gastrostomy tract or using special commercial kits at the time of the original PEG puncture.

Further reading

General

Blades EW, Chak A, eds. *Upper Gastrointestinal Endoscopy*. Gastrointestinal Endoscopy Clinics of North America, Vol. 4(3) (series ed. Sivak MV). Philadelphia: WB Saunders, 1994.

Greene FL, Ponsky JL. *Endoscopic Surgery*. Philadelphia: WB Saunders, 1994.

Hawes RH, ed. *Experimental and Investigational Endoscopy*. Gastrointestinal Endoscopy Clinics of North America, Vol. 4(2) (series ed. Sivak MV). Philadelphia: WB Saunders, 1994.

VanDam J, ed. *The Oesophagus*. Gastrointestinal Endoscopy Clinics of North America, Vol. 4(4) (series ed. Sivak MV). Philadelphia: WB Saunders, 1994.

Wyllie R, ed. *Pediatric Endoscopy*. Gastrointestinal Endoscopy Clinics of North America, Vol. 4(1) (series ed. Sivak MV). Philadelphia: WB Saunders, 1994.

Dysphagia

Boyce GA, Boyce HW. *Endoscopic Management of Gastrointestinal Tumors.* Gastrointestinal Endoscopy Clinics of North America, Vol. 2(3) (series ed. Sivak MV). Philadelphia: WB Saunders, 1992.

Earlam R, Cunha-Melo J. Benign oesophageal strictures: historical and technical aspects of dilatation. *Br J Surg* 1981;**68**:829–36.

Earlam R, Cunha-Melo J. Malignant oesophageal strictures: a review of techniques for palliative intubation. *Br J Surg* 1982;**69**:61–8.

Lightdale CJ. Staging of esophageal cancer I: endoscopic ultrasonography. *Semin Oncol* 1994;**21**:438–46.

Pasricha PJ, Fleischer DE, Kalloo AN. Endoscopic perforations of the upper digestive tract; a review of their pathogenesis, prevention and management. *Gastroenterology* 1994;**106**:787–802.

Pass HI. Photodynamic therapy in oncology: mechanisms and clinical use. *J Natl Cancer Inst* 1993;**85**:443–56.

Payne-James JJ, Spiller RC, Misiewicz JJ, Silk DBA. Use of ethanol-induced tumor necrosis to palliate dysphagia in patients with esophagogastric cancer. *Gastrointest Endosc* 1990;**36**:43–6.

Vermeijden JR, Bartelsman JFWM, Fockens P *et al.* Self-expanding metal stents for palliation of esophagocardial malignancies. *Gastrointest Endosc* 1995;**41**:58–63.

Foreign bodies

American Society for Gastrointestinal Endoscopy. *Guideline for Management of Ingested Foreign Bodies.* ASGE Publication 1026. Manchester: American Society for Gastrointestinal Endoscopy, 1995.

Greene FL. Endoscopic management of gastrointestinal tract foreign bodies. In: Greene FL, Ponsky JL, eds. *Endoscopic Surgery.* Philadelphia: WB Saunders, 1994.

Webb W. Management of foreign bodies of the upper gastrointestinal tract. *Gastroenterology* 1988;**94**:204–16.

Upper gastrointestinal bleeding

Binmoeller KF, Soehendra N. 'Super glue'; the answer to variceal bleeding and fundal varices? *Endoscopy* 1995;**27**:392–6.

Chung SCS, Leung JWC, Sung JY, Lo KK, Li AKC. Injection or heat probe for bleeding ulcer. *Gastroenterology* 1991;**100**:33–7.

Cook DJ, Guyatt GH, Salena BJ, Laine LA. Endoscopic therapy for acute nonvariceal upper gastrointestinal hemorrhage; a meta-analysis. *Gastroenterology* 1992;**102**:139–48.

Fardy JM, Laupacis A. A meta-analysis of prophylactic endoscopic sclerotherapy for esophageal varices. *Am J Gastroenterol* 1994;**89:**1938–48.

Freeman ML, Cass OW, Peine CJ, Onstad GR. The non-bleeding visible vessel versus the sentinel clot: natural history and risk of rebleeding. *Gastrointest Endosc* 1993;**39**:359–66.

Goff JS. Gastroesophageal varices: pathogenesis and therapy of acute bleeding. *Gastroenterol Clin North Am* 1993;**22**:779–800.

Infante-Rivard C, Esnaola S, Villeneuve JP. Role of endoscopic variceal sclerotherapy in the long-term management of variceal bleeding: a meta-analysis. *Gastroenterology* 1989;**96**:1087–92.

Laine L, Peterson WL. Bleeding peptic ulcer. *N Engl J Med* 1994; **331**:717–27.

Laine L, El-Newihi HM, Migikovsky B *et al.* Endoscopic ligation compared with sclerotherapy for treatment of bleeding esophageal varices. *Ann Intern Med* 1993;**119**:1–7.

National Institutes of Health Consensus Conference. Therapeutic endoscopy and bleeding ulcers. *Gastrointest Endosc* 1990;**36**:S1–S65.

Steele RJC, Chung SCS, Leung JWC. *Practical Management of Acute Gastrointestinal Bleeding*. Oxford: Butterworth-Heinemann, 1993.

Swain P. What should be done when initial endoscopic therapy for bleeding peptic ulcer fails? *Endoscopy* 1995;**27**:321–8.

Westaby D, ed. *Variceal Bleeding*. Gastrointestinal Endoscopy Clinics of North America, Vol. 2(1) (series ed. Sivak MV). Philadelphia: WB Saunders, 1992

Endoscopic band ligation of varices. *Gastrointest Endosc* 1993;**39**:877–8.

Nutrition/percutaneous endoscopic gastrostomy

Ponsky JL. *Percutaneous Endoscopic Gastrostomy*. Gastrointestinal Endoscopy Clinics of North America, Vol. 2(2) (series ed. Sivak MV). Philadelphia: WB Saunders, 1992.

ASGE guidelines and technology assessments

Therapeutic Gastrointestinal Endoscopy. Manchester: American Society for Gastrointestinal Endoscopy, 1990.

Appropriate Use of Gastrointestinal Endoscopy. Manchester: American Society for Gastrointestinal Endoscopy, 1992.

The Role of Endoscopy in the Management of Non-variceal Acute Gastrointestinal Bleeding. Manchester: American Society for Gastrointestinal Endoscopy, 1992.

Endoscopic Feeding Tubes. Manchester: American Society for Gastrointestinal Endoscopy, 1994.

Balloon Dilatation of Gastrointestinal Tract Strictures. Manchester: American Society for Gastrointestinal Endoscopy, 1994.

ERCP—Diagnostic Technique
Endoscopic Retrograde Cholangiopancreatography

6

Endoscopic retrograde cholangiopancreatograpy (ERCP) has many applications in patients with known or suspected biliary and pancreatic diseases. The techniques are complex and carry some risk. Optimal results require teamwork between a skilled endoscopist, trained gastrointestinal (GI) nurse/assistants and interested radiology staff.

The experience needed for training, and to maintain competence thereafter, is such that endoscopists should not all expect to practice ERCP. The therapeutic developments (e.g. sphincterotomy, stenting) have become more important than the purely diagnostic studies. There are risks in performing a diagnostic ERCP in the presence of biliary or pancreatic obstruction without being able to provide immediate endoscopic drainage. Thus, ERCP and its therapeutic applications should be considered together. Training in diagnostic ERCP alone is no longer appropriate.

Equipment

Endoscopes

Cannulation is performed with side-viewing instruments. These allow face-on views of the papilla which cannot be achieved with standard forward-viewing endoscopes (Fig. 6.1). There is little to choose between the duodenoscopes of different companies. All have wide-angle lenses to facilitate orientation and a working channel of at least 2.8 mm. Endoscopes with larger channels (3.8–4.2 mm) are needed for stenting (see Chapter 7), and can be used for *all* ERCP procedures (except in young children). As in other areas, video-endoscopes are supplanting fibreoptic duodenoscopes. Videoscopes provide excellent images and working conditions for ERCP. The slightly longer tip of some first-generation videoscopes was a disadvantage (e.g. when attempting to cannulate from within a diverticulum).

Catheters

Standard catheters are simple Teflon tubes with an outer diameter of at least 5 French gauge (1.7 mm), with distal markings to help judge the depth of insertion (Fig. 6.2). The tip should be slightly rounded and radio-opaque (with metal or special paint) to assist orientation during fluoroscopy. The lumen should be sufficient to allow the passage of a standard 0.035-inch

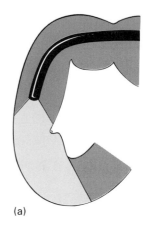

(a)

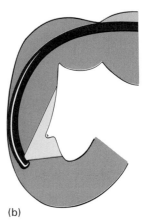

(b)

Fig. 6.1 (a) Inadequate view of the papilla with a forward-viewing endoscope . . . (b) . . . and a face-on view with a side-viewer.

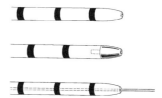

Fig. 6.2 Catheters in routine diagnostic use: standard (above); metal tip (centre); catheter with 0.035-inch guidewire (below).

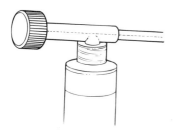

Fig. 6.3 A Luer–Lock syringe attachment to an ERCP catheter with a stiffening stilette.

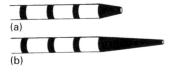

(a)

(b)

Fig. 6.4 (a) Short taper catheter. (b) Very fine taper catheter.

guidewire. The proximal end of the standard catheter has two orifices: one to accommodate a stiffening metal stilette (or guidewire), the other with a Luer fitting at the side for injection of contrast with a syringe (Fig. 6.3).

Innumerable varieties of catheter designs are available, with different sizes, tips and lumens. Double-lumen catheters have the advantage that contrast can be injected relatively easily while maintaining the position with the guidewire. A tip with a short taper (but still a 0.035-inch capable lumen) is often helpful in difficult cases (Fig. 6.4), but very fine tapers (Fig. 6.4) are rarely useful — except at the accessory papilla (see below) — and can easily cause a false passage and some submucosal injection of contrast.

Guidewires

Guidewires are an essential part of diagnostic and therapeutic ERCP. Usually they are 400–480 cm in length to allow complete exchange of catheters over the wire. The most commonly used diameter is 0.035 inch; the distal 3 cm or so of which is 'floppy'. Standard guidewires have a spiral design and a central stilette, and are Teflon-coated. Hydrophilic-coated guidewires are extremely slippery when wet. Although more expensive, they certainly facilitate entry into and around tortuous strictures and many endoscopists use them almost exclusively. Some wires are made with the hydrophilic coating only over the distal 70 cm or so, so that the part being handled by the assistant is not so slippery. Standard guidewires have straight (but floppy) tips. However, wires are also made with a slight preformed curve, or a tight J-tip, designed to 'back through' difficult areas. Smaller diameter guidewires (e.g. 0.028, 0.021 and 0.018 inch) are available for use with smaller catheters. Inevitably they kink more easily, and the tip may be somewhat more traumatic if used clumsily.

Disinfection of equipment

ERCP, more than any other endoscopic technique, carries a significant risk of introducing infection into closed spaces (i.e. obstructed ducts and pseudocysts). There have been many reported outbreaks of serious hospital-acquired infections (especially of *Pseudomonas*) traced to the use of contaminated equipment. Disinfection procedures are therefore of paramount importance. The endoscopes are disinfected in the standard manner (see Chapter 3), not only after use, but also *before* each case. Everything that can be autoclaved or gas-sterilized should be, including all catheters. Single-use accessories are increasingly popular but add significantly to the cost. We use a newly autoclaved water bottle for each case, and sterile water.

X-ray facilities

Diagnostic ERCP is a radiographic procedure initiated by an endoscopist. It is essential to have optimal X-ray equipment and rapid film processing. Some endoscopy units are fortunate enough to have their own radiology facilities. Those who have to borrow a room in the X-ray department know of the potential problems this can bring. Most endoscopists use a standard fluoroscopy or 'barium' suite, but modern digital C-arm units provide excellent screening quality and have hard-copy capabilities.

Room layout is important. There must be enough room for the endoscopist, radiologist (and/or technician) and nurse assistants (and all of their equipment). Most X-ray tables are installed close to one wall. If the patient is put on the table in the standard position for a barium examination, the endoscopist and his assistants are cramped into a corner (Fig. 6.5). Therefore, it is usually better to work with the patient's position reversed. As a result, the endoscopist and radiologist are on the same side of the table, and both can see the fluoroscopy (and video) monitor placed across from them (Fig. 6.6). When working in this position, check

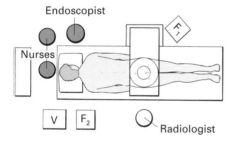

Fig. 6.5 Do not use the X-ray room in the standard 'barium' position. Nurses and the endoscopist are cramped; only the radiologist has space and can see the fluoroscopy monitor (F_1) in its usual position. The endoscopist would need an extra fluoroscopy monitor (F_2) and the radiologist cannot see the video monitor (V).

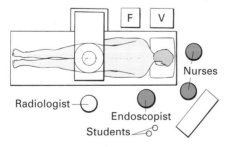

Fig. 6.6 Turn the patient so that the radiologist (or technician) and endoscopist work side by side. They, and the assisting nurse, can easily see both monitors. There is more space for the gear and students. F, fluoroscopy monitor; V, video monitor.

that the table top can travel far enough so that the patient's upper abdomen can be brought into fluoroscopic view; and also that the X-ray image can be reversed. The table should be capable of tilting at least 30° up and down.

Patient preparation

Diagnostic ERCP is performed routinely as an out-patient procedure, but post-examination observation may need to be more prolonged than after other endoscopies to detect the earliest signs of complications, such as pancreatitis.

Prior to starting the examination, the endoscopist should review the indication carefully, taking into account the latest clinical radiological and laboratory information. The aims, hazards and alternatives of the procedure are discussed fully with the patient (and relative or friend where appropriate). It is helpful to provide printed information as part of the education and consent process.

The patient should be asked about any allergy to iodine. Despite the fact that there have been no published reports of anaphylactic reactions to contrast agents during ERCP, and that there is little evidence that specific precautions are helpful, a patient's history of contrast 'allergy' should not be ignored. The procedure to be followed in this circumstance should be determined jointly by the endoscopist (or his director) in collaboration with the appropriate radiologist—and documented in the unit policy manual. Our policy in subjects believed to be iodine allergic is to use non-ionic contrast, and pre-treat with oral steroids for at least 12 h. Other details of general risk factors and precautions are given in Chapter 3.

Antibiotics should be given intravenously 1 h prior to the procedure in any patient with evidence or suspicion of duct obstruction or pseudocyst. For years we have used gentamicin with ampicillin (or vancomycin if the patient is penicillin-sensitive). Other broad spectrum regimens are acceptable.

Patients are kept 'nil by mouth' for at least 4 h before procedures, usually overnight. An intravenous line is established, preferably in the right arm (since the patient will lie partially on the left arm), and appropriate monitoring is initiated (see Chapter 3).

Procedure

The patient lies on the X-ray table with the left arm behind the back, to facilitate rotation subsequently into the prone position (Fig. 6.7). A plain radiograph is taken (in the prone position) to check exposures, to document any soft-tissue shadows (e.g. pancreatic calcification) and to ensure that the field is clear of previous contrast, monitoring wires etc.

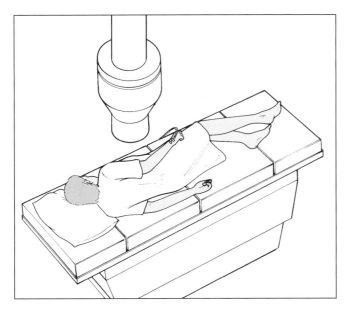

Fig. 6.7 Starting position of the patient for an ERCP.

Most patients receive standard sedation, i.e. diazepam/mida-zolam with pethidine (Demerol). General anaesthesia may be necessary for children and for some difficult patients and complex therapeutic procedures. Once the duodenum has been entered, it is necessary to suppress duodenal and sphincter motility. Buscopan (hyoscine *n*-butylbromide) is effective given in increments of 20 mg i.v. Glucagon is a reasonable alternative (in increments of 0.25 mg) when Buscopan is not available.

As always, check all functions of your instrument before starting.

Passing the endoscope to the papilla

Lateral-viewing instruments are easy to swallow because they have rounded tips. However, passage through the pharynx and upper oesophagus is virtually blind, so the instrument must not be pushed forcibly when there is any resistance; *gentle* pressure during swallowing should be sufficient. When intubation proves difficult, the instrument should be withdrawn and the situation reviewed. It may be wise to use a forward-viewing instrument to check for a problem (e.g. a diverticulum). Rarely, a barium study may be necessary.

Although a tunnel view is not obtained, most of the distal oesophagus can been seen with a lateral-viewing instrument if air is insufflated and the tip angled slightly down whilst pushing in or pulling out (Fig. 6.8). Excessive angulation may be haz-ardous and force should not be used. Slight resistance is nor-

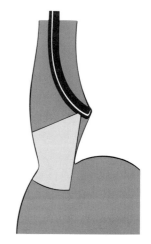

Fig. 6.8 Examination of the oesophagus is possible with a side-viewer by angling down, but take care.

mally felt at the cardia (38–40 cm from the teeth), followed by a characteristic 'give' as the tip is advanced through it with gentle pressure.

Through the stomach and into the duodenum

1 Angle the tip down in the proximal stomach to view forwards; aspirate any gastric pool and insufflate air to obtain a view.

2 Advancing through the body of the stomach with the tip angled down provides axial views similar to those of a forward-viewing instrument (Fig. 6.9).

3 Rotate to obtain face-on views of all four wall of the proximal stomach when necessary (Fig. 6.10).

4 Pass the endoscope to the greater curvature and angle up to see the cardia (Fig. 6.11).

Passage of a lateral-viewing endoscope through the pylorus is partially a blind manoeuvre but provides no difficulty with experience.

1 Advance the tip through the antrum with a slight 'down' tip deflection to keep the pylorus in view (Fig. 6.12), whilst sliding the shaft inwards and around the greater curvature of the stomach.

2 When close to the pyloric ring, angle the tip 'up' into the neutral position (or slightly beyond it) and advance (Fig. 6.13, top). The ideal view of the pylorus during the manoeuvre is described as the 'setting sun' (Fig. 6.13, bottom).

3 Sometimes it may be necessary to slide over the pylorus (i.e.

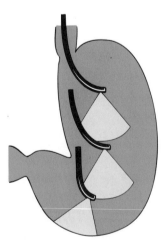

Fig. 6.9 Angle down to give a forward view before advancing the side-viewer.

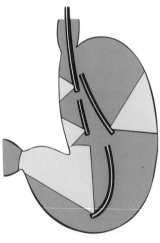

Fig. 6.10 Rotating the side-viewer gives face-on views of the whole stomach.

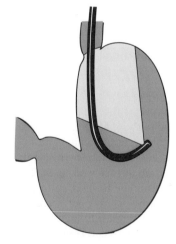

Fig. 6.11 Rotate to the greater curve and angle up to see the cardia with a side-viewer.

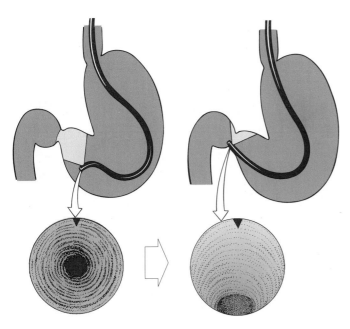

Fig. 6.12 Angle down to see the pylorus . . .

Fig. 6.13 . . . then angle up to let the tip enter the pyloric canal with a 'setting sun' view.

lose the view of it), and then angle the instrument tip sharply downwards, so as to enter the duodenum blindly.

Passage through the pyloric ring is felt rather than seen; success depends upon having the instrument in the central axis of the antrum. Check the orientation, if in difficulty, by withdrawing and angling the tip up. The angulus should be seen square-on, not obliquely, so that further upward angulation would show the instrument shaft passing down the midline of the greater curvature of the gastric body (Fig. 6.14). The lateral angling controls or shaft twist should be used to achieve the correct midline axis.

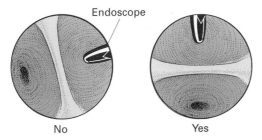

Fig. 6.14 Use twist or the lateral control to square up the angulus before passing into the pylorus . . .

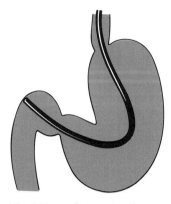

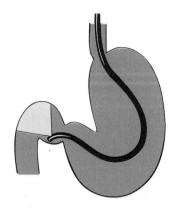

Fig. 6.15 . . . after passing the pylorus the endoscope tip tends to impact the duodenal wall.

Fig. 6.16 Angle the tip down and withdraw into a hooked position to see the duodenum and cap . . .

When the instrument passes the pylorus, the springiness of the redundant loop in the stomach propels the tip inward to the distal bulb (as with forward-viewing endoscopes) (Fig. 6.15) and results in a 'red-out'. Withdraw the instrument slightly, angling the tip sharply down and insufflating some air; the tip is then virtually hooked beyond the pyloric ring, and the view is similar to that obtained with a forward-viewing endoscope (Fig. 6.16). The roof of the bulb is seen face on, and lateral tip deflection and rotation provide views of the anterior and posterior walls. The inferior part or floor of the bulb is more difficult to survey; there is a tendency to fall back into the antrum during the necessary acute clockwise rotation.

Passing the superior duodenal angle

Passing the superior duodenal angle into the descending duodenum requires a corkscrew 'right twist and pull' manoeuvre as used with forward-viewing instruments. From the bulb-viewing position the tip is angled up towards the neutral position and advanced until it is over the superior duodenal angle at the entry of the descending duodenum (Fig. 6.17). The tip is then angled acutely right and up at the same time as the instrument is rotated about 90° clockwise (Fig. 6.18). This corkscrew rotation produces a tunnel view of the upper part of the descending duodenum (Fig. 6.19) and often of the telltale bulge of the pre-papillary fold. Further tip advance can be achieved simply by pushing, but—as with forward-viewing scopes — this is *much better achieved by pulling back*, to shorten the loop in the stomach (Fig. 6.20). When the shaft has been straightened (with less than 70 cm of instrument inside the patient), the tip will lie beyond the papilla of Vater. The descending duodenum is surveyed during gradual withdrawal, using tip manipulation and rotation.

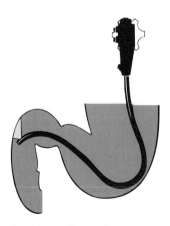

Fig. 6.17 . . . then angle up again to advance over the superior dudodenal angle . . .

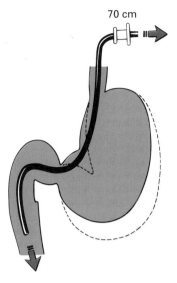

70 cm

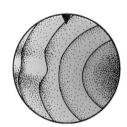

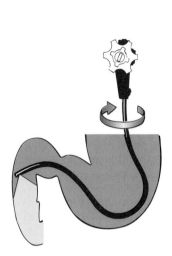

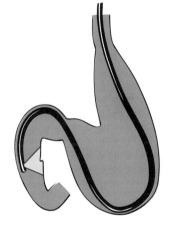

Fig. 6.18 . . . and rotate 90° clockwise, whilst angling right and up, to view the descending duodenum.

Fig. 6.19 A tunnel view of the papillary region from above.

Fig. 6.20 Withdrawal helps to advance the scope into the second part of the duodenum.

Getting the instrument shaft straight is the key to cannulation success. Most beginners simply push, steer and rotate as appears visually appropriate to advance over the superior duodenal angle, and then into the second part of the duodenum. This technique is known as the 'long route' (Fig. 6.21). It obviates the risk of falling back into the stomach, but is unpleasant for the patient and control of the distal tip is greatly reduced. Straightening is achieved by pulling, when the tip of the duodenoscope is hooked beyond the superior duodenal angle. This manoeuvre is similar to a straightening procedure in the colon (Fig. 6.22).

The sequence of moves should become combined and automatic with practice.

Fig. 6.21 The 'long route'.

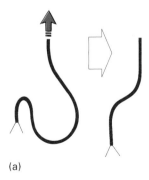

(a)

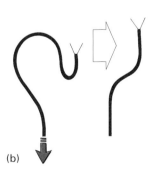

(b)

Fig. 6.22 Straightening maneouvre in (a) the duodenum, and (b) the colon. The duodenum is the inverse of the colon.

1 Advance the tip to engage the superior duodenal angle.
2 Rotate yourself (and therefore the scope) to the *right*.
3 Angle the instrument tip fully to the *right* and fix it there (with the brake).
4 Angle the tip *up*, and withdraw the instrument slowly maintaining clockwise rotation. The instrument shaft will be straight in the 'short route' position (Fig. 6.23a) when the 60–70 cm mark is at the mouth (Fig. 6.23b).
5 Once the shaft is straight, the up/down and left/right control wheels can usually be released towards their neutral positions, and the patient rotated prone. The endoscopist can then turn back slightly to the left, so as to face more towards the patient. It should then be easy to find the papilla close by.

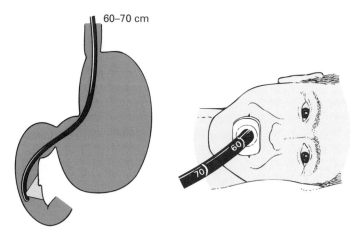

Fig. 6.23 The 'short route': (a) withdraw the tip and angle up to see the papilla … (b) … the 60–70 cm mark is at the patient's mouth.

Gastroduodenoscopy en route?

It is not difficult to examine the entire stomach and proximal duodenum with a side-viewing duodenoscope, and good views can be obtained of the distal oesophagus if the instrument tip is angled down (with care) and air insufflated. The endoscopist should decide before starting an ERCP examination whether formal gastroduodenoscopy is indicated, and must make it clear in the report whether or not it has been performed. It is remarkably easy to miss substantial lesions in the stomach and proximal duodenum when hurrying to the papilla. For the beginner, who is likely to be rather slow, there are disadvantages in attempting to be comprehensive. Prime cannulating time and conditions will be lost. However, an expert should be able to provide a complete survey and will usually wish to do so.

Finding the papilla

With the short route (Fig. 6.23), the papilla is usually in view when the straightening manoeuvre is completed. The lens automatically faces the medial wall of the descending duodenum if the patient is prone and the endoscopist is facing the patient (with the buttons facing upwards). If the papilla is not in view, the tip is usually beyond it, in the third part of the duodenum (Fig. 6.24). If in doubt, check with fluoroscopy. The shaft is withdrawn slowly (and rotated slightly from left to right) to scan the medial wall. Coming up from below the papilla, the first landmark is the angle dividing the second and third parts of the duodenum (Fig. 6.25). Above this is a bare shelf of mucosa without transverse folds. A longitudinal fold, or several oblique folds of differing size, lead over the shelf directly up to the papillary structure (Fig. 6.26).

The *normal papilla* varies considerably in size, shape and appearance. Its colour (often pinker than its surroundings) and surface characteristics (usually rough or matt compared to the shiny duodenal mucosa) make it stand out to the trained eye (Plate 6.1). It is most commonly an oval shape approximately 8 mm wide and 10–12 mm long (sometimes much smaller), tailing off below into a longitudinal fold or folds (Fig. 6.26). The course of the bile duct may be obvious as a longitudinal bulge into the lumen for 1–2 cm above the papilla. Often a horizontal 'hooding' fold crosses just above the papilla, and may sometimes hide the orifice. The orifice is at the apex of the papillary nipple. It may be patulous with several fleshy 'fronds' of protruding mucosa, or quite obscure; peripapillary diverticula are common, especially in the elderly.

Although anatomy books state that the papilla can occur in any part of the duodenal loop (and even in the stomach), it is very rarely found outside the second part of the duodenum — occasionally it is found just in the third part. If the papilla is elusive, go back to first principles with the endoscope straight. Start with the tip at the junction of the second and third parts of the duodenum (check with fluoroscopy) and then withdraw slowly again. Beginners often do not withdrawal far enough, for fear of falling back into the stomach. If the endoscope does fall back into the stomach, re-passage of the pylorus may be facilitated by temporarily returning the patient to the left lateral position.

Cannulation of the papilla

Duodenal conditions must be ideal. If foaming obscures the view, infuse 20 ml of water containing a few drops of a silicone suspension down the instrument channel, and suck it back again. Further increments of Buscopan or Glucagon should be

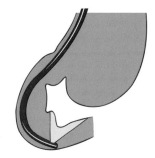

Fig. 6.24 The scope tip in the entrance of the third part of the duodenum.

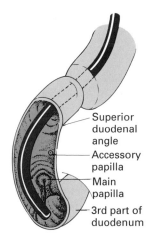

Superior duodenal angle

Accessory papilla

Main papilla

3rd part of duodenum

Fig. 6.25 Landmarks in the duodenal loop.

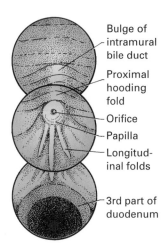

Bulge of intramural bile duct

Proximal hooding fold

Orifice

Papilla

Longitudinal folds

3rd part of duodenum

Fig. 6.26 The medial wall.

given intravenously if peristalsis is a problem. Cannulation should *not* be attempted until the papilla is seen properly face-on.

The aim is to pass the catheter through the papillary orifice in the same horizontal and vertical axes as the desired duct system — and this is the key to success. Tangential thrusts are certain to fail. Only when a reasonable face-on position has been achieved, with the patient prone and the duodenum relaxed, is the catheter passed through the instrument. To avoid injecting the air up the ducts, the catheter should be preflushed with contrast and attached to a large syringe reservoir (20–50 ml). Flushing contrast into the duodenum should be avoided because it stimulates peristalsis.

Sometimes it may be difficult to pass the catheter tip over the elevator, especially when using the long route (when the control wires are stretched). If in difficulty, straighten the instrument and insert the catheter initially with the elevator *raised*. The catheter is advanced until it abuts against the elevator; gentle forward pressure should allow the catheter tip to pass into the field of view as the elevator is gradually lowered (using the left thumb to roll the control wheel towards the operator).

It is unusual to see an actual hole in the papilla (except after surgery or stone passage), but the orifice is *always* at the apex of the nipple. Excessive fronds may make it difficult to judge the central axis of the structure. Occasionally the nipple and orifice are partly hidden by the proximal transverse fold; then the catheter tip should be used to lift the fold away (Fig. 6.27).

Before poking the papilla, the instrument tip should again be manoeuvred face-on, looking directly up the papillary axis. It may be helpful to use the brake to fix the left/right-angling control in a neutral position. Minor left/right adjustments are then achieved by rotating the instrument.

The cannula is placed within the orifice of the papilla, but not pressed too hard. Concentrate on trying to imagine the axis of the required duct, and swing the endoscope tip around (and advance and withdraw the instrument slightly) so as to cannulate in this axis (Fig. 6.28). Pushing the catheter may actually lose the axis due to exaggerating the curve in it (Fig. 6.29).

Contrast is injected in small increments (1–2 ml) during fluoroscopy in order to check when a duct has been entered. The endoscopist must control these injections very carefully, either by handling the syringe personally or through clear and firm ('military') instructions to an assistant. If the desired duct is visualized, more contrast is injected until optimum opacification is achieved.

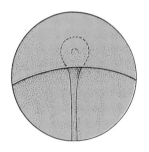

Fig. 6.27 (a) The papilla is obscured by the transverse fold …

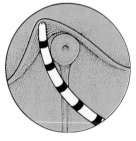

(b) … use the catheter to evert the fold.

Selective cannulation

The most difficult part of ERCP is learning to select the relevant duct (or ducts), and to change where necessary from one to the other. Most endoscopists find pancreatography significantly easier to achieve than cholangiography, but success should reach at least 95% for both with good technique and practice.

Selective cannulation becomes easier as manipulative co-ordination increases. ERCP is always easier the quicker it is performed, before the staff, endoscopist, patient, duodenum and papilla all become tense. Clumsily directed pokes probably induce papillary muscle spasm as well as oedema. Further small increments of Buscopan or Glucagon may help, but medication is no substitute for thoughtful gentle manipulation and, especially, remember to get the catheter into the correct axis.

Almost all patients have a single orifice for the pancreatic and biliary ductal systems, with a common channel of 1–10 mm long. Both ducts may fill simultaneously if contrast is injected when the catheter tip is only just within the orifice. However, opacification of one or both ducts may be suboptimal in this position, and contrast will also reflux back into the duodenum. *The best radiographs are obtained with deep selective cannulation.* Again, this depends on finding the correct axis, so that the catheter tip does not impact within the papilla in a fold of mucosa (Fig. 6.29). Inject only very small quantities of contrast (preferably yourself), since repeated inadvertent pancreatography increases the risk of pancreatitis. It may be possible to tell which duct has been entered without further injection if contrast is still present in the pancreas. Movements of the catheter tip will distort the distal pancreatic duct (on fluoroscopy). A catheter which passes easily for at least 5 cm is usually in the bile duct. However, this should not be assumed, since injuries can occur if contrast is forcibly injected into a side branch of the pancreas. If the catheter is deeply in the bile duct, aspiration will usually produce yellow bile (seen in the catheter under endoscopic view).

Pancreatography is more likely to result if the catheter enters the orifice perpendicular to the duodenal wall, or pointing only slightly upwards, and at approximately 1 o'clock (Figs 6.28 & 6.30). When attempting *cholangiography*, the orifice should be approached from below, and slightly from the right (aiming the catheter towards the 11 o'clock axis) (Figs 6.28 & 6.30). The idea is to enter the roof of the orifice (and common channel) when aiming for the bile duct, and to enter the floor of the orifice when seeking the pancreatic duct. Once the catheter tip has just entered the orifice, it should be lifted (or lowered) to achieve this aim (Fig. 6.31). This is more effective than approaching the papilla from too far below (Fig. 6.32). Withdrawing the scope slightly may be helpful (Fig. 6.33).

The commonest problem is changing from the pancreatic duct to the bile duct.

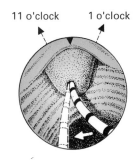

Fig. 6.28 Imagine the axis of the required duct and swing the tip around as necessary.

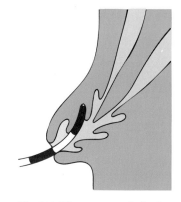

Fig. 6.29 The wrong vertical axis for deep cannulation.

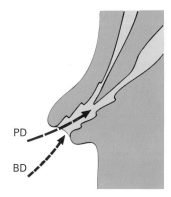

Fig. 6.30 The vertical axes for selective cannulation. BD, biliary duct; PD, pancreatic duct.

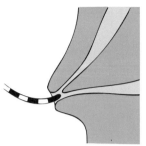

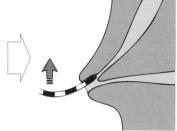

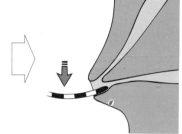

Fig. 6.31 (a) From the central catheter position . . .

(b) . . . lift up for the bile duct . . .

(c) . . . and drop down for the pancreatic duct.

The difficult bile duct

What can be done if these standard techniques are not effective? If the procedure has been prolonged and pancreatography repeated, it may be wise to desist. If the indication remains strong, the examination can be repeated at a later date or by another endoscopist. Here are the tricks we use, in the usual sequence.

1 *Push in and angle up.* Distorting the lateral duodenal wall may give a better view of the papilla (Fig. 6.34).

2 *Back off with the tip of the scope.* The natural curl of the catheter can help achieve the upward axis if the papilla is approached from a greater distance (Fig. 6.35).

3 Alternatively, *get very close*—the 'kissing technique':

(a) have the catheter protruding minimally and the elevator lifted fully;

(b) place the tip in the orifice using up angulation and scope withdrawal;

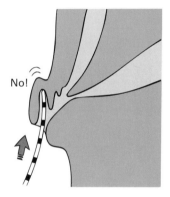

Fig. 6.32 Too much emphasis on pushing up from below is counterproductive.

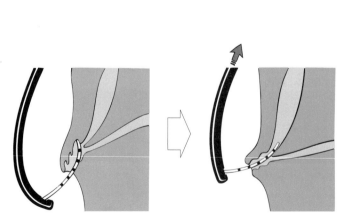

Fig. 6.33 Pull the scope back to correct the axis for bile duct cannulation.

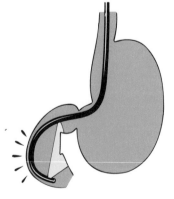

Fig. 6.34 With the scope in the straight position, angle the tip up.

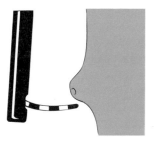
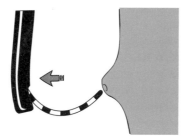

Fig. 6.35 Biliary access may be facilitated by approaching the papilla from a greater distance; the natural curl of the catheter helps orientation.

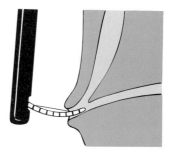

(c) rotate the scope shaft sharply to the left to lift the tip of the catheter into the 11 o'clock position in the roof of the common channel and inject contrast.

4 *Use a (double-lumen) sphincterotome.* This makes it possible to change the angle of approach by bowing the tip (Fig. 6.36). The stiffness of the instrument also facilitates the 'lifting' manoeuvre.

5 *Try a tapered-tip catheter — carefully.* Inadvertent submucosal injection can give alarming endoscopic and radiological appearances (Fig. 6.37); usually it has no adverse clinical consequences but makes completion of the procedure more difficult, at least for several days.

6 *Use a guidewire (preferably hydrophilic) — carefully.* Sharp wires can be traumatic, but the technique is probably safer than repeated pancreatography:

(a) the assistant holds the accessories so that the guidewire protrudes about 6 mm from the catheter tip (Fig. 6.38);

(b) probe the roof of the common channel under fluoroscopy. If the pancreatic duct still contains contrast, the guidewire can be seen *either* to enter the pancreas (the duct moves on probing) *or* to advance easily in a different direction; then it must be in the bile duct;

(c) advance the catheter into the duct over the wire, remove the wire, aspirate bile and then inject contrast.

7 Combine techniques 4 and 6 using a sphincterotome and a guidewire.

8 Pre-cutting (with a needle knife, see Chapter 7) is popular with some experts. However, there are risks involved; we recommend pre-cutting only for strong indications and not for diagnostic cholangiography alone.

The difficult pancreatic duct

When pancreatography is elusive, retrace the techniques required for obtaining the correct ductal axis.

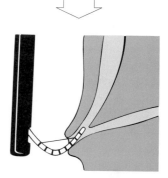

Fig. 6.36 Use the sphincterotome bowing to achieve the correct axis and push further to gain a better bile duct axis.

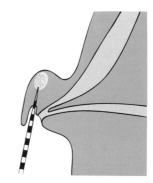

Fig. 6.37 Submucosal injection can be easily done by mistake with a sharp taper-tipped catheter.

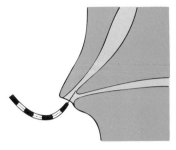

Fig. 6.38 Cannulating with a guidewire.

1 Place the catheter tip in the lower margin of the orifice, press it downwards by lowering the elevator and aim slightly more to the right (1–3 o'clock position).
2 Try the same technique with a tapered catheter.
3 Use a hydrophilic guidewire.

'Failure' may be due to the congenital anomaly of the pancreas divisum, where the main (or only) drainage is via Santorini's duct and the minor papilla. Sometimes a very small ventral pancreas can be identified only if radiographs are taken during contrast injection (Fig. 6.39) even when nothing can be seen on fluoroscopy.

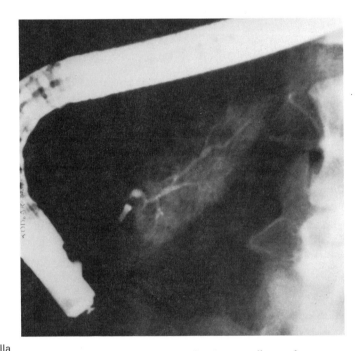

Fig. 6.39 Endoscopic pancreatogram showing a small ventral pancreas.

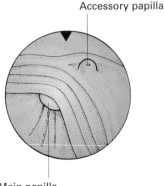

Accessory papilla

Main papilla

Fig. 6.40 Position of the accessory and main papillae.

Cannulation of the accessory (minor) papilla

This should be attempted when contrast injection through the main papilla does not provide the required pancreatogram, and when it shows only a separate ventral pancreas. The minor papilla can be identified in virtually all patients, approximately 2 cm above and slightly to the right of the main papilla (as seen at endoscopy), lying just below the superior duodenal angle (Plate 6.1). Its size varies considerably, from a tiny blind nodule to a major structure which can be mistaken for the main papilla. Unlike the main papilla, it does not have any distinct longitudi-

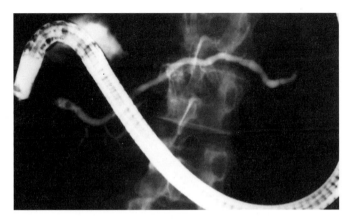

Fig. 6.41 The endoscope in the 'semi-long' position often provides the best face-on access to the minor papilla.

nal structure, being solely a hemispherical nipple found characteristically at the junction of two transverse folds (Fig. 6.40). A face-on position for cannulation of the minor papilla is best achieved using a 'semi-long route' (Fig. 6.41).

1 Bring the endoscope back into the duodenal bulb with the shaft straight.

2 Push it again whilst angling to the *left* to wedge the tip and prevent it advancing over the superior duodenal angle.

3 When the shaft is 'half-long', slight right rotation of the instrument and right angulation will corkscrew the tip over the superior duodenal angle, and will usually reveal the minor papilla.

The papilla can be made more prominent and the orifice visible if the pancreas is stimulated with secretin (give 25–50 units i.v. and wait 3 min). A problem with using secretin is that contrast must then be injected against a flow of juice. Whilst this does not appear to be dangerous, it may prove difficult to outline the entire duct system without using excessive pressure.

Minor papilla cannulation is best attempted with fine-tipped catheters; we prefer a short metal tip. Alternatively we use a 0.018-inch guidewire protruding from a taper-tipped catheter, after secretin injection. Once the guidewire is inserted, the catheter tip is slid into the orifice. The guidewire is removed and contrast is injected. However, there will be air in the catheter after removal of the guidewire, so the pancreatogram may be incomplete.

Dorsal duct cannulation should succeed in over 80% of cases. However, pancreas divisum (or dominant Santorini drainage, whether congenital or acquired) can be diagnosed without opacification of the dorsal duct by giving secretin; clear juice flows from the minor papilla, occasionally like a fountain.

Radiographic technique

The slickest cannulation is of no avail (and may be a disservice to the patient) without good radiological technique. It is not necessary to have a radiologist present throughout all the procedures, but some collaboration with radiology staff is essential. A specially trained radiology technician can help achieve the goal of providing high-quality studies and can ensure the maintenance of X-ray safety standards. Physical layout and the issues of contrast allergy have already been discussed. Standard water-soluble contrast agents are used, as for urography (e.g. Renografin, Urografin, Conray, Angiografin). This is no evidence, as yet, that non-ionic contrast agents are safer. We start with full strength (in a 20 or 50 ml syringe attached to a pre-flushed catheter), but change to a less dense mixture (15–25%) when filling dilated ducts. This reduces the risk of missing small stones (or even quite large stones in a very dilated system), and makes it easier to see catheters and guidewires on fluoroscopy. The optimum amount of contrast is judged solely by fluoroscopy and intermittent radiographs; injection continues until the relevant ducts are fully outlined without overdistension. The total volume of contrast is irrelevant; this depends upon which system is being filled and how much is spilled into the duodenum.

Pancreatography

Radiographs always show more detail than fluoroscopy (depending on the equipment). By the time the pancreatic duct tail can be seen on fluoroscopy, radiographs usually show filling of all major branches. Opacification of the parenchyma (acinarization) should be avoided. The appearance of a urogram during ERCP is a sign that a large volume of contrast has been injected (and absorbed); there is then an increased risk of pancreatitis.

Contrast leaves the normal pancreatic duct system rapidly and is often completely cleared within 5 min. Radiographs should therefore be taken during contrast injection with the instrument and catheter in place. The prone position is convenient, and a 'straight scope' does not usually overlie the pancreas (as would a long scope) (Figs 6.42 & 6.43). Oblique films may be necessary to clarify local duct changes and to separate areas of interest from the vertebral column. Lateral views are rarely necessary and are often confusing.

Cholangiography

Many cholangiograms produced by beginners are inadequate for interpretation. The whole biliary tree (and gallbladder when present) must be filled, and views taken in appropriate posi-

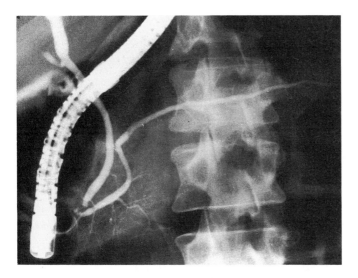

Fig. 6.42 A normal pancreatogram (and part cholangiogram) with the instrument in the 'short scope' position.

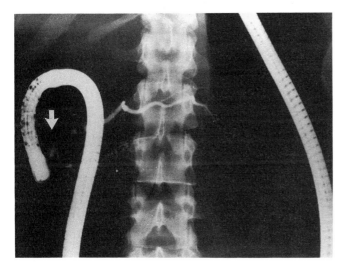

Fig. 6.43 Instrument with a long loop in the stomach (the 'long route'). The papilla of Vater is arrowed.

tions. In the prone position the right intrahepatic ducts fill last (because they are 'uphill') (Fig. 6.44), and the gallbladder fundus may not be seen.

After cholecystectomy the biliary tree may be completely 'full' with bile in the resting state. Contrast injection may result in pain though overdistension, even before adequate opacification is achieved. Thus, it is good practice to aspirate bile once deep biliary cannulation has been achieved. We try to exchange

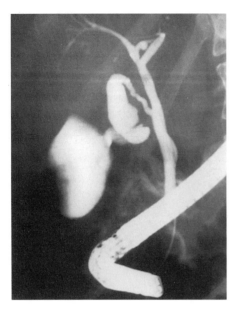

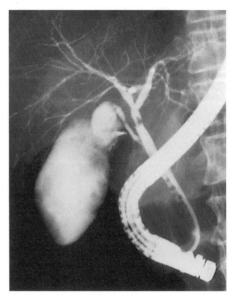

Fig. 6.44 Retrograde cholangiography showing poor filling of the right intraheptic ducts during injection in the prone position.

Fig. 6.45 Further injection after occluding the common hepatic duct with a balloon gives better intrahepatic filling.

contrast for bile, volume for volume. This is particularly important in the presence of infected bile, since increasing the biliary pressure can provoke bacteraemia. When the gallbladder is present, it acts as a reservoir and may (because it fills preferentially) prevent adequate views of the upper biliary tree. To provide good intrahepatic cholangiograms it is usually necessary to inject when the tip of the catheter is above the cystic duct orifice. Even better and selective filling of the biliary tree can be achieved by the *balloon occlusion technique*. A balloon-tipped catheter (as used for stone retrieval) is placed in the common hepatic duct, if necessary with the use of a guidewire. Contrast is injected after the balloon is inflated (Fig. 6.45).

To obtain good views of the whole biliary tree it may also sometimes be necessary to rotate the patient (usually to the right), tilt the table and temporarily push the endoscope in deeper to form a loop in the stomach, so as to expose the mid-duct which is otherwise overlain by the catheter (Fig. 6.46). We also usually take radiographs after the scope has been removed, with the patient supine and rotated slightly to the right (to separate the bile duct from the vertebral column). These and other views are necessary to provide a full perspective of the gallbladder (when present), facilitate study of the sphincter zone in contraction and relaxation (Fig. 6.47) and to help differentiate stones from air bubbles.

Delayed films may sometimes be helpful. When gallbladder

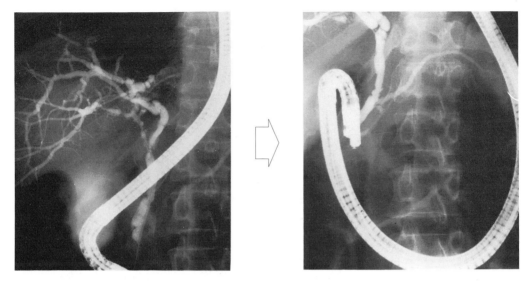

Fig. 6.46 Changing the position of the endoscope may provide better views of the common bile duct.

disease is suspected, delayed radiographs should be taken at 1–2 h, at which time the patient can be moved around more easily and contrast mixing is more complete. Small gallstones can be detected in the fully erect position and compression views may also be helpful. Abnormalities of gallbladder emptying can be detected by serial films taken at 30 and 60 min after i.v. injection of cholecystokinin (25–50 units) (Fig. 6.48). Some experts routinely take *drainage films* if sphincter dysfunction is suspected in a patient who has previously undergone cholecystectomy. Lack of complete duct drainage after 45 min is often considered

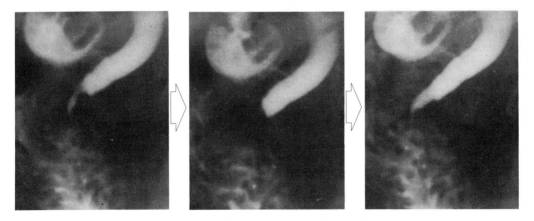

Fig. 6.47 Sequential views of the bile duct termination during relaxation and contraction.

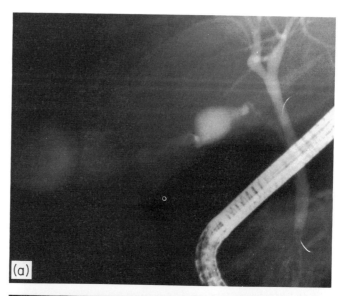

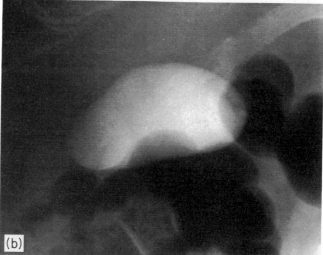

Fig. 6.48 (a) Initial filling of the gallbladder (with contrast streaming) at retrograde cholangiography. (b) Inadequate emptying and asymmetrical shape of the gallbladder after injection with cholecystokinin.

abnormal. However, control data are scarce and the drainage must be influenced by the medication employed as well as the trauma of a difficult cannulation.

ERCP in children

Experimental small paediatric instruments are available, but the standard duodenoscope can be used (with the straight scope technique) down to the age of about 1 year. Success in neonates has been reported. Small-diameter, more flexible taper-tipped catheters preformed with a tight distal curve are easier to manoeuvre in the close confines of the infant duodenum. Actual cannulation is usually easy, often with simultaneous filling of both duct systems. We use general anaesthesia up to the mid-teens, since it is essential for the patient to remain still. General anaesthesia eliminates normal warnings of discomfort, and care must be taken to avoid unnatural manipulations and the excessive use of air and contrast.

Cannulation problems

Problems due to local disease

Diverticula. Diverticula close to and surrounding the main papilla are the commonest pathological reasons for cannulation difficulty. They occur frequently, especially in elderly patients with duct stones. Small diverticula are shallow caves, most frequently seen above the papilla at the 9–11 or 1–3 o'clock positions, when seen face-on (Fig. 6.49). Larger diverticula may override the papillary mass and eventually 'swallow' it, so that the orifice actually lies within the diverticulum. The papilla can sometimes be persuaded out of the diverticulum by probing the folds radiating towards it with the cannula, and then using a combination of endoscope tip manipulation and duodenal deflation. Once the orifice is visible, it is often helpful to 'hook' the papilla out of the diverticulum using the tip of a sphincterotome (with or without a guidewire). Occasionally it is necessary to place the tip of the duodenoscope actually within the diverticulum, but this must be done very carefully. Diverticula are sometimes also seen around the accessory papilla.

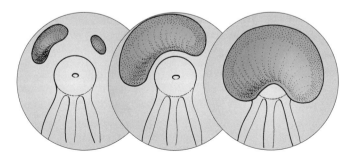

Fig. 6.49 Diverticula around the papilla.

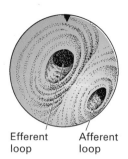

Fig. 6.50 Usual orientation in Billroth II gastrectomies and gastroenterostomies.

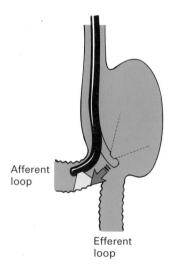

Fig. 6.51 'Backing in' to the afferent loop.

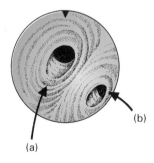

Fig. 6.52 (a) Usual approach. (b) Approach for access to the afferent loop.

Malignancy. Malignancy of the papilla or periampullary region can also cause difficulty (Plates 6.2 and 6.3). Pancreatic tumours may simply distort the anatomy or ulcerate through the floor of the bulb or the medial wall of the descending duodenum. The endoscopic appearance of an ulcerating malignancy is fairly characteristic, and biopsy specimens should confirm the diagnosis. When the tumour remains submucosal, the endoscopic appearances of oedema and irregularity are similar to those seen in patients with active pancreatitis. A large mass lesion in the pancreas (tumour or pseudocyst) often makes it more difficult to straighten the endoscope.

Most primary tumours of the papilla are obvious endoscopically, and the diagnosis is easily confirmed by biopsy and/or brush cytology. The orifice is usually in the centre of the tumour mass. Look carefully for clues (especially for any trace of bile) before touching the papilla, which often bleeds easily.

Deformity. Deformity of the papilla can occur for other reasons. The apex of the papilla may appear lumpy, oedematous and congested in the absence of tumour or previous surgery. Impacted stones cause a prominent oedematous papilla, and the orifice may be obscured below it (Plate 6.4). Cannulation is often most easily achieved with a sphincterotome, used to 'hook' it upwards. Impacted stones may cause a fistula at the apex of the oedematous papilla (above the normal orifice), as may surgically and percutaneously placed catheters (Plate 6.5). The orifice may be lax and ragged soon after the passage of a stone.

Problems due to previous local surgery

Billroth II gastrectomy. This is the commonest anatomical problem for ERCP. The orifice of the afferent loop is usually less obvious than that for the efferent loop, and more difficult to enter. The correct orifice is usually (but not always) found in the 2–5 o'clock sector when viewing the stoma (Fig. 6.50). Entry to this loop can often be achieved by 'backing in' (Fig. 6.51), a similar technique to that used to enter the ileum at colonoscopy. The tip of the endoscope is placed over the orifice and angled sharply downwards. It may also be helpful to approach the stoma from about 3 o'clock, rather than the usual 6 o'clock position (Fig. 6.52).

Once in a loop, there are no useful landmarks until the papilla is recognized. To see increasing amounts of bile (or resulting bubbles) whilst advancing is encouraging. Fluoroscopy is somewhat helpful, but only in the negative sense of being sure the scope is in the 'wrong' (efferent) loop when fluoroscopy shows the endoscope tip to be deep within the pelvis. When confident of being in the *wrong* loop, it may be helpful to take a few biopsies just below the stoma, to leave a little blood as a marker of the

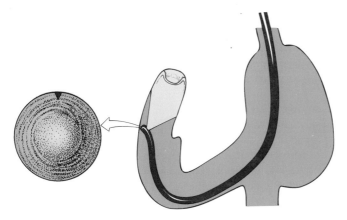

Fig. 6.53 An invaginated duodenal stump may resemble a polyp.

wrong route. Once in the afferent loop, it may be possible to recognize the telltale bare shelf (or longitudinal fold) below the papilla in the distal half of the second part of the duodenum. The other landmark is the blind termination of the duodenal loop, which (because invaginated) may resemble a smooth polyp (Fig. 6.53).

Be careful as excessive stretching of the loops can result in perforation, especially in elderly patients.

Cannulation in Billroth II patients is more difficult because everything is upside down (Plate 6.6); the natural curl of standard catheters is counterproductive (Fig. 6.54). For the same reason, cholangiography is much more difficult to achieve than pancreatography. Several techniques are helpful in trying to overcome this problem of orientation.

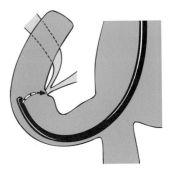

Fig. 6.54 The natural curl of the catheter is unhelpful.

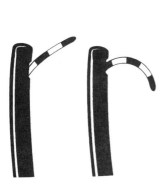

Fig. 6.55 A new catheter tends to curl less than an old one.

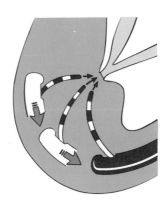

Fig. 6.56 Withdrawing the scope produces a better catheter axis but a more distant approach.

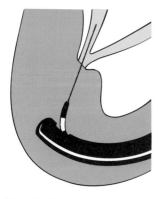

Fig. 6.57 Cannulating with a guidewire.

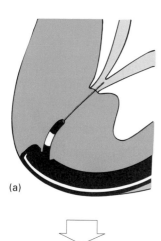

(a)

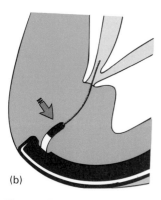

(b)

Fig. 6.58 (a) Having placed the tip of the guidewire in the orifice, (b) its direction can be changed by altering the catheter direction with the elevator.

A new catheter tends to go straighter than an old one (Fig. 6.55). Pulling the scope back to the junction of the second and third parts of the duodenum can change the angle of attack appropriately, but it may then be necessary to attempt cannulation from a distance (Fig. 6.56). Our favoured method involves the use of a 0.035-inch guidewire, protruding from the tip of a standard catheter or inner 'guiding' catheter of a stent set. The guidewire travels in a straight line (until it reaches the papilla). Its angle of approach can be altered by changing the length of guidewire protruding from the catheter, as well as by use of the elevator (Fig. 6.57). Once the tip of the guidewire has been impacted in the orifice of the papilla, its direction can be altered somewhat by looping manoeuvres (Fig. 6.58).

Some experts favour an end-viewing instrument for Billroth II cannulation. In theory, the lens looks directly into the axis of the papilla (Fig. 6.59). However, the lack of an elevator often makes detailed cannula movements more difficult, and we prefer the standard side-viewing duodenoscope. A long floppy (paediatric) colonoscope may be helpful in patients with a very long afferent limb, or when attempting cannulation up a rouxen-Y loop. Cannulation in the latter situation is almost impossible without a combined percutaneous-endoscopic approach (see Chapter 7).

Billroth I gastrectomy, pyloroplasty and gastroenterostomy. These should not interfere with ERCP (provided the pylorus is patent).

Surgery of the papillary region. Surgery of the papillary region may produce confusing appearances. Duodenotomy results in a puckered scar on the lateral wall of the duodenum, which may slightly reduce its lumen and affect endoscopic manoeuvrabil-

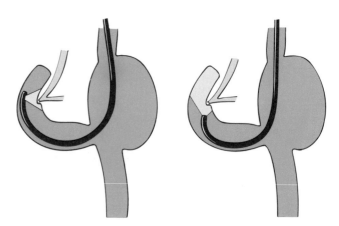

Fig. 6.59 Some experts prefer a forward-viewing scope to obtain better alignment at the papilla, especially for the bile duct.

ity; these scars can be misdiagnosed as polyps and tumours by the unwary. Papillary appearances after surgical sphincterotomy vary from normal to a wide-open biliary orifice. Standard surgical sphincteroplasty results in a gaping hole, dribbling bile and blowing bubbles; the pancreatic duct orifice is usually visible in the floor of the sphincteroplasty (Fig. 6.60).

Choledochoduodenostomy stoma. This is usually easy to find in the roof or left lateral wall of the duodenal bulb, but can escape detection when stenosed. Cannulation of a tight stoma may require a guidewire. When the orifice is widely patent, a balloon occlusion catheter technique will provide good radiographs. It may be necessary to use a guidewire to facilitate selective cannulation of the upper and lower limbs.

Operations on the pancreas. These do not usually involve the papillary region and cannulation is unaffected. The standard Whipple procedure usually takes the biliary and pancreatic duct orifices out of endoscopic reach. The site of a pseudocystogastrostomy looks like a ragged pale gastric ulcer (which usually heals completely within a few weeks).

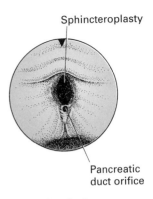

Fig. 6.60 Standard sphincteroplasty.

Specimen collection

Pure bile and pancreatic juice. These can be collected by aspiration after deep cannulation of the relevant duct. Very little pancreatic juice is obtained without an intravenous injection of secretin. Bile can be inspected for microcrystals, and pancreatic juice analysed for bicarbonate. More complex analyses are experimental. The results of juice cytology (both pancreatic and biliary) have been disappointing; yields are higher with direct intraductal brushing.

Brush cytology specimens. These can be taken from deep within the ductal systems using a dual-channel sleeve passed over a guidewire (Figs 6.61 and 6.62).

Biopsies. Biopsies can be taken in the standard manner from lesions of the papilla and surrounding structures. Large specimens can be taken from proliferative tumours using diathermy snare loops (Plates 6.2 and 6.3). Some tumours confined within the papilla are detected only after a sphincterotomy has been performed for apparently benign papillary stenosis.

Biopsy samples can be taken from within the biliary and pancreatic ducts under fluoroscopic guidance with standard or smaller forceps. These can be passed through the normal papilla, but are easier to manipulate after a sphincterotomy or through a preplaced covering sleeve. Biopsies can also be taken under

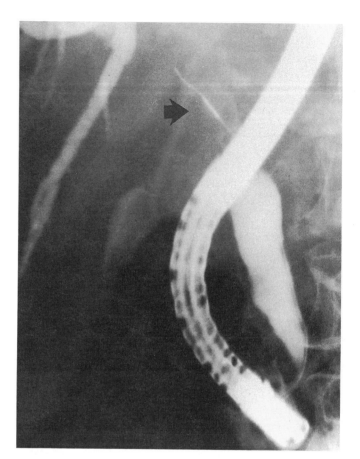

Fig. 6.61 A cytology brush (arrowed) passed deep into the common hepatic duct.

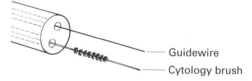

Guidewire

Cytology brush

Fig. 6.62 Double-lumen brush cytology device.

direct vision from within the duct systems, using a 'mother and baby' choledochoscope (Fig. 6.63; Plate 6.7).

Needle-aspiration specimens. These can also be obtained from within the ductal systems, or even directly through the wall of the duodenum into a submucosal mass.

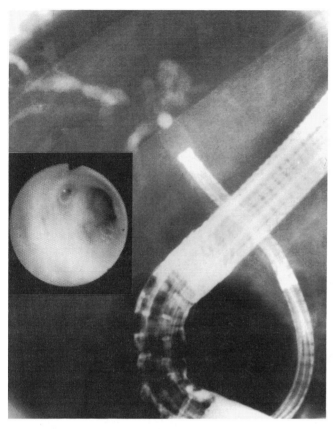

Fig. 6.63 Radiography showing the 'baby' choledochoscope passed up the bile duct through the 'mother' instrument.

Sphincter of Oddi manometry

Dysfunction of the sphincter of Oddi can cause biliary pain (especially in the post-cholecystectomy situation) as well as recurrent pancreatitis. ERCP has brought the problem of 'papillary stenosis' into closer focus by making it easier to rule out other causes, such as stones or tumours. Pressures can be measured in the ducts and sphincter zones by standard manometric techniques, using a triple-lumen perfused catheter system at the time of ERCP (Fig. 6.64). Endoscopic manometry is often difficult for the endoscopist and the patient since medication must be minimized. Interpretation of the tracings is often subjective (Fig. 6.65). Furthermore, manometry appears to increase the risk of pancreatitis above that expected for standard ERCP. For these reasons, sphincter of Oddi manometry is restricted to a few special centres, and attempts are being made to obtain similar diagnostic information by less invasive methods.

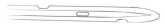

Fig. 6.64 Triple-lumen catheter tip for manometry.

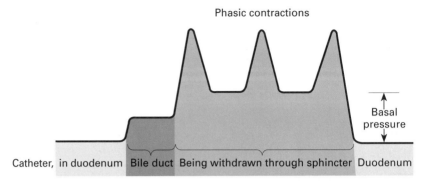

Phasic contractions

Basal
pressure

Catheter, in duodenum | Bile duct | Being withdrawn through sphincter | Duodenum

Fig. 6.65 (a) Stylized manometry trace.

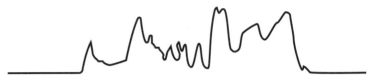

(b) Actual tracing from a patient showing potential difficulties in interpretation.

Radiographic interpretation and artefacts

Cholangiograms are relatively familiar, and retrograde studies resemble those obtained by other techniques. Specific artefacts caused by layering and streaming of contrast, and also by the introduction of air bubbles, can be recognized and eliminated by good technique. There should be relatively few problems of interpretation. Bile duct size remains a controversial issue (especially after cholecystectomy). There is little evidence that the bile duct increases in size after cholecystectomy (in the absence of pathology); thus a 'dilated' duct cannot be interpreted as indicating obstruction unless it is known that the bile duct was smaller at the time of surgery. The appearance of the terminal bile duct is very variable, and overinterpretation is more common than the reverse. Numerous views taken during emptying may resolve diagnostic problems (see Fig. 6.47). It can be difficult to decide whether a distal biliary stricture is due to pancreatitis or carcinoma, but coincident pancreatography may help. Radiographic distinction between sclerosing cholangitis and cholangiocarcinoma may be impossible, and the diagnostic specificity of changes in the intrahepatic biliary tree remains controversial. Beginners are often surprised by the low insertion of the cystic duct, but this is very common. Failure to opacify the gallbladder indicates pathology only if sufficient contrast has entered the biliary system to demonstrate the entire intrahepatic tree.

Pancreatograms are less familiar than cholangiograms, and are often more difficult to interpret than to obtain. The course of

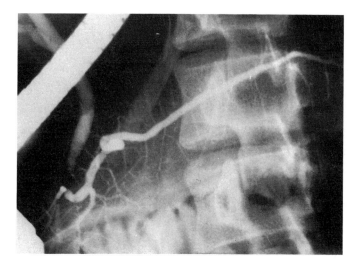

Fig. 6.66 Good-quality normal pancreatogram.

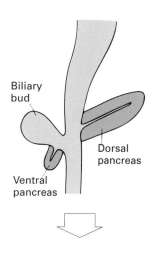

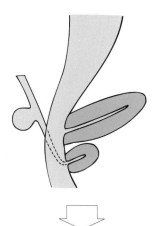

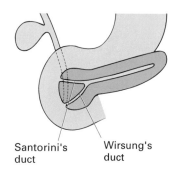

the main duct varies considerably. It usually ascends almost vertically in the head; after a sharp turn or loop at the neck it crosses the vertebral column horizontally or slightly upwards towards the tail. No diagnostic significance can be attributed to odd shapes of the pancreatic duct. The mean diameters of the main duct in the head, body and tail of the normal pancreas are approximately 4, 3 and 2 mm, respectively, but the upper limits of normality are closer to 6, 4 and 3 mm. These figures are corrected for the radiographic magnification (usually about 30%) by checking the apparent endoscopic diameter on the radiographs. There is some increase in pancreatic duct diameter beyond middle age. First and second order branches are usually visible throughout the gland (with good technique), but the distribution and course of these branches is variable (Fig. 6.66). There are fewer branches over the vertebral column where the pancreas is thinner.

Congenital variations in the duct relationships in the head of the pancreas are predictable from their embryological derivation. There is often a narrowing in the main duct close to the junction with Santorini's duct — an appearance which should not be misinterpreted as pathological. The absence of upstream dilatation should provide reassurance. Complete non-union of the ventral and dorsal segments gives rise to pancreas divisum (Fig. 6.67). Cannulation of the main papilla then shows only the ventral pancreas (see Fig. 6.39). This may be very small or even absent. The dorsal duct becomes dominant and drains the bulk of the pancreas through Santorini's duct and the accessory papilla (Fig. 6.68). Santorini's duct may be dominant even when union occurs—the partial pancreas divisum (Fig. 6.69).

Fig. 6.67 Embryonic development of the pancreas. Arrest at mid-phase results in pancreas divisum.

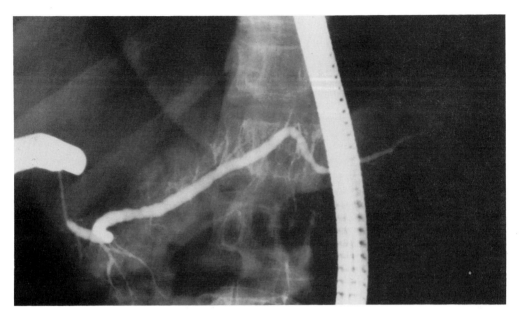

Fig. 6.68 Normal dorsal pancreatogram achieved by cannulating the accessory papilla and filling the body and tail of the pancreas through Santorini's duct.

Pancreatograms are usually grossly abnormal in patients with ductal adenocarcinoma, showing complete obstruction or a tight stricture with upstream dilatation. Tumours which do not arise in the ductal system are less apparent, and tumours of

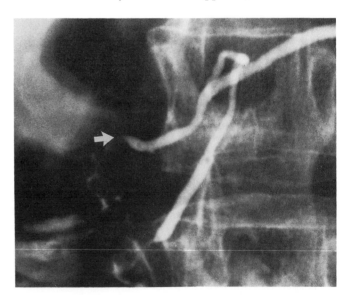

Fig. 6.69 A dominant Santorini duct discharging at the accessory papilla (arrowed).

the uncinate process can be missed altogether. A normal pancreatogram (of good quality, i.e. showing branches throughout the gland) has a specificity of about 95% in ruling out pancreatic cancer.

The pancreatogram is often normal in patients with recurrent attacks of acute pancreatitis. Abnormalities are classified by the Cambridge system (Table 6.1). In *marked* chronic pancreatitis, the main or branch ducts are usually diffusely and irregularly dilated (Fig. 6.70), and often contain filling defects which eventually calcify and cause duct obstruction. Without calcification,

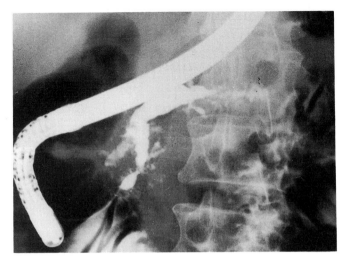

Fig. 6.70 Chronic pancreatitis with disorganization of the duct system, multiple strictures and areas of dilatation.

Terminology	Main duct	Abnormal side branches	Additional features
Normal	Normal	None	
Equivocal	Normal	Fewer than 3	
Mild	Normal	3 or more	
Moderate	Abnormal	More than 3	
Marked	Abnormal	More than 3	One or more of: large cavity, obstruction filling defects, severe dilatation or irregularity

If pathological changes are limited to one-third or less of the gland they are said to be 'local', and are designated as being in the head, body or tail; if more than one-third is affected, they are diffuse.

Table 6.1 Classification of pancreatograms in chronic pancreatitis (Cambridge system).

the radiographic appearances of duct obstruction due to pancreatitis may resemble those seen in cancer — indeed the two diseases may occasionally coexist. Radiographically, *moderate* pancreatitis is characterized by less impressive variation in the main pancreatic duct and its branches. The earliest changes in *mild* pancreatitis are seen in the branch ducts alone. The clinical significance of minor branch duct changes remains controversial, but there are correlations with functional abnormalities and clinical follow-up. However, similar abnormalities in the branch ducts can occur with advancing age. Radiographs are interpreted as 'equivocal' when less than three branches appear abnormal.

The ERCP report should be the combined opinion of the endoscopist and the radiologist, in the full knowledge of the clinical context and other imaging studies.

Further reading

See further reading list in Chapter 8.

ERCP—Therapeutic Technique

7

Endoscopic sphincterotomy and stone extraction was first reported in 1974. Satisfaction with the results and familiarity with the methods has led to widespread use and an expansion of indications. It has been followed by many other therapeutic techniques, including balloon dilatation of strictures, placement of stents and nasobiliary drains and increasing interest in the endoscopic management of pancreatic as well as biliary problems.

These procedures are amongst the most worthwhile that endoscopists attempt, but also the most difficult and hazardous. The indications and risks are reviewed in Chapter 8. It is essential to be properly trained and to have a volume of work sufficient to maintain and develop expertise. The therapeutic endoscopist must work in close association with surgical colleagues, forming a team approach which involves other specialists (including radiologists and pathologists). Complex procedures should be performed only in institutions with facilities adequate to deal rapidly with major complications, such as bleeding. Likewise, the importance of trained gastrointestinal (GI) nurses/assistants cannot be overemphasized. A minimum of two are required; one to ensure the patient's comfort and safety during the procedure, the other to assist the endoscopist and manage the complex equipment. The quality of this assistance can make the difference between success and failure, triumph and disaster.

Biliary sphincterotomy

Sphincterotomy is performed with standard side-viewing duodenoscopes, appropriate sphincterotomes and an electrosurgical source. Electrosurgical units used for polypectomy are suitable; operating room electrosurgical units are unnecessarily powerful and can be hazardous if used without expert knowledge. Familiarity with a single source is probably more important than the precise specification. Most experts prefer equipment which allows the application of blended coagulation and cutting current. Regular maintenance of electrosurgery equipment and attachments is essential.

Sphincterotomes

There are many varieties, most based on the original Demling–Classen ('pull-type') design (Fig. 7.1). The main differ-

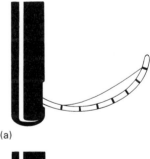
(a)

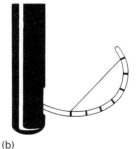
(b)

Fig. 7.1 Standard 'pull-type' sphincterotome: (a) relaxed, and (b) bowed.

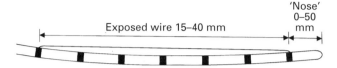

'Nose'
0–50
mm

Exposed wire 15–40 mm

Fig. 7.2 Length variables of sphincterotomes.

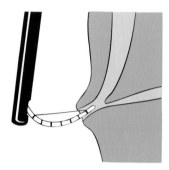

Fig. 7.3 The sphincterotome bow is used to obtain the correct axis for bile duct cannulation.

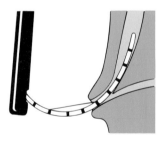

Fig. 7.4 A long-nose sphincterotome in place.

ences are the length of the exposed diathermy wire, the length of the nose (Fig. 7.2) and the number of lumens.

A relatively short nose (5–8 mm) is convenient for cannulation. The tip can be engaged in the papilla without the wire interfering, and tension on the wire can be used to bow the tip into the correct axis (Fig. 7.3). This bowing facility is lost with sphincterotomes with longer noses (2–5 cm beyond the wire), since the diathermy wire (tensing on which causes the bow) inevitably remains inside the endoscope until deep cannulation has been achieved. The sole advantage of the long-nose sphincterotome is that cannulation is not lost while it is being withdrawn during the process of sphincterotomy (Fig. 7.4). Sphincterotomes without any protruding nose are sometimes used for pre-cutting; the diathermy wire extends into the tip of the catheter (Fig. 7.5).

The length of exposed wire in the original standard sphincterotomes was about 35 mm. Now versions are available ranging from 15 to 40 mm. Since most endoscopists perform sphincterotomies with only 5–8 mm of wire in contact with the tissues, it seems illogical to have a much longer wire, especially since it is essential to avoid touching and damaging the endoscope tip with the proximal end of the wire during the application of diathermy current. Unfortunately, a persistent problem of short-wire sphincterotomes is that most have a tendency to flip sideways, towards the 3 o'clock position (Fig. 7.6). The longer wire sphincterotomes (e.g. 35 mm) follow the natural curve of the

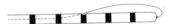

Fig. 7.5 A 'pre-cut' sphincterotome.

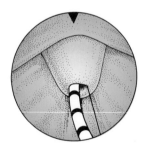

Fig. 7.6 Bad orientation—a common problem with short-wire sphincterotomes.

endoscope and elevator, and are more likely to enter the papilla in the correct orientation (11–1 o'clock). All sphincterotomes behave better if 'trained' before use. The tip should be curled so that the wire enters and leaves the catheter along its left side (Fig. 7.7). Assistants must appreciate that sphincterotomes with short wires require less movement of the control handle to produce a bow; uninformed excessive 'tightening' will result in permanent kinking. Manufacturers are still seeking the magic formula for a '12 o'clock' sphincterotome. The diathermy wire can be monofilament or braided. It is suggested that bleeding is more commonly associated with the former, and pancreatitis with the latter. We prefer monofilament wires.

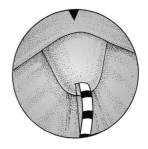

Fig. 7.7 The correct position of the wire, which enters and leaves the *left* side of the catheter.

The original sphincterotomes had only a single lumen for the diathermy wire. Contrast injected down this lumen exits from the wire ports which is unhelpful unless deep cannulation has been achieved. Most sphincterotomes now have a second separate lumen for the injection of contrast (out of the tip) or for passage of the guidewire (Fig. 7.8). Some sphincterotomes have three lumens so that contrast can be injected without removing the guidewire.

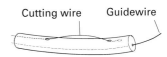

Fig. 7.8 Double-lumen sphincterome. The channel for the guidewire (or contrast) insertion is separate from the cutting wire.

Sphincterotomes with a sigmoid shape (reverse bow) are available for patients with a Billroth II anatomy (Fig. 7.9). Unfortunately they rarely orientate as intended.

The needle-knife sphincterotome consists simply of a bare diathermy wire protruding 3–5 mm from the end of a catheter (Fig. 7.9). 'Push-type' and 'shark-fin' sphincterotomes are variants in which the wire is pushed out to form a bow (Fig. 7.9). These have little application.

Patient preparation

Patient checks, preparation and sedation are broadly similar to those used for diagnostic ERCP. Detailed discussion of the aims, risks and alternatives must take place for the patient's consent to be truly informed. An information leaflet helps this process (see Chapter 3). Coagulation status is usually checked but the relevance of doing so has been questioned in the absence of any suggestive prior history.

Most experts give antibiotics prophylactically before therapeutic ERCP procedures, especially if there is any evidence of duct obstruction. Broad spectrum antibiotic coverage is appropriate. We use gentamicin with ampicillin (with vancomycin as a substitute in patients who are penicillin-sensitive). Other regimens are acceptable. We emphasize again the importance of well-trained assistants and of good disinfection practice. Other aspects of preparation, risks and indications are discussed in Chapters 3 and 8.

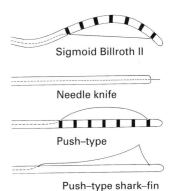

Fig. 7.9 Specialized sphincterotomes.

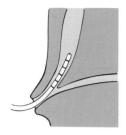

Fig. 7.10 (a) When deep
cannulation has been
achieved . . .

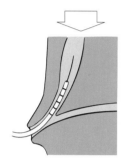

(b) . . . the guidewire is
inserted . . .

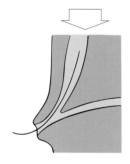

(c) . . . the catheter is removed . . .

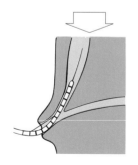

(d) . . . and the sphincterotome is
slid over the guidewire.

Technique of biliary sphincterotomy

Most endoscopists use a standard catheter to perform cholangiography before considering and initiating sphincterotomy.
When deep cannulation has been achieved (especially when it
has been difficult), the catheter can be exchanged for a sphincterotome over a guidewire (Fig. 7.10).

Frequently nowadays we use a double-lumen sphincterotome
for the initial cannulation, especially when the indication for
sphincterotomy is strong. Deep cannulation is often easier to
achieve with a sphincterotome than with a standard catheter; the
tip is somewhat stiffer and the axis of approach can be changed
by bowing the wire (see Chapter 6). The sphincterotome tip is
inserted into the roof of the orifice, angling and bowing up
slightly. Deep cannulation is usually best achieved by lifting the
sphincterotome tip up with the elevator and *withdrawing* the
endoscope somewhat, thus pulling the tip up into the duct axis
(Fig. 7.11a–c). Attempting to achieve deep cannulation by simply
pushing the sphincterotome is usually unsuccessful (and counterproductive), since the curved tip is forced around into the
'duodenal' wall of the bile duct or between mucosal folds in the
sphincter itself (Fig. 7.11d). Confirmation that the sphincterotome is in the bile duct can be achieved by aspirating bile or
injecting contrast. If pancreatography has been performed
already, the position of the sphincterotome can be established by
'wiggling' it; the pancreatic duct will be seen to move (on fluoroscopy) if the tip is within it.

Once a sphincterotome is placed deeply in the bile duct and
the indication for sphincterotomy is confirmed, it is time to
check that the electrosurgical equipment is properly connected
and to assess the anatomical constraints on the procedure. The
size of the papilla, the size of any stone and the shape of the
distal bile duct, can all determine the appropriate and safe
length of incision. It is usually wise to place (or leave) a
guidewire through the sphincterotome during the incision. This
adds stability and prevents the embarrassment of falling out
completely at a crucial moment. With standard guidewires there
is some concern about leakage currents between the guidewire
and the diathermy wire (particularly if a sphincterotome is
reused and the channel has been damaged). We employ an insulated guidewire designed specifically for this purpose.

When everybody and everything is ready, the sphincterotome
is withdrawn slowly under visual and fluoroscopic control until
half of the cutting wire is visible outside the papilla. The wire
should be pointing between 11 and 1 o'clock, preferably at 12
o'clock (Fig. 7.12). Sphincterotomy should not be performed if
the wire cannot be placed within these limits, since perforation is
more likely, especially if it swings laterally beyond the 3 o'clock
position. One way to coax the wire anticlockwise is to push the
endoscope tip more deeply into the duodenum whilst angling

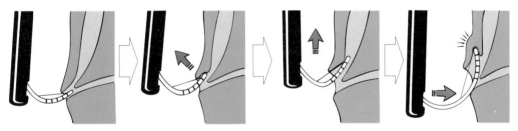

Fig. 7.11 A sphincterotome can be used to achieve deep cannulation. (a) Insert the tip into the orifice . . .

(b) . . . bow the sphincterotome to achieve the bile duct axis . . .

(c) . . . and withdraw the scope.

(d) Simply pushing usually does not advance the tip into the duct.

up; another is to 'lean' to the left while cutting. If good orientation cannot be achieved by manipulating the endoscope tip, it may be necessary to change to a different sphincterotome.

Experts have evolved different methods for the actual incision, but most use only slight bowing of the sphincterotome and a short (5–8 mm) length of wire in contact with the mucosa (Fig. 7.13). The principle of incision should be 'hot and slow', which is achieved by lifting the sphincterotome upwards progressively to provide the necessary pressure between the wire and tissue. The principal aim is to use the sphincterotome as a short hot wire, which is 'walked up' from the tip of the papillary orifice (Fig. 7.13). The roof of the ampulla peels open progressively and under control, to expose the distal bile duct mucosa.

Electrical settings vary with experts and electrosurgical machines. In general we use blended current at 50–60 W. However, the effectiveness and safety of sphincterotomy depends much more on the length of wire in contact with tissue (the current density) than the precise settings. The commonest error is to have too much wire inside the papilla (partially for

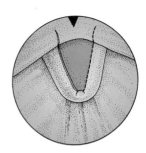

Fig. 7.12 The correct sphincterotomy sector.

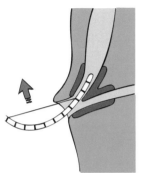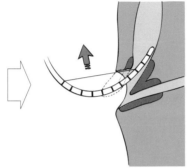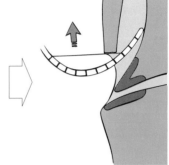

Fig. 7.13 (a) Use an up-angle and a short wire contact . . .

(b) . . . to cut the papilla in steps . . .

(c) . . . and to 'walk up' the bile duct.

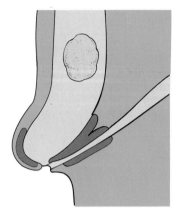

Fig. 7.14 An easy sphincterotomy with a swollen papilla, a big duct and a 'square' termination.

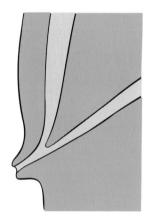

Fig. 7.15 A more dangerous sphincterotomy with a small papilla and a small tapering duct.

fear of falling out), and to apply too much bowing tension; nothing will happen when current is applied — or only slow coagulation will result—which increases the risk of subsequent pancreatitis. There is then a temptation to increase the current settings and pressure, which will eventually and suddenly cut through the coagulated area at alarming speed with a risk of significant bleeding (the so-called 'zipper'). If nothing appears to be happening when current is applied during sphincterotomy, it is much better to reduce the length of wire in contact with the mucosa, which increases the current density and should initiate the incision.

Sphincterotomy size

The size of the sphincterotomy should be tailored to the size of the bile duct and stone, and will be influenced somewhat by the shape and direction of the terminal bile duct in relation to the duodenum. The simplest, and probably safest, sphincterotomies are those performed in patients who have (or have had) a stone impacted above the orifice; the papilla is large and oedematous, and cuts easily without bleeding; the bile duct termination is often somewhat 'square' (Fig. 7.14). Sphincterotomy is more hazardous in patients with a relatively small papilla and a duct which is either not dilated or tapers distally (Fig. 7.15). Probably for this reason, the risk of perforation is significantly greater when sphincterotomy is performed for papillary stenosis.

When to stop cutting

This is a crucial question, for which there is no easy answer. Some endoscopists rely on external landmarks, stating that it is safe to cut up to, but not beyond, the proximal hooding fold. Unfortunately, this fold varies in size and position, and bears little relationship to the underlying anatomy. More important is the size of the papilla itself, and whether or not any of the intramural bile duct can be seen from the duodenum. It is usually safe to cut as far as the duodenal wall; although this may produce an impressively long cut on the surface it may not reach the upper part of the biliary sphincter (Fig. 7.16). It is usually necessary to cut some more on the inside (Fig. 7.17). For this reason, measurements of sphincterotomy length are of limited relevance. Often the sphincterotome 'jumps' into the bile duct as the upper sphincter is broached, and bile flows out of the incision. *A good sign of an adequate sphincterotomy is when the partially bowed sphincterotome slides easily to and fro through the orifice.* The size of the orifice can be estimated with balloon-tipped catheters.

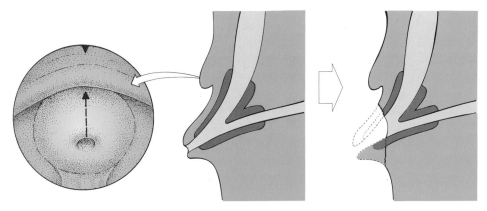

Fig. 7.16 It is probably safe to cut down to the estimated duodenal wall — but the upper sphincter is not necessarily divided.

Difficult sphincterotomies

There are certain circumstances in which bile duct access and sphincterotomy may be more difficult, and where additional skills and judgement may be required.

Peripapillary diverticula. These are common, especially in elderly patients with duct stones. Cannulation and sphincterotomy may be extremely difficult when the papilla is actually inside the diverticulum. It can usually be found by following the longitudinal fold upwards (Fig. 7.18). The papilla is then teased out of the diverticulum by aspirating air to collapse the duodenum partially and/or by pressing firmly sideways (with a catheter or sphincterotome) to pull on the duodenal folds which flow into the diverticulum (Fig. 7.19). Sometimes it is necessary to use two accessories at the same time to hold the position while cannulating.

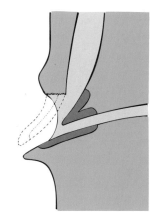

Fig. 7.17 It is usually necessary to cut inside to ablate the biliary sphincter.

There is no evidence that sphincterotomy is more dangerous in the presence of a diverticulum. The direction of the bile duct is somewhat unpredictable (unless it can be seen traversing the floor of the diverticulum) but the sphincterotome, once inserted, necessarily follows the bile duct direction.

Billroth II gastrectomy. This turns the anatomy of the papilla 'upside down'. The diathermy wire needs to be pointing at 6 o'clock rather than 12 o'clock. Sigmoid-loop sphincterotomes designed to achieve this position do not always succeed in practice (Fig. 7.20). Our routine method is first to place a short 7 French gauge stent in the bile duct, which is easily done since cannulation is usually effected with a guidewire (see Chapter 6). A needle knife is then used to perform a cut-down sphinctero-

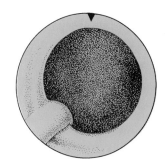

Fig. 7.18 A papilla within the diverticulum—only the longitudinal fold shows.

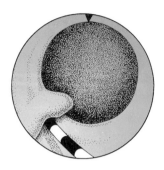 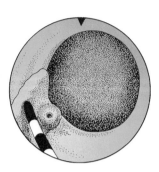

Fig. 7.19 (a) Push with the catheter or sphincterotome to evert the papilla from the diverticulum . . .

(b) . . . further pressure laterally brings the orifice into view.

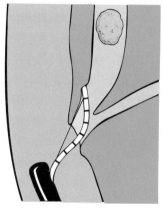

Fig. 7.20 A sigmoid-loop sphincterotome used in Billroth II patients.

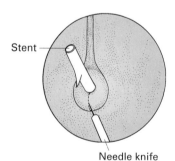

Stent

Needle knife

Fig. 7.21 A needle-knife sphincterotomy over a stent in a Billroth II patient (papilla upside down).

tomy on to the stent (Fig. 7.21); the stent is then removed. Sometimes a standard (long-nose) sphincterotome can be persuaded into the correct position by deft endoscopic manoeuvring.

Impacted stones. These can cause the papilla to bulge into the duodenum and displace the orifice downwards (Fig. 7.22). Cannulation can be achieved with a bowed sphincterotome, 'hooking' the tip into the orifice (Fig. 7.23a). Alternatively, a needle knife can be used to incise the face of the papilla over the stone (Fig. 7.23b).

Pre-cutting

Pre-cutting means starting an incision from within the common channel (or even pancreatic duct) without having achieved deep biliary cannulation. This can be done with a 'no nose' variant of the standard sphincterotome where the cutting wire extends to the tip (see Fig. 7.5), but the needle-knife sphincterotome (see Fig. 7.9) has become more popular. The bare wire is inserted into the papillary orifice and diathermy applied in short bursts with upward pressure in the 11–12 o'clock direction (Fig. 7.24). The bile duct orifice can usually be identified in the floor of this incision, either immediately or on a subsequent day (often most easily achieved by probing with the tip of a hydrophilic guidewire). A needle knife can be used also to make a direct 'drill' incision above the papilla into a dilated bile duct, or into the face of a papilla swollen by an impacted stone or choledochocele.

Pre-cutting is more dangerous than a standard sphincterotomy. It should not be used as a substitute for proper training and experience in standard techniques, and should be reserved for use by experts in high-risk patients with a strong indication for sphincterotomy when standard techniques have been

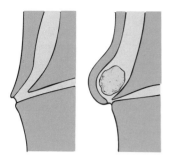

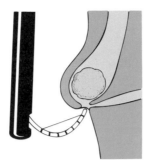

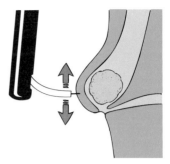

Fig. 7.22 Compared to the normal anatomy, an impacted stone forces the orifice downwards.

Fig. 7.23 (a) Use a bowed sphincterotome to cannulate . . .

(b) . . . or a needle knife to incise over the stone.

exhausted. Pre-cutting cannot be recommended purely for diagnostic access to the bile duct.

Combined endoscopic-radiological procedure

An alternative to pre-cutting when standard sphincterotomy fails is to work over a guidewire previously positioned through the papilla (from above) by an interventional radiologist (or surgeon at cholecystectomy). The endoscopist can simply slide a double-lumen sphincterotome over the guidewire and pass it deep into the duct (Fig. 7.25). This procedure is more commonly employed for the insertion of stents and it is described in more detail on p. 160.

Stone-extraction techniques

Although most stones (at least those <1 cm in diameter) (Plate 7.1) will pass spontaneously in the days or weeks following an adequate sphincterotomy, most experts prefer to extract them directly. This immediately clarifies the situation and reduces the risk of impaction, cholangitis and/or pancreatitis. Stones can be removed using balloon-tipped catheters or baskets.

Balloon catheters

Balloon catheters are useful for extracting large numbers of relatively small stones and for sweeping the duct after extraction procedures to demonstrate that it is clear. Balloon diameters vary from 8 to 20 mm. The catheter shaft should be 7 French gauge (to provide some rigidity), with a central lumen for a guidewire or injection of contrast. Some balloon catheters have a third lumen which provides a useful injection port below the balloon.

The balloon catheter is advanced to the hilum of the liver.

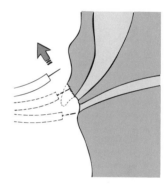

Fig. 7.24 Pre-cutting up from the orifice with a needle knife.

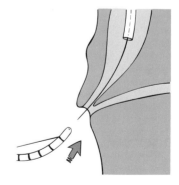

Fig. 7.25 A combined procedure where a sphincterotome is slid over the percutaneously placed guidewire.

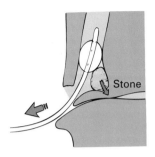

Fig. 7.26 Difficulties may arise using a ballon for stone extraction: traction on the balloon may simply force the stone sideways against the duct wall.

This is best done over a guidewire, which makes it possible to run the balloon repeatedly down the duct without losing access. Contrast is injected and the balloon is inflated to the duct diameter, and then pulled back slowly under fluoroscopic control. It is important to check the location of the catheter tip before inflating the balloon since damage can be caused if it is inflated in a narrow duct (e.g. pancreatic duct, cystic duct or intrahepatic biliary tree). Many endoscopists prefer balloons to baskets because they cannot become impacted. Unfortunately, they are less effective for extracting larger stones, probably because the force is applied tangentially; the balloon may slip past the stone or simply force it sideways against the duct wall (Fig. 7.26). Balloons are also fragile and relatively expensive.

Basket extraction

Basket extraction is more reliable in most cases. Standard baskets have four wires in an elongated diamond shape (Fig. 7.27). They are described by their length and maximum open dimensions, commonly 30 by 15 mm. Variants such as the three-wire and spiral baskets have not become popular. Baskets with a guidewire leader may be helpful when access is difficult.

The basket catheter is passed beyond the stone before it is fully opened, taking care not to push the stone into the intrahepatic ducts. It may be necessary to 'jiggle' the basket to trap a stone within it. The basket is then trawled down the duct in the fully or partially open position. Attempting to close the basket fully may eject the stone or, worse, impact the wires within it. Usually there is resistance when the basket and stone reach the sphincterotomy orifice; pulling harder simply drags the endoscope tip onto the papilla. The final stage of extraction is best done under fluoroscopic control using a 'flip-down' manoeuvre. Holding the basket position steady at the papilla, the endoscope tip is angled sharply down and rotated to the right; this applies force in the correct biliary axis and is usually successful in extracting the stone (Fig. 7.28). When a stone cannot be extracted, it can sometimes be embarrassingly difficult to release it from the basket. Try pushing the open basket high in the common hepatic duct and forcing a loop (Fig. 7.29).

Difficult and big stones

Many factors (not least the experience of the endoscopist) determine the success of stone extraction. Amongst the most important is stone size. A useful guide is the size of the endoscope, which measures 13–15 mm on the radiographic film (because of magnification); increasing difficulty must be expected with stones larger than the endoscope. Stones of up to 25 mm in

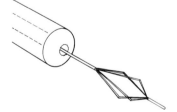

Fig. 7.27 Standard diamond-shaped stone extraction basket.

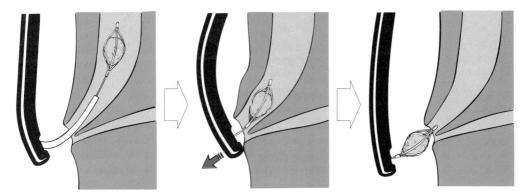

Fig. 7.28 Stone extraction by the 'flip down' technique.

diameter can be extracted (or may even pass spontaneously) after endoscopic sphincterotomy, but the risks of bleeding and perforation increase with sphincterotomy size. Stones over 25 mm have caused gallstone ileus when released into the duodenum.

The importance of the shape of the distal bile duct has already been emphasized in relation to the safety of sphincterotomy. It is much easier to remove a large stone when the lower end of the bile duct is relatively 'square' (see Fig. 7.14) and it is foolish to attempt to pull it out intact when there is a long distal taper. Stones may be difficult to retrieve from unusual positions such as the cystic or intrahepatic ducts. A balloon catheter can usually be placed beyond such stones after careful manipulation with appropriate guidewires. Stones located above strictures can be removed only if the stricture is first dilated satisfactorily. Flat (coin-shaped) stones may be difficult to trap in a basket (or trawl in front of a balloon), and angulated stones may resist transit through the sphincterotomy. Stones which are 'sausage shaped' are the easiest to remove, partly because they are usually relatively soft, brown pigment stones. The most difficult are the large square stones which fill the bile duct lumen like a piston (Fig. 7.30). Baskets usually deform around such stones and fail to engage them—which is sometimes just as well since their size and shape make them difficult to extract through the sphincterotomy.

Mechanical lithotripsy techniques should be used when standard methods fail. In essence, the mechanical lithotriptor is simply a stronger (often larger) basket with a metal, spiral sheath. The basket wires should be strong enough to open vigorously, and designed so that the basket does not become trapped in the duct if they break. The metal sheath is sometimes difficult to manipulate into the duct directly, which has led to the development of 'three-layer' lithotriptors (Fig. 7.31). The basket is

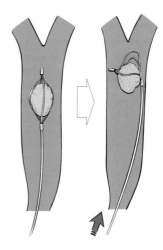

Fig. 7.29 Releasing the stone by advancing and distorting the basket.

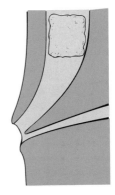

Fig. 7.30 The 'piston'-shaped stone which is difficult to grasp and extract.

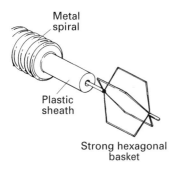

Fig. 7.31 The 'three-layer' lithotripsy basket system.

placed deep in the duct through a standard plastic sheath, over which the metal sleeve is then passed.

Mechanical lithotripsy is used also when a stone and standard basket have become stuck in the duct. The basket handle is cut off and the endoscope is removed gently, leaving the basket in place, preferably with the plastic sleeve over it. A flexible spiral metal 'crushing sleeve' (Soehendra lithotriptor) is then advanced over the basket wires to the papilla, under fluoroscopic control, whilst pulling on the basket wires. The wire is then tightened with a reel mechanism or pliers (Fig. 7.32). Usually the stone will crush; alternatively, the basket wires will break and the stone will be released.

Failed stone extraction

When stones cannot be removed with standard balloon and basket techniques (including mechanical lithotripsy), it is time to review other options. These involve a delay, during which stone impaction may cause cholangitis. It is therefore wise to provide temporary drainage in this context, using a nasobiliary drain or stent (see below). A nasobiliary drain is preferred if the patient is septic and when further intervention (endoscopic or surgical) is likely to take place within a few days. A stent is usually favoured when the patient's condition is stable and when there may be a significant delay before further attempts are made by specialist

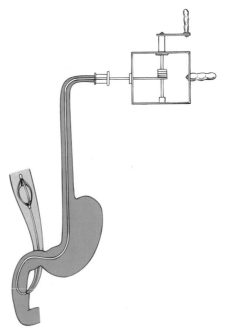

Fig. 7.32 The reel mechanism for tightening the basket wires.

techniques (see below), particularly if these are to be at another institution.

Options for patients with big stones include *surgical interven-tion*, which may well be appropriate in younger and fitter patients (and certainly those with the gallbladder still in place). Large stones can be fragmented within the bile duct using *endo-scopically directed shockwaves* (using pulsed lasers and electrohy-draulic techniques). Because of the risk of damage to the bile duct wall, these should be employed only under direct choledo-choscopic vision using a 'mother and baby' system or a percuta-neous transhepatic approach. Options are discussed further in Chapter 8.

Infusion of *solvents* through nasobiliary drains has proved dis-appointing, largely because most of the big stones are not choles-terol rich. Solvent techniques (using mono-octanoin or methyl *tert*-butyl ether) are also time-consuming and not without hazard.

Extracorporeal shockwave lithotripsy (ESWL) has been used successfully, but further endoscopic manipulation is usually required to remove the fragments.

Removing bile duct stones without sphincterotomy

Stones of less than 5 mm diameter can be extracted from the bile duct through the intact papilla using a standard basket catheter. Larger stones can be removed after balloon dilatation of the papilla (to 6 or 8 mm), with or without the addition of mechani-cal lithotripsy. Specialized equipment for this technique is being developed. Whether balloon dilatation is safer than sphinctero-tomy in the short and long term remains to be proven. When stone extraction has proved to be difficult, it may be wise to place a nasobiliary drain overnight.

Nasobiliary drainage

Nasobiliary catheters are simply long polyethylene tubes (5 or 7 French gauge), at least twice the length of the endoscope, with multiple distal side holes. The tip is moulded to prevent it falling out. Several designs are available, including terminal pigtails, right-angle bends, mid-duct pigtails and a variety with a pre-formed loop in the duodenum (Fig. 7.33). The advantage of those without distal pigtails is that they can be inserted directly into the bile duct, without the need of a straightening guidewire. If a standard catheter is already in the bile duct when the decision is made to leave a nasobiliary drain, it is easiest to perform an exchange over a guidewire.

Once the distal tip has been placed in the correct position high in the biliary tree (and above any retained stone), the endoscope

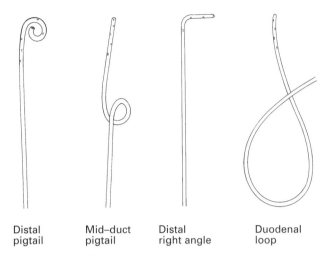

Distal	Mid–duct	Distal	Duodenal
pigtail	pigtail	right angle	loop

Fig. 7.33 Designs of nasobiliary catheters.

must be removed gradually without dislodging the catheter. It is easiest for an assistant to withdraw the endoscope slowly, while the endoscopist pushes the catheter and monitors the position by fluoroscopy (Fig. 7.34).

After the endoscope has been removed, the proximal end of the drain must be rerouted from the mouth to the nose. A short plastic tube is passed through a nostril into the pharynx, grabbed by a surgical forceps (or fingers) and brought out through the mouth. The top of the biliary drain is then fed back through it; both are withdrawn at the nose until the drain lies straight in the pharynx. The drain should be strapped to the patient's face and connected to a bag with an injection/aspiration side-port.

Nasobiliary drains are usually well tolerated for several days, and have been left in place for weeks. Their essential role is to provide effective drainage; therefore, the output should be monitored and the catheter flushed (and the position checked by fluoroscopy) if there is any question of dislodgement. The drain can be used for check cholangiography, flushing and infusion of chemical solvents.

Dilatation of biliary strictures

Biliary dilatation techniques were developed from those used in angioplasty. Sausage-shaped balloon catheters are slid over standard guidewires. For most purposes, it is convenient to use a balloon which is 8 mm in diameter and 2 cm long, mounted on a 7 French gauge shaft. Radiographic metal markers are incor-

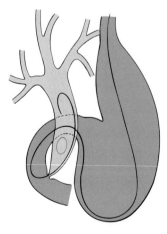

Fig. 7.34 Nasobiliary drainage.

porated (Fig. 7.35). Smaller balloons are used for tight strictures. Once placed through the stricture over a guidewire, the balloon is inflated to a predetermined pressure and the procedure is monitored under fluoroscopy for the disappearance of the 'waist' (Fig. 7.36). Dilatation may be painful and often cannot be maintained for more than 30 s. Repeated dilatations may be necessary. Most strictures recur quickly after simple dilatation; it is therefore customary to leave a stent (or stents) in place for several months.

Dilatation of strictures which are so tight that they will not accept a balloon catheter can be achieved using 'stepped' dila-

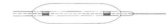

Fig. 7.35 A dilating balloon placed over a guidewire; the radio-opaque metal markers show up.

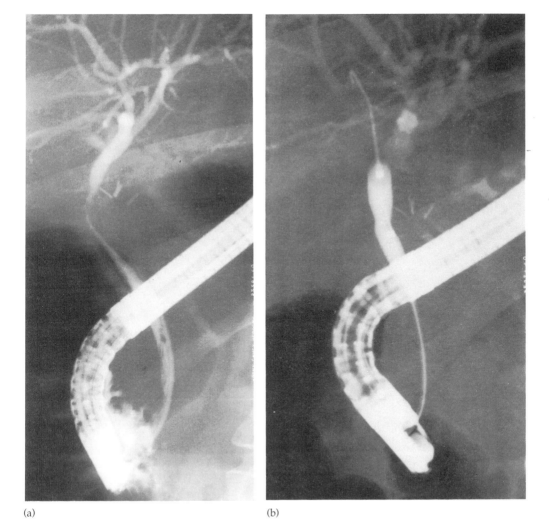

(a)   (b)

Fig. 7.36 (a) Postoperative stricture. (b) Balloon dilatation over a guidewire.

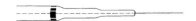

Fig. 7.37 Tapered 'stepped' dilator for use in the bile (or pancreatic) duct over a guidewire (note metal marker).

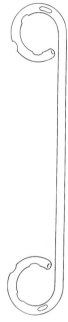

Fig. 7.38 A pigtail stent.

tors over a guidewire (Fig. 7.37). Various sizes are available; the commonest have three steps at 5, 7 and 9 French gauge. These dilators are most commonly used in patients with malignant strictures, prior to stenting (see below).

Biliary stenting

Endoscopic biliary stent placement is now well established, especially for palliation of malignant obstructive jaundice. Precise indications in this and other contexts are discussed in Chapter 8. Stents made of plastic (usually polyethylene) are most commonly used, but various types of expandable metal mesh stent are becoming more popular. These are discussed later.

Patient preparation

The patient's focal problem and general status are reviewed in detail, and appropriate informed consent is obtained (see Chapter 3). The biggest specific risk of stenting is infection. This occurs mainly because of inadequate drainage, but it is essential to ensure that endoscopes and accessories are disinfected rigorously. Prophylactic antibiotics are given routinely. Stent placement requires high-quality fluoroscopy and two well-trained nurses or assistants.

Plastic stent design

Plastic stents and introducing sets are produced by several manufacturers, with little variation in precise design. Stents of 7 French gauge can be placed through a standard diagnostic duodenoscope, and are appropriate in some contexts. How-

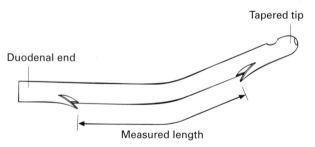

Tapered tip

Duodenal end

Measured length

Fig. 7.39 The anatomy of an Amsterdam-type stent.

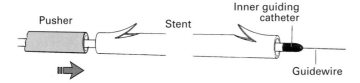

Fig. 7.40 Standard three-layer system for stent insertion.

ever, most indications (especially malignant disease) require the use of larger stents (10–12 French gauge), for which a large-channel therapeutic duodenoscope is mandatory. The larger stents (e.g. 11.5 French gauge) are more awkward to use and have no proven advantage; most experts use 10 French gauge stents routinely. Stents with pigtails (Fig. 7.38) are still used occasionally, e.g. in patients with unremovable stones. The vast majority of stents, however, are of the 'Amsterdam' type, i.e. slightly curved with flaps near each end to prevent migration (Fig. 7.39). Stent length is traditionally measured between the flaps. Numerous variants have been produced (different plastics, side holes and flaps) without any proven advantage, as yet.

Stenting requires a long 0.035-inch diameter guidewire with a radio-opaque tip and most experts prefer hydrophilic wires. Stents of 7 French gauge are inserted directly over the wire (once it has been placed through the stricture), using a 7 French gauge pushing catheter. Larger stents require a three-layer system (Fig. 7.40). The stent is slid with a pushing tube over a 6–7 French gauge inner guiding catheter, which itself lies over the guidewire.

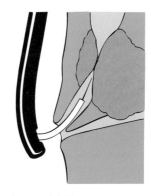

Fig. 7.41 (a) The assistant protrudes the guidewire 2 cm beyond the catheter . . .

Techniques of stent insertion

Some endoscopists used to perform the initial ERCP procedure with a standard-sized duodenoscope and changed to the more cumbersome larger-channel instrument once the indication for stenting had been confirmed (usually after performing a small sphincterotomy). However, modern large-channel endoscopes are simple to use from start to finish.

Cannulation is initiated with a standard catheter or with the inner catheter of a stent set. Contrast is injected to define the anatomy but without overdistending the biliary tree. A guidewire is inserted through the catheter to engage and pass through the stricture (Fig. 7.41). Independent manipulations of the catheter and guidewire may be necessary to achieve the correct angle (Figs 7.42 & 7.43). Once the guidewire has passed through the stricture, the catheter can be slid over it and further

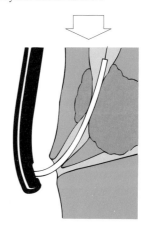

(b) . . . then the catheter and guidewire are advanced together to engage and pass the stricture.

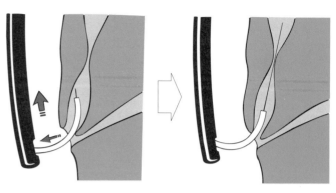

Fig. 7.42 (a) Pull back the scope and catheter . . .

(b) . . . to improve the angle for guidewire advancement.

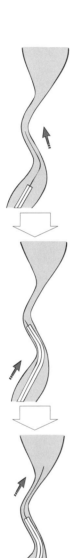

Fig. 7.43 Advance through tortuous strictures one bend at a time, first the guidewire and then the catheter.

radiographs obtained. The guidewire can be left in place whilst cytology specimens are taken. In addition, the wire can be used for placement of a sphincterotome. An alternative approach is to start the procedure with the double-lumen sphincterotome through which the guidewire can be threaded after cholangiography.

Sphincterotomy before stenting? Most endoscopists perform a *small* sphincterotomy as part of the stenting procedure. Although it is possible to pass stents of up to 11.5 French gauge through the intact papilla, a sphincterotomy facilitates this process and makes it possible to place more than one stent when required (e.g. in hilar lesions), and probably facilitates subsequent stent replacement. Sphincterotomy has also been advocated to prevent the bile duct stent from compromising the pancreatic orifice (and causing pancreatitis); however, this risk appears to be very small, even without sphincterotomy.

Stricture dilatation before stenting? Benign strictures are dilated before stenting since the stent is used simply to maintain the initial dilatation. Most malignant strictures can be stented without dilatation but difficulty may be experienced in hilar lesions, perhaps particularly because less force can be applied at a distance. Under these circumstances, it is convenient to use a stepped dilator (5, 7 and 9 French gauge) over the guidewire (see Fig. 7.37).

Stent placement

The correct stent length is chosen so that the top flap will be above the stricture and the bottom flap just outside the papilla (usually leaving a margin of about 1 cm for movement and tumour growth, but remember that ERCP radiographs have a magnification of about 30%). Some 'inner guide' catheters for stenting have radio-opaque markers to facilitate precise measurements (Fig. 7.44).

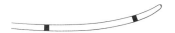

Fig. 7.44 Radio-opaque markers on the stent insertion catheter.

The guidewire and inner guiding catheter (for a 10 French gauge stent or larger) should be placed well above the stricture, preferably in a main intrahepatic duct. Make sure that you are not in the cystic duct. The stent is passed over the guide catheter and into the biopsy port. The proximal flap of the stent is flattened into the biopsy channel; usually this can be done with the finger, but an introducing sleeve is provided. The 'pusher tube' is then used to guide the stent down through the endoscope. There is considerable friction in this system, so that movement of the pusher will tend also to advance the inner guide catheter (and its contained guidewire). This tendency can be minimized by attempting to 'grasp' the inner guide catheter with the endoscope elevator. Maintenance of the correct position of the guidewire and catheter in the liver should be monitored repeatedly by fluoroscopy. The assistant should inform the endoscopist as soon as the inner catheter appears out of her end of the pusher; she can then help the passage of the stent by pulling back on the inner catheter, against the pusher tube. In fact, this merely maintains the inner guide catheter and guidewire in the same position in the liver as the stent advances. Close collaboration between the endoscopist and assistant is essential.

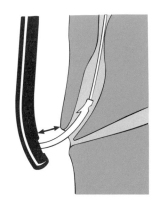

Fig. 7.45 Good scope position, close to the papilla.

The endoscopist can feel when the tip of the stent reaches the elevator. It is important to work carefully and deliberately at this stage. The tip of the endoscope should be kept *close to the papilla*, without allowing any significant bow in the catheter (or stent) (Fig. 7.45). The position of the inner catheter and guidewire are checked again. Once everything and everyone is prepared the following steps are performed.

1 Lower the elevator and push the stent tip 1–2 cm into the endoscopic view (Fig. 7.46).

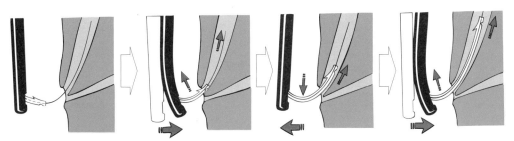

Fig. 7.46 (a) Advance the stent tip until just visible . . .

(b) . . . insert the stent tip into the bile duct by angling the scope tip up and lifting the elevator . . .

(c) . . . then back off the scope slightly (angle down), drop the elevator and advance the stent slightly . . .

(d) . . . then push the stent into the bile duct by angling the scope tip and lifting the elevator.

2 Advance the stent tip into the papilla by lifting the elevator and angling the endoscope up.

3 The assistant maintains traction on the inner catheter against the pusher tube, whilst the process is monitored on fluoroscopy.

4 Insert the stent further in small moves, remembering that the stent cannot be withdrawn once it has been extended too far.

5 Repeat the sequence: elevator down, stent out 1–2 cm and elevator and endoscope tip up to push the stent inwards.

6 The assistant may need to withdraw the inner catheter slightly before the sequence is repeated (Fig. 7.46).

7 Stop once the bottom flap abuts the papilla.

8 If necessary, take further radiographs after removing the guidewire and injecting contrast.

9 Remove the inner catheter and guidewire together, holding the stent in place.

10 Watch the gratifying rush of bile as the stent and pusher separate (Plate 7.2).

Straightening and 'jerk back' manoeuvres. Usually there is resistance to stent passage when the tip enters the stricture. Pushing the stent simply results in a loop in the duodenum (Fig. 7.47a). If this is allowed to continue, the situation becomes irremediable and it will be necessary to remove the endoscope completely (grasping the stent in the elevator) and to start the procedure over again. To avoid this predicament, the endoscope is advanced further into the duodenum so as to straighten the stent (Fig. 7.47b). The tip of the endoscope is then angled sharply

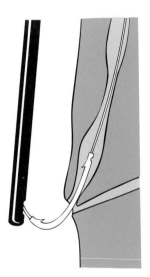
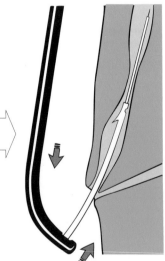
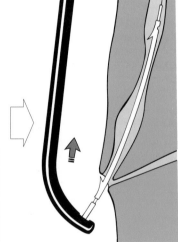

Fig. 7.47 Getting out of loop trouble. (a) If there is too much stent in the duodenum . . .

(b) . . . advance the scope and angle it up to get the stent straight . . .

(c) . . . then pull back on the scope to force the stent inwards.

upwards, and the whole instrument withdrawn or 'jerked back' (Fig. 7.47c). This usually produces enough force in the correct axis to advance the stent through the stricture.

Bifurcation lesions (and double stenting)

Type 1 hilar strictures (not involving the bifurcation) can be managed with a single stent. Management of type 2 and 3 lesions (involving the bifurcation or higher branches) is more difficult technically, and provides less satisfactory results. The strictures are often tortuous and sclerotic and further away from the fulcrum provided by the duodenoscope tip.

Jaundice can be relieved if about one-third of the liver can be drained. The main problem is the risk of sepsis in undrained segments. Whether or not it is necessary to attempt to drain all obstructed ducts in every case remains controversial; in fact, this is often impossible. A single stent provides good palliation of jaundice in most hilar lesions (provided an appropriate segment is selected), with an early cholangitis rate of less than 10%. When sepsis does develop, it is essential to provide drainage of the obstructed ductal system (urgently). This can be done by a second endoscopic procedure, a primary percutaneous approach or a combined endoscopic-radiological technique (see below).

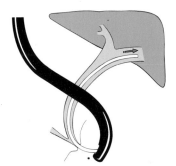

Fig. 7.48 The natural curve of the catheter takes it into the right intrahepatic duct preferentially (patient prone).

Steering into the intrahepatic ducts

Catheters usually enter the right intrahepatic ductal system preferentially, because of their natural curl (Fig. 7.48). It is sometimes necessary to select the left intrahepatic system; several methods may be useful in this situation. If the catheter is brought down low in the bile duct, the guidewire (which always goes straight) may be aimed towards the left side (Fig. 7.49). Another method involves the use of a catheter with a preformed bend (or side hole) near the tip (Fig. 7.50). It is also possible to use a torque-stable guidewire with a bent tip. This is placed below the stricture and rotated into the correct axis. The friction in the long catheter systems often prevents this method working optimally.

When attempting to insert two stents in different parts of the liver, it is wise to start by placing the two guidewires; it is often not possible to place a second wire once a stent has been inserted.

Failed stent insertion

The commonest reason for failure of stenting is difficulty in deep biliary cannulation, caused by distortion of the anatomy by tumour impression or actual involvement of the papilla. Failure

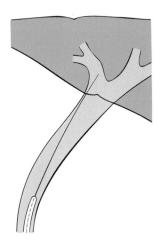

Fig. 7.49 Pulling the inner 'guiding' catheter down the duct directs the straight guidewire into the left intrahepatic duct (patient prone).

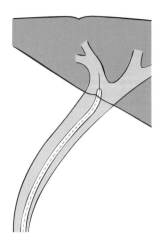

Fig. 7.50 A preformed catheter can be used for selective entry into the left duct (patient prone).

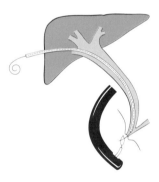

Fig. 7.51 The combined procedure where the endoscopist catches the radiologically placed guidewire and pulls it back through the scope.

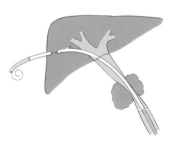

Fig. 7.52 A danger is to advance the stent too far, so that it no longer drains . . .

puts the patient at risk for cholangitis, especially if contrast has been injected above the stricture. Alternative drainage techniques must be employed within days and preferably within hours (certainly once sepsis has developed). Drainage can be provided by direct percutaneous transhepatic radiological intervention or by a combined procedure.

Combined endoscopic-radiological stenting ('rendezvous' procedure)

The use of a transhepatically placed guidewire has been mentioned as a method for facilitating bile duct access for sphincterotomy. Combined procedures are used for the insertion of stents when the initial cannulation fails and in patients with hilar lesions when it proves necessary to drain more than one liver segment.

In units with combined endoscopic-radiological facilities and excellent collaboration, combined procedures can often be performed immediately when the indication arises—provided that the patient's consent has been obtained beforehand. However, in most centres, combined procedures are done in stages. The first stage (after failure of endoscopic access) is to perform a standard percutaneous transhepatic drainage procedure, leaving the catheter through the stricture if possible. Radiologists usually prefer to do these procedures in their own specialized suites.

Once the patient is stable (and whilst continuing antibiotics), he is brought back to the ERCP department. The radiologist places a long standard 0.035-inch diameter guidewire through the patient's catheter into the duodenum, and the endoscopist passes the therapeutic duodenoscope opposite the papilla. The radiologist pulls the catheter back until it is only just protruding from the papilla and the guidewire is projecting 1–2 cm from it. The endoscopist grasps the tip of the wire with a snare loop and draws it back slowly through the endoscope channel (Fig. 7.51). The radiologist holds the catheter in place and helps by pushing the guidewire at the skin surface. It is important to maintain the catheter in position in order to prevent the wire traumatizing the liver. The guidewire is pulled at least 2 cm out of the endoscope, and is then used in the standard way to insert the stent using the three-layer system already described (Fig. 7.40). As the endoscopist's inner catheter advances through the papilla, it pushes the radiologist's catheter back to a position above the stricture. A significant danger with the combined procedure is advancing the stent too far, so that the tip is impacted in liver tissue and is no longer draining a duct (Fig. 7.52). One way to prevent this happening (after the radiologist has inserted a second wire) is for the endoscopist to withdraw the first guidewire until its tip is just above the stricture, and then advance it into an appropriate large duct (Fig. 7.53).

Once the stent is in place, it is customary to leave the percutaneous drainage catheter in for at least one night and to do a check cholangiogram on the following day. The catheter can then be removed if the stent is functioning. Sometimes, with high lesions, there may be little room for the percutaneous catheter above the stent. This is another advantage of placing two guidewires percutaneously (through a common sleeve). One guidewire is used by the endoscopist for the stent insertion, the other subsequently by the radiologist to place a temporary external drainage tube.

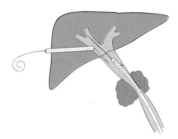

Fig. 7.53 . . . to avoid this the endoscopist can pull the guidewire back and then place it in a large duct.

A variant of the combined procedure utilizes a forward-viewing endoscope to retrieve the guidewire from the duodenum. The stent is passed through the mouth over this wire, and pushed into place with an endoscope or under radiological control using a pusher tube. These methods allow the insertion of very large stents since they do not have to be passed through the instrument channel. The techniques have not become popular because it is difficult to pass the stent through the stricture and to judge when the stent is in the optimal position.

The combined procedure stenting techniques were developed to reduce the risk of passing a large stent through the liver substance. However, these techniques are now used less frequently as endoscopists have become more skilled, and, particularly, with the development of expandable metal mesh stents which can be placed percutaneously by a radiologist through a smaller catheter.

Post-stenting care

Most stent procedures are straightforward and well tolerated. Overnight observation is wise after the first stent procedure, but may not be necessary for any subsequent elective stent exchange. Antibiotics are continued overnight and the patient is discharged on a normal diet the next morning if there are no adverse developments. Stool and urine colour should return to normal within 1 week, and improvement in liver function tests can be monitored.

Stent malfunction

This is indicated by the failure of jaundice to resolve or the recurrence of obstruction. Inadequate drainage is usually followed by sepsis, which can be life-threatening. Although stent patency can be investigated by plain abdominal radiographs and scans (to check for air in the biliary tree and duct dilatation) and by dynamic isotope scans, the only way to clarify the situation completely is to repeat the ERCP procedure. Early stent dysfunction may be due to a poor position. The stent may have been placed too high with the tip impacted in a small hepatic radical, or even inadvertently in the cystic duct. Occasionally stents can be blocked by blood clots. If the stent appears to be in the correct position, patency can be checked by injecting contrast through the tip (gently so as not to increase intrahepatic pressure in the presence of sepsis).

Delayed stent dysfunction may be due to migration, usually downwards. The tip becomes impacted in the duodenal wall and can rarely cause ulceration or bleeding. Most delayed occlusion is due to the accumulation of bacterial and biliary debris, which is inevitable eventually. Stents of 10–11.5 French gauge can be expected to remain patent for 3–6 months; 7 French gauge biliary stents rarely stay patent for more than 3 months.

Life-threatening sepsis can develop rapidly after stent occlusion. Patients and their care-givers should be warned about the early symptoms (especially chills), and advised to return to specialist care immediately when these develop. Because of the potential for severe complications, consideration should be given to changing stents electively. Most experts recommend that stents should be routinely changed about every 3 months (with 10 French gauge stents) in patients with benign strictures. The value in patients with malignant disease remains to be proven, since most patients die before stent occlusion.

Stent removal and exchange

The simplest way to remove a blocked (or migrated) stent is to grasp the tip in the duodenum with a snare loop or basket, and pull it out through the mouth. The duodenoscope is replaced and a new stent inserted. It is wise to note the endoscopic appearances of the papilla before withdrawing the stent, since removal may cause bleeding and an embarrassing difficulty in locating the orifice. Because of occasional problems in recannulating or re-accessing the stricture, methods have been developed for removing (then replacing) stents over a guidewire. Even when a stent is clogged with biliary material, it is usually possible to cannulate it with a wire. It can then be withdrawn through the endoscope using a small snare (Fig. 7.54) or the Soehendra extraction screw (Fig. 7.55).

Stents which have migrated downwards and impacted the duodenal wall can be dislodged with grasping forceps. Those which have migrated upwards into the biliary system are more difficult to extract, since the tip is no longer visible within the duodenum. It is often possible to grasp the tip by fishing with a basket under fluoroscopy, or to pull the stent down again by inflating a retrieval balloon alongside or above it. If these methods fail, it is usually satisfactory to place another stent alongside the old one.

Should stent reinsertion fail, an alternative drainage procedure must be arranged immediately. The risk of life-threatening sepsis is substantial.

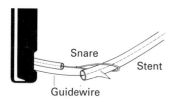

Fig. 7.54 Removing a stent through the scope using a small snare over a guidewire.

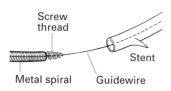

Fig. 7.55 Using the Soehendra 'screw' stent extractor over a guidewire.

Expandable metal stents

The problem of plastic stent clogging has led to the development of devices which expand to a greater diameter *in situ*. Current models are all variants on a metal mesh (Fig. 7.56). Stents are supplied compressed within the tip of a 10 French gauge delivery catheter. When released, the stents expand up to a maximum diameter of 10 mm. Most expandable metal stents shorten significantly during deployment. This field is developing so rapidly, that further details are likely to become obsolete.

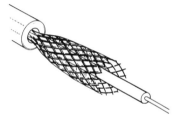

Fig. 7.56 A metal mesh stent expanding as it is released from the compressing sleeve.

Most expandable metal stents are easier to insert than standard plastic stents, since the introducing system is 'continuous'. The device is simply inserted slowly over a guidewire and into the correct position across the stricture. It is probably wise to perform a brief dilatation (with stepped dilators), before committing yourself to stenting. It is also important to control the stent position carefully (under fluoroscopy) during deployment. Full expansion may not occur for 1 or 2 days (Fig. 7.57).

Randomized controlled trials indicate that expandable metal stents remain patent longer than standard plastic stents—but not forever. Stent malfunction is usually due to ingrowth of tumour through the mesh and appears to be more common with larger meshes. Expandable metal stents with plastic covering may overcome this problem, but there is concern that a sleeved stent may occlude duct branches (e.g. cystic ducts, intrahepatic ducts). Expandable metal stents are considerably more expensive and cannot be removed.

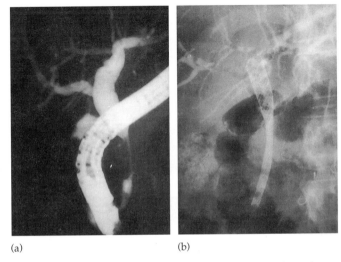

(a)   (b)

Fig. 7.57 (a) A bile duct tumour, and (b) a partially expanded metal stent.

Golden rules for stenting

1 Make sure everyone understands what is being attempted before the procedure, including the patient and GI and radiology assistants.
2 Maintain sterility as much as possible.
3 Do not hurry. This can lead to inadvertent withdrawal of the guidewire or to the development of loops in the duodenum — both of which often mean that the procedure has to be restarted.
4 Make certain that the patient has adequate drainage at the end of the procedure.

Failure of drainage, either initially or after stent occlusion, places the patient at grave risk of serious sepsis. It is essential to use broad coverage parenteral antibiotics and to provide adequate drainage — by further stent insertion, nasobiliary catherization or percutaneous or surgical techniques.

Gallbladder techniques

There are very few indications to approach the gallbladder endoscopically. However, it is technically possible to traverse the cystic duct using floppy hydrophilic wires and to place nasogallbladder drains or stents. Once the guidewire is in place, dilatation and stenting techniques are the same as for bile duct strictures.

Pancreatic techniques

The success of endoscopic biliary treatment has encouraged endoscopists to explore their potential in patients with pancreatic diseases. The techniques are variants of those used in the biliary tree.

Pancreatic sphincterotomy

Pancreatic sphincterotomy is performed with a standard sphincterotome or needle knife. Most experts perform a biliary sphincterotomy first in order to clarify the anatomy. The pancreatic duct is then recannulated and a cut of 5–8 mm is made in the 1 o'clock direction, over a guidewire. Pure cutting current may reduce the risk of pancreatitis. An alternative technique is to place a short (2 cm long) 5 or 7 French gauge stent into the pancreatic duct (after biliary sphincterotomy), and then to use a needle knife to perform the septotomy. There is no clear indication which technique is preferable. If a stent is used, it is removed after 1–4 weeks. The stent/needle-knife technique is preferred when performing a sphincterotomy of the minor papilla (Fig. 7.58).

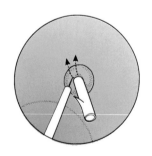

Fig. 7.58 Needle-sphincterotomy of the minor papilla over a stent.

Pancreatic stone extraction

Pancreatic stone extraction can often be achieved using standard baskets and balloon catheters after pancreatic sphincterotomy. Soft and small (less than 5 mm) stones located in the pancreatic head are relatively easy to remove. Other stones may require multiple procedures and adjuvant techniques such as ESWL.

Pancreatic stricture dilatation

Stricturing of the pancreatic orifice or duct can be dilated using a small (4–6 mm diameter) balloon, or graduated stepped dilators, over a guidewire. Hydrophilic wires are particularly useful in the tortuous pancreatic duct. Stents are usually placed after dilatation.

Pancreatic duct stenting

The techniques for placing stents in the pancreatic duct (and minor papilla) are similar to those for biliary applications. Stents selected are usually smaller (7 or 5 French gauge). Most endoscopists remove pancreatic stents after only a few weeks because they can cause duct damage, particularly at the inner tip (Fig. 7.59). To reduce this risk, the stent shape should conform to the duct configuration. Stents which have migrated into the pancreatic duct can be very difficult to remove. For this reason, many stents designed for pancreatic use have an extra external flap or a pigtail.

Nasopancreatic drainage

Nasopancreatic drainage can be provided when necessary, particularly in the short-term management of pancreatic fistulae and after a difficult stone extraction. Commercially available drains have a straight tip with multiple side holes and a curl corresponding to the shape of the duodenum.

Pseudocyst puncture

Pseudocysts adjacent to, and compressing, the wall of the duodenum or stomach can be drained by direct endoscopic puncture (Plate 7.3). Although this can be performed with a standard needle knife, it is wise to use a device which maintains access after the incision (e.g. a needle knife through a sleeve) and the possibility of track coagulation (using a specially designed diathermy puncture set). This is relevant since the major risk of this procedure is serious bleeding from dilated gastric vessels. Endoscopic ultrasound has been used to detect large vessels (and varices) and to confirm the exact cyst relationships.

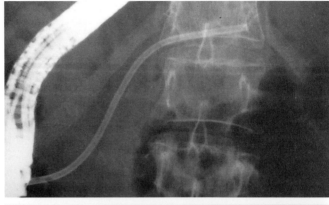

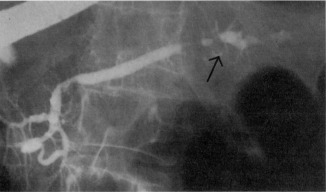

Fig. 7.59 Pancreatic duct damage due to a stent (arrowed).

After puncturing the cyst, a nasocystic drain should be left in place for a few days for aspiration, flushing and subsequent check radiology. In some circumstances, a 10 French gauge (double pigtail) stent is placed through the orifice to maintain patency for a few weeks (Plate 7.4).

Further reading

See further reading list in Chapter 8.

ERCP and Therapy

Risks and Indications

8

The techniques of diagnostic and therapeutic endoscopic retrograde cholangiopancreatography (ERCP) have been described separately in previous chapters. However, it is logical to discuss their application together. There are very few indications for ERCP which may not sometimes lead to a therapeutic manoeuvre. For this reason, we do not support training in diagnostic ERCP alone.

ERCP is perhaps the most rewarding endoscopic procedure performed by gastroenterologists. It is also the most dangerous. Consideration of its role involves careful balancing of its risks and benefits, with full knowledge of the alternative management methods, especially interventional radiology and surgery. Which technique to use is also influenced considerably by the stage of the disease (e.g. the extent of the tumour) and by the general health of the patient. Some general aspects of risks are covered in Chapter 3 and outcome definitions in Chapter 12.

This chapter discusses the place of ERCP in pancreatic and biliary diseases (as viewed in 1996). First, the known risks associated with ERCP procedures are reviewed.

Complications

ERCP carries the same (rare) risks associated with all endoscopic procedures, including medication reactions, cardiopulmonary accidents and intestinal perforation. Risk factors for some of these complications and patient safety aspects related to prevention are detailed in Chapter 3. Attempted duct cannulation can cause pancreatitis and sepsis. Therapeutic procedures add additional risks, especially retroduodenal perforation, bleeding, stone impaction and stent dysfunction.

The incidence of complications depends on many factors, including the definitions which are used (see Chapter 3). Many patients have some discomfort after pancreatography and the serum amylase is usually raised; what constitutes pancreatitis? Equally, some oozing of blood is not unusual after sphincterotomy; when is it called 'bleeding'? Consensus definitions and stratification for severity have been published (Table 8.1).

Many older series of sphincterotomy reported complication rates of approximately 10%, with 1% fatality rates. Recent publications indicate a lower overall complication rate of about 5%, of which 3% are mild, 1% moderate and 1% severe. In expert hands,

	Mild	**Moderate**	**Severe**
Bleeding	Clinical (i.e. not just endoscopic) evidence of bleeding Haemoglobin drop < 3 g, and no need for transfusion	Transfusion (4 units or less), no angiographic intervention or surgery	Transfusion 5 units or more, or intervention (angiographic or surgical)
Perforation	Possible, or only very slight leak of fluid or contrast, treatable by fluids and suction for 3 days or less	Any definite perforation treated medically for 4–10 days	Medical treatment for more than 10 days, or intervention (percutaneous or surgical)
Pancreatitis	Clinical pancreatitis, amylase at least three times normal at more than 24 h after the procedure, requiring admission or prolongation of planned admission to 2–3 days	Pancreatitis requiring hospitalization of 4–10 days	Hospitalization for more than 10 days, or haemorrhagic pancreatitis, phlegmon, or pseudocyst, or intervention (percutaneous drainage or surgery)
Infection (cholangitis)	> 38°C for 24–48 h	Febrile or septic illness requiring more than 3 days of hospital treatment or endoscopic or percutaneous intervention	Septic shock or surgery
Basket impaction	Basket released spontaneously or by repeat endoscopy	Percutaneous intervention	Surgery

Any intensive care unit admission after a procedure grades the complication as severe. Other rarer complications can be graded by length of needed hospitalization.

Table 8.1 Grading system for the major complications of ERCP and endoscopic sphincterotomy.

the very rare deaths occur only in patients with severe co-morbidities (e.g. patients already septic and in intensive care). There has been particular concern about the risks in younger patients and in those with smaller ducts. Data concerning sphincterotomies (for stones only) were collected prospectively from seven centres in the USA recently (Table 8.2). The results are somewhat reassuring. Contrary to some opinions (and one paper related mainly to sphincter of Oddi dysfunction), sphincterotomy did not appear to be more dangerous in small ducts; short-term complications in younger patients were rare (Table 8.2).

Pancreatitis

Pancreatitis is the commonest complication of diagnostic and therapeutic ERCP procedures. Using the agreed definitions, the

	All patients (%)	Patients < 60 years with ducts < 9 mm
Total no. patients	**1921**	**238**
Complications	112 (5.8)	10 (4.2)
Mild	70 (3.6)	7 (2.9)
Moderate	26 (1.3)	2 (0.8)
Severe	12 (0.6)	1 (0.4)
Fatal	4 (0.2)	0 (0)

Table 8.2 Complications of sphincterotomy for stone; prospective study of seven centres in the USA, 1994.

incidence is around 3% in most series. Most attacks are mild, settling within a few days with conservative management, but life-threatening complications can develop and deaths have resulted. Pancreatitis can occur even without pancreatography, but it is clear that the incidence increases with repeated injections of contrast. The risk is definitely increased in the context of sphincter dysfunction, is slightly higher in patients with a prior diagnosis of pancreatitis, and is lower when Santorini's duct is patent. Surprisingly, one study showed that the risk was not significantly higher in patients who had already experienced an attack of ERCP-induced pancreatitis. Randomized studies have shown no prophylactic benefit from non-ionic contrast agents or various prophylactic medications (e.g. Glucagon, somatostatin).

Sepsis (cholangitis and septicaemia)

Sepsis can result from cholangiography in the presence of infected bile. The risk can be minimized by avoiding excessive bile duct pressure (exchanging bile for contrast) and by prior use of antibiotics. However, the most important factor is relief of obstruction by removing stones or providing nasobiliary or stent drainage. When these fail, percutaneous or surgical intervention may be necessary as a matter of urgency.

Serious sepsis (due to *Pseudomonas* and *Serratia*) has resulted from contaminated endoscopes and accessories (such as the water bottle). Any such incident should result in an immediate review of disinfection procedures. Nosocomial sepsis is more common in the presence of duct strictures or pseudocysts, but deaths have occurred after a normal-appearing ERCP. The risk of performing ERCP in the presence of a pseudocyst has been overstated; ERCP is indicated (with proper disinfection regimens) when information about the ductal systems will affect management decisions.

Retroduodenal perforation

Retroduodenal perforation is reported in less than 1% of endoscopic sphincterotomies. It may be recognized immediately by the unusual endoscopic and radiographic appearances; the earliest sign is a diffuse leak of contrast behind the duodenum (Fig. 8.1). Further manipulation will drive air into the retroduodenal space, which may be recognized immediately on fluoroscopy or subsequently on plain radiology.

The risk of perforation is presumably greater with longer incisions. Patients with 'papillary stenosis' are at higher risk, but the assumption that small ducts are more dangerous has not been substantiated recently. Some series show that needle-knife pre-cut sphincterotomy carries an increased risk.

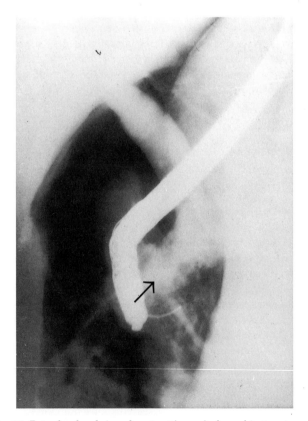

Fig. 8.1 Retroduodenal air and contrast (arrow) after sphincterectomy perforation.

Perforation should be considered in any patient who develops abdominal pain within hours of sphincterotomy although pancreatitis is far more common. A relatively normal serum amylase level in the presence of patient distress is an added pointer. If a plain abdominal film shows no air, computed tomography (CT) scanning is a very sensitive method for detecting perforation.

The management of perforation calls for early detection and a measured therapeutic approach in collaboration with a surgical colleague. Immediate operation is rarely indicated and most retroduodenal perforations after sphincterotomy have been managed conservatively. If the patient still has a problem of biliary obstruction when the perforation is recognized (e.g. with stones in the duct and gallbladder), it may be logical to proceed directly to surgery to clear the duct, place a T-tube and drain the retroperitoneal space. When there is no residual biliary disease or obstruction, most patients have been treated successfully using gastric suction, 'nil-by-mouth' and antibiotics. Some experts suggest adding nasobiliary drainage, but this is not of proven benefit. The patient's progress should be monitored carefully by the endoscopist and surgical colleague at least once a day. Conservative management should be continued only so long as the patient appears to be responding. A gastrografin swallow showing no continuing leak may be reassuring. Patients who develop a retroperitoneal abscess will require percutaneous or surgical drainage.

Bleeding

Bleeding after sphincterotomy sufficient to require blood transfusion is now very rare—possibly because smaller sphincterotomies are made and/or because of the increased use of coagulation/blended current. Bleeding most often results from cutting too quickly (the 'zipper'). The incision should be made slowly with adequate coagulation of the margins. Most bleeding stops spontaneously. A small ooze can be controlled by flushing adrenaline (epinephrine), at a dilution of 1:100000 over the sphincterotomy site. If bleeding continues, we inject adrenaline (epinephrine), at a dilution of 1:10000 into the sides of the raw sphincterotomy using a standard sclerotherapy needle. Alternatively, a stone-retrieval balloon is inflated in the bile duct above the sphincterotomy, and then pulled down firmly to tamponade the bleeding site against the face of the endoscope.

Bleeding sufficient to obscure the view within 1–2 min is unlikely to stop spontaneously. Skilled angiographic embolization is usually effective. Unfortunately, bleeding may recur after surgical oversewing alone; the use of non-absorbable sutures and ligation of the major feeding vessel have been recommended.

Stone impaction

Stone impaction can nowadays be avoided by the use of lithotripsy sleeves and baskets (see Chapter 7). If a stone and basket do become impacted and cannot be removed by standard means, it may be permissible to observe the patient overnight; spontaneous disimpaction has sometimes occurred.

Stent dysfunction

Stent dysfunction occurs when stents migrate (up or down) or become blocked with biliary debris. Patients present with obstructive cholangitis. Details are provided in Chapter 7.

Delayed complications

Most complications of diagnostic and therapeutic ERCP are obvious within 12 h, but there are potential delayed problems, about which patients and their physicians should be advised. These include late bleeding, gallstone ileus (after removing very large stones), cholangitis (if stones have been left in place) and acute cholecystitis in patients with gallbladders.

Follow-up studies at 5–15 years after sphincterotomy demonstrate that 15–25% of patients develop late biliary problems — usually new stones, with or without sphincterotomy stenosis. Most of these cases have been managed endoscopically. Gallbladder symptoms sufficient to warrant cholecystectomy occur in about 20% of patients in whom the gallbladder is left in place for follow-up periods of 5–10 years.

Alternatives

The first ERCP treatments (such as sphincterotomy for stones) were developed at a time when surgical intervention was hazardous. Improvements in anaesthesia and perioperative care (as well as the laparoscopic revolution) have reduced the risks considerably. Similarly, interventional radiology techniques have developed markedly over the last two decades. Although transhepatic puncture remains uncomfortable and potentially hazardous, the use of smaller catheters and expandable metal stents has reduced this negative aspect of percutaneous biliary work. Application of ERCP is also affected by developments in noninvasive imaging. Magnetic resonance cholangiopancreatography (MRCP) can provide excellent images (Fig. 8.2). Its impact on reducing (or even increasing) the use of ERCP has yet to be determined.

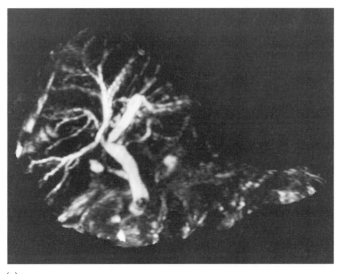

(a)

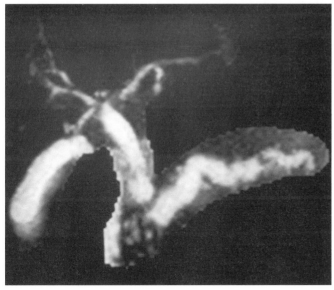

(b)

Fig. 8.2 Magnetic resonance cholangiography and pancreatography.
(a) Dilated bile duct (post-cholecystectomy) showing a distal stone
above a stricture—previously failed ERCP. (b) Small tumour in
pancreatic head causing double duct dilation.

Influence of disease stage and co-morbidities

Our management approach to biliary and pancreatic problems is greatly influenced by the stage of disease and the general condition of our patients. There are many patients in whom anaesthesia and surgery are hazardous (e.g. severe sepsis, recent myocardial infarction, extensive malignancy). There are scales which can be used to measure co-morbidities, e.g. the American Society of Anesthesiology (ASA) grades. These are rather crude and more sensitive measures are needed. There are also specific risk factors for different therapeutic approaches; for example, percutaneous transhepatic procedures are more hazardous in patients with coagulopathy.

The role of ERCP techniques will be discussed in broad clinical contexts.

Clinical role of ERCP and therapy

Jaundice and malignancy

The patient presenting with jaundice is at the intersection of many disciplines, and a plethora of tests and treatments are available. This is a prototype challenge to multidisciplinary collaboration and the development of cost-effective care and algorithms.

Patients with jaundice used to be classified as 'medical' or 'surgical'. The latter category is now better called 'obstructive' since most obstructions are not treated surgically. Making the distinction between hepatocellular and obstructive jaundice is the crucial first task, which can usually be achieved early with percutaneous ultrasound scanning. This is usually (and reasonably) the first-line imaging test. However, as usually performed, CT scanning gives more information, particularly concerning surrounding organs (e.g. liver metastases). Bile duct dilatation may not be detected at an early stage in some patients with obstruction, especially when this occurs at the liver hilum, or in rarer conditions such as sclerosing cholangitis. A negative scan therefore does not rule out an obstructive aetiology. This can only be done by invasive cholangiography at the present time, although magnetic resonance cholangiography is making astonishing progress.

Cholangiography can be obtained in the jaundiced patient by ERCP or by percutaneous transhepatic cholangiography (PTC). Where both of these techniques are available, ERCP is usually preferred. It provides more diagnostic information (including a view of the papilla and pancreas as well as the bile duct) and has a broader therapeutic spectrum, e.g. in the management of stones and tumours. Certainly, the patient suspected of having obstructive jaundice due to stones (on clinical and ultrasound evidence) should go straight to ERCP for definitive diagnosis and management.

When the clinical situation and initial scans strongly suggest malignant obstruction, other considerations come into play, especially the potential for surgical cure. This depends on two important but separate factors — the extent of the tumour and the health of the patient. Surgery (and perioperative care) have made remarkable strides, but it is still not logical to consider a major resection (e.g. a Whipple procedure) in an elderly patient with severe co-morbid disease. If the patient is not an operative candidate on health grounds alone, there is no need to spend time and money on investigating the second important question — whether or not the lesion is potentially resectable. In general, this depends on whether the tumour is still localized or whether it has spread locally or metastasized.

Numerous techniques are now available to help in the staging process and it is not difficult to consume a great deal of time (and money) in staging a tumour.

Staging

Staging is unnecessary in patients who are not fit for surgery. It is also less important in young and fit patients in whom a trial of surgery may be the correct approach. However, staging is crucial in the middle-ground patients who are acceptable, but not good, operative candidates. Surgery is appropriate in elderly patients when the tumour is certainly localized (e.g. in' the papilla of Vater), but not when there is good radiological evidence of local vessel involvement. Here there are more tools than maps. Techniques available include ultrasound scanning with Doppler, CT, magnetic resonance imaging, endoscopic ultrasonography and laparoscopy. CT is the simplest and most readily available way of detecting major tumour spread. Endoscopic ultrasound appears to be the most sensitive staging tool in expert hands.

The decision whether or not to operate depends on integrating data on health status and tumour staging. Some patients may require surgery because of duodenal obstruction.

Preoperative stenting

The value of preoperative drainage has been debated vigorously. With careful selection of patients (and earlier operations), the risks of attempted resection are now so low that it would be difficult to prove that preoperative endoscopic stenting provides any benefit. However, when ERCP is performed in a patient with malignant biliary obstruction, it seems reasonable to place a stent even if resection may be attempted later. This eliminates the risk of obstructive cholangitis and starts the treatment should the patient prove not to be a surgical candidate. The argument that preoperative stenting makes the surgery more difficult does not seem to be universally accepted by surgical experts.

Tissue diagnosis

When the decision has been made *not* to operate on a patient with presumed malignancy, there is a strong obligation to prove the diagnosis. Occasionally, localized inflammation, islet cell tumours and lymphoma can mimic malignancy on imaging studies. If ERCP is part of the treatment protocol, the diagnosis can usually be confirmed by taking brush biopsy or needle samples up the bile or pancreatic duct. Tissue can also be obtained by fine-needle aspiration cytology under ultrasound or CT guidance. However, many surgeons planning to operate on a patient with malignant obstructive jaundice do not now advocate preoperative percutaneous tissue confirmation. A negative result will not change the approach, and there is some concern about tumour seeding.

Palliation

Approximately only 20% of patients with malignant obstructive jaundice are nowadays operated on (at least at specialist centres). Half of these will undergo resection, the others some form of palliative bypass. This leaves 80% of the patients to be managed by non-operative methods. For low lesions, stenting at ERCP is the preferred method, using standard polyethylene stents. The role of expandable metal stents is not yet fully established. Although they stay patent longer than plastic stents, the additional duration may not be worth the cost (depending on the patient prognosis). This situation is more difficult in patients with tumours obstructing the liver hilum. More than one stent may be needed and the results may be better by the percutaneous transhepatic route (Fig. 8.3). A randomized trial is in progress.

Surgical bypass remains a legitimate palliative technique, and is certainly appropriate when there is any evidence of duodenal obstruction. A recent randomized trial confirmed that endoscopic stenting was safer and cheaper than surgical intervention, although more patients needed to return after a few months because of recurrent jaundice (due to stent clogging). Laparoscopic bypass of the biliary tree is a potential new player. Laparoscopic anastomosis of the gallbladder to jejunum is technically simple, but indications are few, since most tumours involve the cystic duct. Laparoscopic choledochojejunostomy may become technically viable.

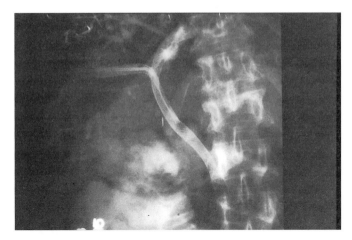

Fig. 8.3 A hilar tumour with bilateral metal stents placed percutaneously.

Laparoscopic cholecystectomy

The rapid and widespread acceptance of laparoscopic cholecystectomy has had a major impact on the practice of ERCP. The indications for ERCP *after* cholecystectomy remain unchanged; the controversy concerns its use *beforehand*. The problem is that most laparoscopic surgeons cannot perform laparoscopic duct exploration. There was a tendency in the early phase for surgeons to request ERCP before operation in most cases, to rule out (or treat) duct stones and also to define aberrant biliary anatomy. This widespread use of ERCP before laparoscopic cholecystectomy is clearly unjustified since the vast majority of examinations are negative; its risks and costs outweigh the benefits.

Most authorities argue for a selective approach, using ERCP before laparoscopic cholecystectomy only when there is a significant suspicion of duct pathology. The problem is to define the level of suspicion. Patients with jaundice and acute biliary sepsis are obvious candidates. Other predictors (abnormal liver tests, dilated ducts and a history of biliary-type pain) have been analysed and it is now possible to allocate a probability score for the presence or absence of a duct stone for most patients. By this means we separate them into three categories: a high-risk group (patients very likely to have duct stones on the basis of jaundice or multiple predictive factors), a low-risk group with no predictive factors (in which unexpected stones are found in less than 3% of cases) and a difficult intermediate-risk group with some suspicion. Here the approach will depend upon the relative expertise with laparoscopy and endoscopy. Paradoxically, ERCP is less necessary before laparoscopy when expertise is high; the endoscopist can (almost) guarantee to clear the duct afterwards if necessary. Surgeons working with less expert endoscopists may tend to 'give it a try' beforehand more often, leaving themselves the option of open duct exploration when necessary.

It is clear that a close collaborative understanding between laparoscopists and ERCP endoscopists is essential in order to provide patients with optimal cost-effective care. It is also obvious that one-stage laparoscopic treatment is preferable, once the techniques have been perfected and disseminated.

A few centres have used ERCP-sphincterotomy actually during laparoscopic cholecystectomy. This is difficult to arrange and to perform, and has not become popular.

Acute biliary sepsis

Spontaneous acute cholangitis is almost always due to a bile duct stone impacted in the papilla (rarely in the cystic duct—the Mirizzi syndrome). Decompression should be performed urgently in patients who do not improve rapidly after a few hours of conservative treatment. Several studies have now indicated that urgent ERCP is the safest drainage method, particularly in patients with suppurative cholangitis. Emergency ERCP can be performed in an intensive care unit where necessary, using only C-arm fluoroscopy. Sphincterotomy and stone extraction is the ideal; however, unstable patients may be managed temporarily with a nasobiliary drain or stent. Percutaneous and/or surgical drainage must be considered if endoscopic management fails. Cholangitis resulting from ERCP intervention (impacted stone or stent dysfunction) requires intervention of equal urgency.

Acute cholecystitis has been managed endoscopically (by placing a stent through the cystic duct). The role of this approach is not yet established. Most patients will be treated surgically, or with temporary percutaneous drainage if seriously unfit.

Problems after biliary surgery

Patients who present after cholecystectomy with pain, fever or abnormalities of liver function tests should undergo ERCP to clarify the situation. Stones can be removed by standard endoscopic techniques in up to 95% of cases. Early postoperative pain may be due to leakage from the cystic duct stump; this has become more common with the widespread use of laparoscopic cholecystectomy. Leakage may be recognized by isotope scanning, and a bile collection documented by ultrasound or CT; percutaneous drainage may be necessary. Cystic duct leaks are best treated by removing any distal obstruction (e.g. stone). However, leakage may persist in the absence of obstruction and can be relieved by removing normal sphincter activity. Although this can be done by sphincterotomy, we prefer to place a short, straight 7 French gauge stent across the sphincter. This is removed as an out-patient procedure after a few weeks. Nasobiliary drainage (with suction) is also effective but may need to remain in place for several days.

Laparoscopic cholecystectomy has also led to an increased incidence of bile duct injuries. Complete transection of the common bile duct or a major branch requires expert surgery. Injuries to the main duct which remain in continuity can be managed by endoscopic stenting, after balloon dilatation of any stricture. The stent is removed after 3–4 months, the stricture is dilated again and *two* stents are then placed if possible. All stents are removed at 8–12 months and the patient is observed carefully. With lesions below the hilum of the liver, the relapse rate appears to be less than 20%. It is important to emphasize that expert surgery provides good treatment for this injury, and that attempts at endoscopic management should not be unnecessarily prolonged; costs and risks multiply. Patients should have the benefit of surgical consultation before a course of endoscopic management is initiated.

Sphincter of Oddi dysfunction

Patients who present with biliary-type pain some months or years after cholecystectomy are often suspected to have papillary stenosis or sphincter of Oddi dysfunction (once stones and other local diseases have been excluded). If sphincter dysfunction exists, sphincterotomy should provide good treatment, but the complication rate is significantly higher than when performed for stones. Thus, it is crucial to select patients carefully — which is the crux of the problem. Most experts pay attention to objective evidence of duct pathology, e.g. abnormal liver function tests in attacks, a dilating bile duct (ducts do not get bigger just because of cholecystectomy unless there is obstruction) or substantially delayed drainage. Endoscopic sphincter manometry is used by many as a gold standard but it is not universally accepted (or practised) — partly because it is difficult for both doctors and patients. Better predictive discriminants are required. Unfortunately, non-invasive imaging studies (e.g. nuclear medicine scans) have not yet proved to be sufficiently sensitive and specific. Temporary stenting is not a good therapeutic trial method; the pancreatitis rate is substantial.

Problems after liver transplantation

Biliary complications occur in up to 25% of patients after orthotopic liver transplantation. Strictures and leaks can be managed by endoscopic balloon dilatation and stenting, which may have to be continued for many months since healing is slow. Stones can develop above anastomotic strictures in this context.

Sclerosing cholangitis

Some strictures are tortuous and very tight, making guidewire passage difficult. Once the guidewire has been placed, it is usually relatively simple to dilate dominant extrahepatic strictures with stepped dilators and balloons. Every effort should be made to reduce the risk of introducing infection. For this reason, we do not routinely perform a sphincterotomy, and use stents sparingly and only for a few weeks. The long-term value of endoscopic manipulation is speculative; however, patients with dominant strictures presenting with recurrent attacks of acute cholangitis can derive useful short-term benefit. Many of these patients have small pigment stones which impact in the strictures.

Biliary obstruction in chronic pancreatitis

Patients with acute biliary obstruction in the context of active pancreatitis (with or without a pseudocyst in the head of the pancreas) can be managed effectively by temporary biliary stenting. Established biliary strictures in end-stage calcific pancreatitis should not be managed endoscopically since the problem will always recur. Surgery should be performed wherever possible.

Endoscopy and pancreatitis

Any patient with pancreatitis whose cause cannot be determined by simpler methods should undergo ERCP to detect or exclude abnormalities of the papilla and ductal systems. Causes include papillary tumours and sphincter dysfunction, congenital anomalies (such as choledochal cysts and pancreas divisum) and gallstones. Examination is traditionally delayed for a few weeks after an acute attack, but the risk of exacerbation appears minimal, even when performed earlier. Indeed some enthusiasts recommend urgent ERCP in all patients with acute pancreatitis, whatever the suspected cause. Most restrict themselves to patients with suspected gallstone pancreatitis.

Gallstone pancreatitis

Many reports indicate that ERCP and sphincterotomy can be performed in the acute phase of gallstone pancreatitis with remarkable safety, and that it is usually easy to remove small impacted stones with impressive clinical recovery. The problem in defining the role for urgent endoscopy is that most patients settle spontaneously within 48h; they are well managed by standard conservative measures, usually leading to elective cholecystectomy. Randomized studies indicate that urgent

ERCP-sphincterotomy is preferable to a standard conservative and surgical approach, at least in patients who had admission characteristics predicting a severe outcome. A reasonable approach is to recommend the ERCP-sphincterotomy if the patient is not improving after 24–48 h, and especially if there is evidence of increasing biliary obstruction and sepsis.

Standard techniques are employed and pancreatography should be performed if no stone is found within the bile duct; occasionally, gallstones migrate into the pancreatic duct.

Pancreatic duct sphincterotomy for stones and stenosis

Solitary stones in the main duct in the pancreatic head can be removed endoscopically with baskets and balloon catheters after pancreatic orifice sphincterotomy; extracorporeal lithotripsy may also be required. Extracting stones appears to be worthwhile in patients suffering from acute attacks of pancreatitis (or pancreatic pain) with spontaneous symptom-free intervals, particularly if the initiating cause (e.g. alcohol) has been removed. Further long-term studies are required. Sphincterotomy is also sometimes performed in patients with idiopathic recurrent pancreatitis judged to be due to sphincter stenosis or dysfunction—but this entity is difficult to define and the results hard to evaluate.

Pancreatic duct strictures

The clinical value of dilatation/stenting of the pancreatic duct (or orifice) has not been established. Currently, experts treat patients suffering from acute recurrent attacks of pancreatitis when there is some evidence of duct obstruction; stents should be left in place only for a few weeks because of the risk of inducing ductal abnormalities. Further research is necessary to establish which (if any) patients obtain long-term benefit.

Pseudocysts and leaks

ERCP may be useful in patients with pseudocysts to define the integrity of the duct system and to show whether or not the cyst is communicating. The risk of introducing infection is minimal if properly disinfected equipment (and antibiotics) are used. If the pseudocyst communicates with an intact duct system, the endoscopist may consider placing a nasopancreatic drain (on continuous low-pressure suction), with subsequent temporary stenting once the cyst has collapsed. Pseudocysts adjacent to, and compressing, the wall of the duodenum or stomach can be managed by direct endoscopic cyst puncture. This method should not be employed unless it is clear that the cyst and gastric or duodenal wall are in intimate contact, as judged by CT scanning or endoscopic ultrasound. Short-term results appear good in selected cases, but there is significant risk of haemorrhage; these techniques should be used only by experts.

Spontaneous pancreatic fistulae and postoperative leaks can be managed by temporary duct decompression (nasopancreatic drain or stent). The analogy with the cystic duct leak is close, and the results appear almost as good. Attempts are being made to close leaks mechanically at ERCP.

Pancreas divisum

The clinical relevance of the congenital anomaly pancreas divisum remains a subject of controversy. The hypothesis that pancreas divisum can result in obstructive pancreatic pain and pancreatitis rests on the assumption that the accessory papilla orifice may be insufficient to allow the full flow of pancreatic juice. This belief has led many endoscopists to attempt treatment by improving drainage at the accessory papilla. Initial attempts at accessory sphincterotomy resulted in an unacceptably high rate of re-stenosis. Currently, selected patients with recurrent acute pancreatitis are being managed by accessory stenting, with or without needle-knife sphincterotomy. The stent is usually removed within a few weeks. Short-term results appear good but long-term efficacy remains to be established.

Obscure abdominal pain

The diagnostic yield of ERCP is small in patients with no abnormalities of abdominal imaging, liver function tests or amylase. Chronic pancreatitis can be detected by duct abnormalities when other tests are negative, but the interpretation of minor abnormalities of the branches remains controversial. It is unusual to detect pancreatic cancer in the presence of a normal CT scan (or good-quality ultrasound study). Even if such scans do not detect the mass lesion itself, they usually show pancreatic duct dilatation upstream, indicating the presence of a lesion. ERCP is of limited value in investigating patients with *known* pancreatic mass lesions, since the duct appearances (obstruction or stricture) may be similar in patients with benign and malignant disease. ERCP may detect pancreas divisum or other rare anomalies which can have clinical significance. ERCP occasionally shows gallbladder stones which had previously escaped detection and the procedure allows sampling of bile for crystals or more sophisticated biochemical analyses.

ERCP in children

The spectrum of problems encountered in children (especially small children and neonates) is different from that seen in adults, but the principles of diagnostic and therapeutic intervention are the same. Congenital anomalies of the biliary tree and pancreas are seen rather frequently; surprisingly, gallstones are not unusual. Several sphincterotomies have been reported in children under the age of 1 year.

Multidisciplinary team work

It is clear from the above brief review that the management of patients with pancreatic and biliary problems continues to evolve and requires a collaborative multidisciplinary approach. Specialist gastroenterologists and surgeons must work together, and in close association with imaging and interventional radiologists, pathologists, oncologists, etc. The extent of this collaboration will determine the quality and efficiency of patient care, and will provide an environment for the objective research which is required.

Further reading

Techniques and general reviews

American Society for Gastrointestinal Endoscopy. *Radiographic Contrast Media used in ERCP*. Technology Assessment Status Evaluation. Manchester: American Society for Gastrointestinal Endoscopy, 1995.

Baillie J. *Pancreatography*. Gastrointestinal Endoscopy Clinics of North America, Vol. 5(1) (series ed. Sivak MV). Philadelphia: WB Saunders, 1995.

Berci G. *Laparoscopic Cholecystectomy and Surgical Endoscopy*. Gastrointestinal Endoscopy Clinics of North America, Vol. 3(2) (series ed. Sivak MV). Philadelphia: WB Saunders, 1993.

Cotton PB. Precut papillotomy—a risky technique for experts only. *Gastrointest Endosc* 1989;**35**:578–9.

Hogan WJ, ed. *Sphincter of Oddi Prime for the Pancreatico-biliary Endoscopist*. Gastrointestinal Endoscopy Clinics of North America, Vol. 3(1) (series ed. Sivak MV). Philadelphia: WB Saunders, 1993.

Kozarek RA, ed. *Endoscopic Approach to Biliary Stones*. Gastrointestinal Clinics of North America, Vol. 1(1) (series ed. Sivak M). Philadelphia: WB Saunders, 1991.

Lambert ME, Betts CD, Hill J *et al.* Endoscopic sphincterotomy: the whole truth. *Br J Surg* 1991;**78**:473–6.

Leung JWC, Cotton PB. Endoscopic nasobiliary catheter drainage in biliary and pancreatic disease. *Am J Gastroenterol* 1991;**86**:389–94.

Lygidakis NJ, Tytgat GNJ. *Hepatobiliary and Pancreatic Malignancies*. Thieme, 1989.

May GR, Cotton PB, Edmunds SE *et al.* Removal of stones from the bile duct at ERCP without sphincterotomy. *Gastrointest Endosc* 1993;**39**:749–54.

Parsons WG, Howell DA. Progress in tissue sampling at ERCP. In: Cotton PB, Tytgat GNJ, Williams CB, eds. *Annual of Gastrointestinal Endoscopy*. London: Current Science, 1995:9–20.

Pott G, Schrameyer B. *ERCP Atlas*. Toronto: Decker, 1989.

Silvis SE, Rohrmann CA, Ansel HJ. *Text and Atlas of ERCP*. New York: Igaku-Shoin, 1995.

Sivak MV. *Gastroenterologic Endoscopy*. Philadelphia: WB Saunders, 1987.

Vaira D, Ainley C, Williams S. Endoscopic sphincterotomy in 1000 consecutive patients. *Lancet* 1989;**2**:431–3.

Stones

Baillie J, Cairns SR, Cotton PB. Endoscopic management of choledocholithiasis during pregnancy. *Surg Gynecol Obstet* 1990;**171**:1–4.

Cotton PB. Endoscopic management of bile duct stones (apples and oranges). *Gut* 1984;**25**:587–97.

Cotton PB. Retained bile duct stones: T-tube in place, percutaneous or endoscopic management? *Am J Gastroenterol* 1990;**85**:1075–8.

Cotton PB. Difficult bile duct stones. In: Kozarek RA, ed. *Endoscopic Approach to Biliary Stones*. Gastrointestinal Endoscopy Clinics of North America, Vol. 1(1) (series ed. Sivak MV). Philadelphia: WB Saunders, 1991:51–63.

Cotton PB, Chung SC, Davis WZ *et al.* Issues in cholecystectomy and management of duct stones. *Am J Gastroenterol* 1994;**89**:S169–76.

Cotton PB, Kozarek RA, Schapiro RH *et al.* Endoscopic laser lithotripsy of large bile duct stones. *Gastroenterology* 1990;**99**:1128–33.

Fan S-T, Lai ECS, Mok FPT *et al.* Early treatment of acute biliary pancreatitis by endoscopic papillotomy. *N Engl J Med* 1993;**328**:228–32.

Hawes RH, Cotton PB, Vallon AG. Follow-up at 6–11 years after duodenoscopic sphincterotomy for stones in patients with prior cholecystectomy. *Gastroenterology* 1990;**98**:1008–12.

Lai ECS, Mok FPT, Tan ESY *et al.* Endoscopic biliary drainage for severe acute cholangitis. *N Engl J Med* 1992;**326**:1582–6.

Neuhaus H, Hoffman NW, Gottlieb K *et al.* Endoscopic lithotripsy of bile duct stones using a new laser with automatic stone recognition. *Gastrointest Endosc* 1994;**40**:708–15.

Strasberg SM, Clavien P-A. Cholecystolithiasis: lithotherapy for the 1990s. *Hepatology* 1992;**16**:820–39.

Benign biliary strictures

Benhamou Y, Caumes E, Gerosa Y *et al.* AIDS-related cholangiopathy. Critical analysis of a prospective series of 26 patients. *Dig Dis Sci* 1993;**38**:1113–18.

Davids PHP, Rauws EAJ, Coene PPLO, Tytgat GNJ, Huibregtse K. Endsocopic stenting for post-operative biliary strictures. *Gastrointest Endosc* 1992;**38**:12–18.

Kozarek RA, Ball TJ, Patterson DJ *et al.* Endoscopic treatment of biliary injury in the era of laparoscopic cholecystectomy. *Gastrointest Endosc* 1994;**40**:10–16.

Lee JG, Schutz SM, England RE, Leung JW, Cotton PB. Endoscopic therapy of sclerosing cholangitis. *Hepatology* 1995;**21**(3):661–7.

Liguory C, Vitale GC, Lefebre JF, Bonnel D, Cornud F. Endoscopic treatment of postoperative biliary fistulae. *Surgery* 1991;**110**:779–84.

Pitt HA, Kaufman SL, Coleman J *et al.* Benign postoperative biliary strictures. Operate or dilate? *Ann Surg* 1989;**210**:417–27.

Qoquo PC, Lewis WD, Stokes K *et al.* A comparison of operation, endoscopic retrograde cholangiopancreatography, and percutaneous transhepatic cholangiography and biliary complications after hepatic transplantation. *J Am Coll Surg* 1994;**179**:177–81.

Vallera RA, Cotton PB, Clavien P-A. Biliary reconstruction for liver transplantation and management of biliary complications. *Liver Transplant Surgery* 1995;**1**(3):143–52.

Malignancy

Ballinger AB, McHugh M, Catnach SM *et al*. Symptom relief and quality of life after stenting for malignant bile duct obstruction. *Gut* 1994;**35**:467–70.

Bismuth H, Castaing D, Traynor O. Resection or palliation: priority of surgery in the treatment of hilar cancer. *World J Surg* 1988;**12**:39–47.

Cotton PB. Management of malignant bile duct obstruction. *J Gastroenterol Hepatol* 1990;Suppl. 1:63–77.

Cotton PB, Schmitt C. Quality of life in palliative management of malignant obstructive jaundice. *Scand J Gastroenterol* 1993;**28**(Suppl. 199): 44–6.

Lai ECS, Mok FPT, Fan ST *et al*. Preoperative endoscopic drainage from malignant obstructive jaundice. *Br J Surg* 1994;**81**:1195–8.

Polydorou AA, Chisolm EM, Romanos AA *et al*. A comparison of right versus left hepatic duct endoprosthesis insertion in malignant hilar biliary obstruction. *Endoscopy* 1989;**21**:266–71.

Smith AC, Dowsett JF, Russell RCG, Hatfield ARW, Cotton PB. Randomised trial of endoscopic stenting versus surgical bypass in malignant low bile duct obstruction. *Lancet* 1994;**344**:1655–60.

Speer AG, Russell RCG, Hatfield ARW *et al*. Randomized trial of endoscopic versus percutaneous stent insertion in malignant obstructive jaundice. *Lancet* 1987;**2**:57–62.

Pancreatic therapy

American Society for Gastrointestinal Endoscopy Technology Assessment. Endoscopic pancreatitis therapy. *Gastrointest Endosc* 1993; **39**:881–4.

Coleman SD, Eisen GM, Troughton AB, Cotton PB. Endoscopic treatment in pancreas divisum. *Am J Gastroenterol* 1994;**89**:1152–5.

Cotton PB. Pancreas divisum—curiosity or culprit? *Gastroenterology* 1985;**89**:1431–5.

Cremer M, Deviere J, Delhaye M, Baize M, Vandermeeren A. Stenting in severe chronic pancreatitis: results of medium-term follow-up in seventy-six patients. *Endoscopy* 1991;**23**:171–6.

Delhaye M, Vandermeeren A, Baize M, Cremer M. Extracorporeal shockwave lithotripsy of pancreatic calculi. *Gastroenterology* 1992; **102**:610–20.

Eisen G, Chutz S, Metzler D *et al*. Santorinicele: new evidence for obstruction in pancreas divisum. *Gastrointest Endosc* 1994;**40**: 73–6.

Guelrud M, Mujica C, Jaen D *et al*. The role of ERCP in the diagnosis and treatment of idiopathic recurrent pancreatitis in children and adolescents. *Gastrointest Endosc* 1994;**40**:428–36.

Kozarek RA, Ball TJ, Patterson DJ *et al*. Endoscopic pancreatic duct sphincterotomy: indications, technique, and analysis of results. *Gastrointest Endosc* 1994;**40**:592–7.

Lans JI, Geenen JE, Johanson JF *et al*. Endoscopic therapy in patients with pancreas divisum and acute pancreatitis: a prospective, randomized, controlled clinical trial. *Gastrointest Endosc* 1992;**38**:430–4.

Sphincter dysfunction

Gilbert DA, DiMarino AJ, Jensen DM *et al.* Status evaluation: sphincter of Oddi manometry. *Gastrointest Endosc* 1992;**38**:757–9.

Guelrud M, Mendoza S, Rossiter G *et al.* Sphincter of Oddi manometry in healthy volunteers. *Dig Dis Sci* 1990;**35**:38–46.

Sherman S, Lehman GA. Opioids and sphincter of Oddi. *Gastrointest Endosc* 1994;**40**:105–6.

Complications and outcomes

Asbun HJ, Rossi RL, Heiss FW, Shea JA. Acute relapsing pancreatitis as a complication of papillary stenosis after endoscopic sphincterotomy. *Gastroenterology* 1993;**104**:1814–17.

Cotton PB. Therapeutic gastrointestinal endoscopy. Problems in proving efficacy. *N Engl J Med* 1992;**326**:1626–8.

Cotton PB. Outcomes of endoscopy procedures: struggling towards definition. *Gastrointest Endosc* 1994;**40**:514–18.

Cotton PB, Lehman G, Vennes J *et al.* Endoscopic sphincterotomy, complications and their management. An attempt at consensus. *Gastrointest Endosc* 1991;**37**:383–93.

Neoptolemos JP, Shaw DE, Carr-Locke DE. A multivariant analysis of preoperative risk factors in patients with common bile duct stones. Implications for treatment. *Ann Surg* 1989;**209**:157–61.

Sherman S, Lehman GA. ERCP and endoscopic sphincterotomy-induced pancreatitis. *Pancreas* 1991;**6**:350–67.

Colonoscopy and Flexible Sigmoidoscopy

9

Flexible colonoscopy started, improbably, in 1958 in Japan with Matsunaga's intracolonic use of the gastrocamera under fluoroscopic control, and subsequently Niwa's development of the 'sigmocamera'. Not surprisingly these had application only in the hands of pioneer enthusiasts. Following the development of the fibreoptic bundle, similar determination by Provenzale and Revignas in Italy and Fox in the UK allowed imaging of the proximal colon after pulling it up using a swallowed guide string or pulley system. Overholt in the USA introduced the 'fiberoptic coloscope' in 1966, but its limited angulation and angle of view again restricted the technique to a few hardy spirits. The West was surprised by the production in 1969 by Japanese engineers (Olympus Optical and Machida) of remarkably effective colonic instruments combining the well-developed and torque-stable mechanics of a gastrocamera with superior fibreoptics. These were easy to handle and gave excellent views, although initially limitations of glass-fibre technology and fragile fibres restricted angulation to around 90° and angle of view to 70°. Very rapid developments in both Japan and the USA brought the four-way acutely angling instruments with near 'fish-eye' vision to which we are now accustomed, further enhanced by the introduction in the USA in 1983 of the video-endoscope (Welch-Allyn). Although small-scale colonoscope production continues in Germany, Russia and China, the combined mechanical, optical and electronic know-how of Japanese manufacturers now dominates the market.

Description in Japanese abstracts of intragastric snare polypectomy in 1970 was followed by its performance in the colon in 1971 by Deyhle in Europe and Shinya in the USA. This set the seal on the emergence of colonoscopy as a powerful technique, set to leapfrog barium-contrast technology as the method of choice for intracolonic diagnosis and, with emerging scanning techniques, largely to replace 'diagnostic laparotomy'. Further refinements of handling technique and instrument technology over the years have substantially transformed colonoscopy from an aggressive and somewhat hazardous experience into a socially acceptable and sophisticated methodology. Its unavoidably intrusive nature and the varied mechanical constraints of the individual colon are limiting factors; overcoming these as far as possible is the current challenge to the flexible endoscopist.

Indications, limitations and complications

The exact place of colonoscopy in clinical practice is outside the scope of this book and depends on local circumstances and available endoscopic expertise. Clinical judgement or financial considerations may sometimes determine that flexible sigmoidoscopy alone (limited colonoscopy with limited bowel preparation) is sufficient for the particular clinical purpose. Thus flexible sigmoidoscopy is, on grounds of logistics, safety and patient acceptability, being considered for population screening, whereas total colonoscopy is more appropriate for those at increased risk for colorectal cancer or requiring symptomatic evaluation.

A double-contrast barium enema (DCBE) remains a safe way (one perforation per 25 000 examinations) of showing the configuration of the colon, the presence of diverticular disease and the absence of strictures or large lesions in patients with pain, altered bowel habit or constipation; it also shows extramural leaks or fistulae which are invisible to the endoscopist. However, the limitations of even a high-quality DCBE are well known, and include the ability to miss large lesions because of overlapping loops, to misinterpret between solid stool and neoplasms or between spasm and strictures, with particular inaccuracy for flat lesions such as angiodysplasias or minor inflammatory change and small (2–5 mm) polyps. Single-contrast barium enemas, in particular, have been dismissed as 'a good way to diagnose inoperable cancer', although perversely it is often on the barium-filled segments of a DCBE examination that filling defects are best demonstrated.

However, colonoscopy too has its limitations — failure of proper examination due to failed bowel preparation or an inability to reach the caecum being obvious ones. The lack of definite landmarks, unless the ileocaecal valve is reached and identified, means that gross errors in localization are possible during the insertion of the colonoscope in up to 30% of cases, even for expert endoscopists. Although it is justifiable to consider colonoscopy by an expert endoscopist as the gold standard, any colonoscopist needs to be aware of the potential for blind spots where it is possible to miss very large lesions, especially in the caecum, just around acute bends and in the rectal ampulla. The accuracy for small lesions is probably better than 90% but it is not 100%. The notion of routinely having a prior barium enema 'to show the shape of the colon' is irrelevant to the endoscopist, since short colons with short mesenteries can be difficult and painful to endoscope, whereas some very long colons prove to be painless and easy. Nonetheless, if a contrast examination has previously been performed, the presence of severe diverticular disease or a very redundant colon (a transverse colon which droops down to the pelvic brim in the erect film is particularly discriminant) increase the likelihood that the procedure will be demanding.

The complication rate of colonoscopy is higher (around one perforation per 1700 examinations in published series overall). All colonoscopy complication series to date include early experience with outdated instruments and are certainly too pessimistic. There has been no significant complication during diagnostic examinations in our experience, or that of others performing colonoscopies at St Mark's Hospital, during the past 20 000 examinations. However, this is the experience of a specialist hospital and, whilst showing the potential for the technique, is not representative of what may be happening in the hands of unskilled endoscopists needing to use heavy sedation to cover up for their ineptitude. Any endoscopist performing therapeutic procedures such as dilatations or polypectomies will inevitably experience complications, although these are remarkably infrequent. Fatalities have, however, been reported after oversedation or due to mismanaged colonoscopic perforation. The endoscopist should therefore be on guard that problems *can* occur and should work with the knowledge and co-operation of a backup surgical team.

Colonoscopy achieves more than contrast radiology, partly in greater accuracy and also through its biopsy and therapeutic capabilities. Because of its colour view and biopsy capability, colonoscopy is particularly relevant to patients with bleeding, anaemia, bowel frequency or diarrhoea and, because of pinpoint accuracy and therapy, to any patient at risk for cancer—in whom detection and removal of any adenomas is important for the patient's future. Colonoscopy is thus the method of choice for most clinical patients and for cancer surveillance examinations and follow-up. The proviso must be added that a few patients who are very difficult to colonoscope for reasons of anatomy or postoperative adhesions may be best examined by combining limited left-sided colonoscopy (much more accurate than DCBE in the sigmoid colon) with a barium enema to demonstrate the proximal colon, which can be arranged at the same visit and with the same bowel preparation. Particularly if carbon dioxide (CO_2) insufflation is used during the endoscopy, the colon will be absolutely deflated within 10–15 min and the DCBE can follow immediately. Even after air insufflation, some radiologists report satisfactory DCBE although the proximal colon can be air-filled and difficult to coat adequately with barium. Colonoscopic biopsies with standard-sized forceps are no contraindication to performing a DCBE and prior hot-biopsy or pedunculated polypectomy should not be either; whereas larger biopsies or sessile polypectomy contraindicate the distension pressure required for DCBE.

Limited examination by flexible sigmoidoscopy or left-sided colonoscopy may, therefore, have a significant role in clinically selected patients with minor symptoms such as left iliac fossa pain or spotting on toilet paper. DCBE alone may be considered by some to be adequate in 'low-yield' patients with constipation or minor functional symptoms where the result is expected to be normal or to show minor diverticular disease. Endoscopy is particularly useful in the postoperative patient, either to inspect in close-up (and biopsy if necessary) any deformity at the anastomosis or to avoid the difficulties of barium or air leakage that a stoma presents for the radiologist.

Contraindications and infective hazards

Against this clinical background, there are few patients in whom colonoscopy is contraindicated. Any patient who might otherwise come to diagnostic laparotomy because of colonic disease is fit for colonoscopy, and colonoscopy is often undertaken in very poor risk cases in the hope of avoiding surgery. For a 3-week period after myocardial infarction, it is unwise to perform colonoscopy due to the risk of dysrhythmias. There is no contraindication to colonoscopy (without fluoroscopy) during pregnancy, although, on common-sense grounds, it may be best avoided in those with a history of miscarriage. In any acute and severe inflammatory process, such as ulcerative, Crohn's or ischaemic colitis, where abdominal tenderness suggests an increased risk of perforation, colonoscopy should only be undertaken with good reason and extreme care. If large and deep ulcers are seen, the bowel wall may be weakened and it may be wise to limit or abandon the examination. In the chronic stage of irradiation colitis, a year or more after exposure, the bowel can be perforated even without excessive force; if the diagnosis has been made, and insertion proves difficult, it may be wiser to withdraw.

Colonoscopy is absolutely contraindicated in acute diverticulitis which is due to local sepsis and threatened perforation. It should not be performed in any patient with marked abdominal tenderness, peritonism or peritonitis from whatever cause because of the high risk of causing perforation.

Possible septicaemia or infectivity are a consideration in certain patients. Passage of the colonoscope, and indeed any other agent including air or barium insufflation, causes transient release of bowel organisms into the bloodstream and peritoneal cavity. This constitutes a relative contraindication to endoscopy of patients with known ascites or on peritoneal dialysis. They, and patients with heart-valve replacements, and also marasmic infants or immunosuppressed or immunodepressed adults, should be protected by the prior administration of antibiotics (see p. 34). There is no contraindication to the examination of infected patients (e.g. patients with infectious diarrhoea or hepatitis) since all normal organisms and viruses will be inactivated by routine cleaning and disinfection procedures including a 4 min soak and channel perfusion with 2% glutaraldehyde. Mycobacterial spores, however, require a much longer period and, therefore, after the examination of suspected tuberculosis patients and before and after the examination of AIDS patients who are susceptible to, and possible carriers of, mycobacteria, a 60 min soak of the instrument in glutaraldehyde is recommended (see Chapter 3).

Patient preparation

Most patients can organize their bowel preparation at home, present themselves for examination and walk out shortly afterwards. Management routines depend on national, organizational and individual factors. In some countries (the USA, France, Italy, Germany) patients are prepared to administer their own cleansing enemas; in others this has to be done by the endoscopy nursing staff. Some nationalities (Dutch, German, Japanese) do not expect sedation whereas others (British, American) frequently insist on it. Management is influenced, amongst other things, by cost, the type of bowel preparation and sedation used, the age and state of the patient, the potential for major therapeutic procedures and the availability of adequate facilities and nursing staff for day-care and recovery. Experienced colonoscopists in private practice and large units are motivated to organize streamlined day-case routines, even for patients with large polyps. These variables result in an extraordinary spectrum of performance, from the many skilled colonoscopists who require patients for less than an hour in an office or day-care unit, to others with less experience and a traditional hospital background who feel that hours, or even days, in hospital are essential.

Colonoscopy can be made quick and easy; this requires both a reasonably planned day-care facility and an endoscopist with the confidence and skill to work gently and fast. A few patients are better admitted before or after the procedure; the very old, sick and very constipated may need professional supervision during bowel preparation, and frail patients may merit overnight observation afterwards, especially if their domestic circumstances are not supportive or they live far away. We admit a few patients with large polyps, especially if the lesion is broad-stalked or sessile, or if the patient has a bleeding diathesis or is on anticoagulants or antiplatelet medications (aspirin, dipyrinamide, etc.). However, even such patients, providing they live near good medical support services and are fully informed as to what to do in a crisis, can often be justifiably managed on an outpatient basis.

Bowel preparation

Failures of bowel preparation occur mainly in older patients with diverticular disease and those with colons damaged by colitis. Constipated patients should be primed with senna at bedtime for several nights preceding the normal preparation regimen. Really stubborn constipation, as in cases of megacolon or cystic fibrosis, can be cleared by hourly doses of magnesium sulphate crystals (Epsom salts, 15–30 g) with large volumes of clear fluid, but since this and the subsequent colonoscopy are likely to be unpleasant for all concerned, the experience should be avoided if at all possible (unprepared barium enema is sometimes sufficient to show the pathological colon configuration).

Limited preparation

For limited colonoscopy or flexible sigmoidoscopy in the 'normal' colon, limited preparation should be enough. The patient need not diet and simply has one or two disposable phosphate enemas (e.g. Fleet's Phospho-soda, Fletchers') 20–30 min beforehand. Examination is performed shortly afterwards so that there is no time for proximal bowel contents to descend. The colon is often perfectly prepared to the transverse or hepatic flexure, especially in young patients (except babies, in whom phosphate enemas are contraindicated). Note that patients with any tendency to faint or with functional bowel symptoms (pain, flatulence, etc.) are more likely to have severe vasovagal problems after phosphate enemas; make sure they are supervised or have a call button and that lavatory doors open from and to the outside in case the patient faints against the door. Diverticular disease or stricturing makes preparation more difficult and phosphate enemas are less likely to work for mechanical reasons; if a good view is important (as for apparent stricturing or possible malignancy) we normally recommend full bowel preparation even for a limited examination. If there is a serious possibility of obstruction, per oral preparation is dangerous, even potentially fatal, and in ileus or pseudo-obstruction normal preparation simply does not work; one or more large-volume enemas are administered in such circumstances (up to 1 litre or more can be held by most colons). A contact laxative such as oxyphenisatin (300 mg) or a dose of bisacodyl can be added to the enema to improve evacuation (see below).

For reasons of institutional convenience or patient compliance, it is sometimes found that a dose of oral laxative is a more convenient approach, for instance taken at home late at night to act in the morning before coming for an early flexible sigmoidoscopy appointment.

Full preparation

The object of full preparation is to cleanse the whole colon, especially the proximal parts, which are characteristically coated with surface residue after limited regimens. However, patients and colons vary. No single preparation regimen predictably suits every patient and it is often necessary to be prepared to adapt to individual needs. Constipated patients need extra preparation; those with severe colitis may be unfit to have anything other than a warm saline enema. A preparation which has previously proved unpalatable, made the patient vomit or failed is unlikely to be a success on another occasion. The doctor, nurse or secretary, should talk to the patient to find out about their normal bowel habit (loose or constipated, laxative requirements, results of previous purgatives, etc.) and to explain the need for special diets and purgation. Minutes spent in explanation and motivation may prevent a prolonged, unpleasant and inaccurate examination due to bad preparation. For most people without prior experience of it, anticipation of the indignity, possible pain and/or dreaded result of colonoscopy are much worse than the procedure itself usually turns out to be. Anything which will justifiably cheer them up, as well as motivate them for the period of dietary modification and bowel preparation, is extremely worthwhile.

Diet

Iron preparations should be stopped 3–4 days before colonoscopy, since organic iron tannates produce an inky black viscid stool which interferes with inspection and is difficult to clear. Constipating agents should also be stopped 1–2 days before, but most other medication can be continued as usual, allowing for modification of anticoagulant regimens and the avoidance of aspirin, non-steroidal anti-inflammatory drugs (NSAIDs) and similar platelet-inhibiting agents, if possible, in those of polyp-bearing age. The patient should have no indigestible or high-residue food (including muesli, fibrous vegetables, mushrooms, fruit, nuts, raisins, etc.) for 24h before colonoscopy; staying for 24h on clear fluids is even better if the patient is compliant. Fruit juices or beer may be easier to drink in large quantities than water, and white wine or spirits can also help morale — especially in the fasting phase. Red wine in any quantity can, with tannates, darken the bowel contents and is best avoided. Written instructions are well worthwhile; many patients, anxious to get a good result, find it easier to follow specific instructions and it helps avoid unnecessary telephone calls.

Oral lavage regimens

Oral lavage regimens have supplanted the traditional purge plus enema approach in most practices because they are more effective and cause no pain. On the other hand, some patients will not or cannot drink the 3–4-litre volumes of fluid required, experience uncomfortable distension, become nauseated or vomit, or simply dislike the taste of the chosen solution. Further work is needed to provide the ideal compromise — a powder which can be sent through the post and dissolved to produce an acceptable volume of a pleasant-tasting combination of non-absorbed solutes and electrolytes, and perhaps also containing a physiological gut activator and/or a prokinetic agent to speed transit.

Balanced electrolyte solution. A balanced electrolyte solution, including the requisite amount of potassium chloride (KCl) and bicarbonate to avoid body losses, is physiologically correct, although unfortunately the taste of the additives (especially KCl and $NaSO_4$) is unpleasant. Normal (0.9%) saline is used by some centres, which has the advantage of being very cheap and easy to make up or post, but less physiological than balanced electrolyte solutions.

Balanced electrolyte solution with polyethylene glycol solution (PEG). Polyethylene glycol solution, also simply called PEG or PEG/electrolyte mixture (GoLytely, Nulytely, Colyte, etc.), is widely used, primarily because it has formal (Food and Drug Administration) approval allowing commercial flavouring and packaging and easy prescription by doctors. Although often known as PEG preparation, the PEG component of a PEG/electrolyte mixture contributes only a minority of osmolality (but the majority of the packaged weight and volume) — sodium salts unfortunately being, of physiological necessity, the important component. Even chilled, its taste is mildly unpleasant due to the addition of $NaSO_4$, bicarbonate and KCl to minimize body fluxes. Modification of the original formula (Nulytely), lowering the sodium content by omitting $NaSO_4$ and reducing KCl, only slightly improves the taste. Patient acceptance of electrolyte/PEG oral preparation can be enhanced, without impairing results from the endoscopist's point of view, by the simple expedient of administering the 3–4 litres necessary in two half doses ('split administration', with 2 litres drunk the evening before and 1–2 litres on the morning of the examination). There are conflicting reports about whether adding prokinetic agents or aperients contributes anything, and the consensus is that they do not.

Mannitol. Mannitol (and similarly sorbitol or lactulose) is a sugar for which the body has no absorptive enzymes. In solution it presents an iso-osmotic fluid load at 5% (2–3 litres) or a hypertonic purge at 10% (1 litre) with a corresponding loss of electrolyte and body fluid during the resulting diarrhoea, although this is only of concern in the elderly and normally can be rapidly reversed by drinking. The solution tastes very sweet and can be nauseous to those without a sweet tooth, although this can be much reduced by chilling and adding lemon juice or other flavourings. Children, in particular, tend to vomit it back. Mannitol alone (1 litre drunk iced over 30 min, followed by 1 litre of tap water) is a very useful way of achieving rapid bowel preparation (2–3 h) for those requiring urgent colonoscopy.

There is a potential explosion hazard because colonic bacteria possess the necessary enzymes to metabolize mannitol and other carbohydrates to form explosive quantities of hydrogen. If they have been used in preparation any electrosurgical or laser procedure is hazardous unless CO_2 insufflation has been used, or alternatively all colonic gas is conscientiously several times exchanged by aspiration and re-insufflation of room air.

Picolax. Picolax, a proprietary combination, produces both magnesium citrate (from magnesium oxide and citric acid) and bisacodyl (from bacterial action on sodium picosulphate), tastes acceptable and works well in most patients. Providing enough fluid is drunk, no enema is needed.

Sodium phosphate. This, presented as a flavoured half-strength orally administered equivalent of the phosphate enema (Fleet's Phospho-soda), has received numerous good reports recently. It is considered to be as effective as PEG/electrolyte solution but significantly more acceptable to patients. This is principally because the volume which needs to be ingested is only 90 ml, followed by at least 1 litre of other clear fluids of choice (water, juices, lager, etc.).

Administration of oral lavage

Low-residue diet instructions will have been given. The patient should be advised to use, and preferably supplied with, petroleum jelly or barrier cream (colourless if possible to avoid lens contamination) to avoid perianal soreness. As mentioned above, large-volume PEG/electrolyte solutions are ideally split-administered in two doses, starting on the evening beforehand with the residue on the morning of the examination. If an afternoon examination is scheduled, and the patient does not have a long distance to travel, both doses can be drunk on the day of examination; if in doubt, a purgative (such as senna, 4–6 tablets) can be also be taken at the previous bedtime. The PEG/electrolyte solution should be drunk steadily at a rate of around 1.5 litres/h (250 ml/10 min initially). Chilling mannitol solution makes it taste much less sweet; cooling PEG/electrolyte solution also improves palatability but may overcool the drinker too. Adding sugar-containing flavouring agents, such as fruit cordials, to PEG/electrolyte solution is discouraged on the basis that increased sodium absorption could occur. Sodium phosphate solution is easily downed with a 'chaser' of some more pleasant drink and then 1 litre or more of fluid to follow in the next hour or two.

The patient should be encouraged to carry on with normal activities during the drinking period, rather than sitting still, in order to encourage transit, but should stop drinking temporarily if nausea or uncomfortable distension occur. Bowel actions should start within about an hour, returns are often clear by 2–3 h and colonoscopy can sometimes be started 1–2 h later. The endoscopist may have to aspirate large quantities of fluid during the examination but the patient is spared the dietary changes, cramps and enemas of a purge regimen and the result is usually excellent.

Purgation and enemas

Sufficient contact laxative or purgative must be taken to produce fluid diarrhoea, which shows that unaltered small intestinal contents are emerging and the colonic residue has been cleared. A large dose is given to ensure this but, as the response is individual rather than dose-related, there is no danger. Nonetheless, any agent producing diarrhoea may also cause nausea or abdominal cramps in some patients. It takes only about 8 h for colonic water absorption to reform ileal effluent into solid stool so that, ideally, administration should be judged to cause the diarrhoea to stop only shortly before examination. However, since some people respond to laxatives in 1–2 h and others take as much as 8–10 h, exact timing is difficult. If the patient is to get some sleep and then be able to travel without risk of accident, the best compromise is for the laxative to be taken at 3–5 p.m. on the previous afternoon. For a mid-afternoon colonoscopy, the purge can be taken early the same morning or, alternatively, at bedtime in the expectation that there will be no action until the gut reactivates in the morning.

Purges. Castor oil (30–40 ml) acts on both the small and large intestine, but is disliked by most patients. Its after-taste and oily texture can be masked by mixing it with orange juice or an effervescent drink immediately before drinking, and following with a 'chaser' of orange juice. Senna preparations work equally well providing a large dose is given (140 mg of sennosides), preferably as syrup or granules. Osmotic purges such as magnesium salts (citrate tastes better than sulphate or hydroxide) can also be effective with repeated 1- or 2-hourly doses and high fluid intake until clear diarrhoea results.

Enemas. Enemas, whether tap water, isotonic saline or purgative (bisacodyl or oxyphenisatin) are self- or nurse-administered

1–2 h before the examination until the returns are clear. Two or three enemas, each of 1–2 litres, may be needed. The fluid should reach the caecum; lavage or 'washouts' of the social variety, where small volumes of water are run in and out of the distal colon, are useless. Having got the fluid in it must also be got out, which entails the patient being able to sit relaxed on the lavatory for 15–20 min initially and then to revisit and evacuate at will afterwards. The returns are inspected and, if any solid matter remains, the enema is repeated. Patients with diverticular disease or painful spasm-obstructing enema inflow are given an intramuscular antispasmodic injection (hyoscine *N*-butylbromide 40 mg i.m.; Glucagon 0.5 mg i.m.).

Bowel preparation in special circumstances

Children

Paediatric patients accept pleasant-tasting oral preparations such as senna syrup or magnesium citrate very well. Drinking large volumes is less well accepted and mannitol may cause nausea or vomiting. The childhood colon normally evacuates easily except, paradoxically, in colitis patients who prove perversely difficult to prepare properly. Small babies may be almost completely prepared with oral fluids plus a saline enema (see p. 267). Phosphate enemas are contraindicated in babies because of the possibility of hyperphosphataemia.

Colitis patients

These patients require special care, during and after preparation. Relapses of inflammatory bowel disease are said occasionally to occur after over-vigorous bowel preparation, although they can also be provoked by simple distension during an unprepared barium enema, which perhaps suggests that the cause is mechanical rather than chemical. Magnesium citrate, senna preparations, mannitol, saline or balanced PEG/electrolyte solutions are all generally well tolerated, and the latter is favoured in patients with diarrhoea from active colitis. A simple tap-water or saline enema will clear the distal colon sufficiently for limited colonoscopy. Patients with severe colitis are unlikely to need colonoscopy at all, since plain abdominal X-ray or an unprepared barium enema will usually give enough information; for severely ill patients even a barium enema is risky and colonoscopy positively contraindicated due to the potential for perforation. When the indication for colonoscopy in a patient with colitis is to exclude cancer or to reach the terminal ileum to help in differential diagnosis, full and vigorous preparation is necessary. A patient fit enough for total colonoscopy is fit for full bowel preparation, which is essential because inflammatory change often makes the proximal colon difficult to prepare properly.

Constipated patients

Patients with constipation may, for obvious reasons, need extra bowel preparation. This is very difficult to achieve in patients with megacolon, Hirschsprung's disease, cystic fibrosis, etc., in whom colonoscopy should be avoided if at all possible. Constipated patients should continue any habitually-taken purgatives in addition to the colonoscopy preparation, and preferably in large doses for several days beforehand. The principle is to achieve regular soft bowel actions during the days before taking the main purge, if necessary using additional doses of paraffin emulsion, magnesium citrate/sulphate, etc. Larger than standard doses of senna or other purgatives are unlikely to produce any extra effect, but frequent doses of magnesium salts and large volumes of fluid are guaranteed to move mountains (see above), providing there is no obstruction.

Colostomy patients

The colons of colostomy patients are as difficult to prepare as those of normal subjects (and often more so). The preparation regimen should not be reduced just because the colon is shorter; if anything it should be increased, with a prior 'pump-priming' maximal dose of senna on the night before. Oral preparation with one of the lavage regimens described above is well tolerated, whereas enemas/colostomy washouts are tedious and difficult to perform satisfactorily, unless the patient is accustomed to this and used to performing it personally.

Stomas, pouches and ileorectal anastomoses

These present few problems. Ileostomies are self-emptying and normally need no preparation other than perhaps a few hours of fasting and clear fluid intake. Kock or ileoanal pelvic pouches can be managed either by saline enema or by oral lavage. After ileorectal anastomosis, the small intestine can adapt and enlarge to an amazing degree within some months of surgery, so that if the object of the examination is to examine the small intestine, full oral preparation should be given. For a limited look, a saline or tap-water enema is usually enough.

Defunctioned bowel

A defunctioned bowel, for instance the distal loop of a 'double-barrelled' colostomy, always contains a considerable amount of viscid mucus and inspissated cell debris which will block the colonoscope. Conventional tap-water/saline rectal enemas or tube lavage through the colostomy are needed before examining a defunctioned bowel.

Active colonic bleeding

Blood is a good purgative and some patients requiring emergency colonoscopy need no specific preparation providing examination is started during the phase of active bright-red bleeding. Posturing the patient during insertion of the instrument will shift the blood and create an air interface through which the instrument can be passed; changing to the right lateral position clears the proximal sigmoid and descending colon, which is otherwise a blood-filled sump. Actively bleeding patients requiring preparation for more accurate total colonoscopy are best managed by nasogastric tube or oral electrolyte/mannitol lavage. This allows examination within an hour or two and ensures that blood is washed out distal to the bleeding point, rather than carried proximally with enemas. Blood can be refluxed to the terminal ileum from a left colon source, which makes localization difficult, unless it is being constantly washed downwards by a per oral high-volume preparation. Massively bleeding patients can be examined peroperatively with on-table colon lavage combining a caecostomy tube with a large-bore rectal suction tube (and bucket).

Medication

Sedation and analgesia

At the time that the colonoscopy booking is arranged, the patient should be given a preliminary verbal and written explanation both of bowel preparation and of the procedure. On arrival for colonoscopy, a few minutes of further explanation will reassure and calm most patients and allow the endoscopist to judge whether the particular individual is likely to require sedation, and if so how much. Most people tolerate some discomfort without resentment if they understand the reason for it. Few people expect to be semi-anaesthetized for a visit to the dentist, but on the other hand they understandably expect the intensity and duration of any pain to be within 'acceptable limits' — a threshold which is not always easy to predict before colonoscopy, because both individual anatomy and tolerance of the unpleasant quality of visceral pain vary so much. It is sensible to warn the patient that there can be some stomach ache or air distension during the procedure, but to ask him to complain at once rather than to suffer in silence, and also to ask for extra analgesia if wanted.

Using moderate or no sedation and employing the skills,

changes of position and other 'tricks of the trade' described here-after, the only pain experienced by the patient during a correctly performed colonoscopy in a 'normal' colon should be for the 20–30 s it takes to pass the sigmoid–descending colon junction and then to straighten the instrument back again; during the rest of the procedure there should be little more than a feeling of distension or apparent desire to pass flatus. It is worth pointing out that any pain that does occur is a useful warning to the endoscopist, is not dangerous and can usually be terminated in a few seconds (by straightening out the loop which must have formed to cause it).

The use of sedation has advantages and disadvantages. Without it, the bowel is possibly more tonic, shorter and so easier to examine; more importantly, the patient can co-operate with any changes of position, needs no recovery period and can travel home unaided immediately. The colonoscopist is also forced to develop a good, and gentle, insertion technique. With sedation, the patient is more likely to find the examination tolerable or to have amnesia for it. The endoscopist can be more thorough and is also more likely to achieve total colonoscopy in a shorter time. However, with heavy sedation endoscopists can get away with ham-handed technique, which is a bad investment in the long term, more likely to result in complications and more expensive in instrument repair bills. It is often said that it is dangerous to sedate because the safety factor of pain is removed; this is not strictly true, providing that the endoscopist raises his own threshold of awareness as the patient's pain threshold is raised, responding to restlessness or changes of facial expression as a warning that the tissues are being overstretched. With the heavy sedation wrongly employed by some endoscopists (e.g. diazepam 10 mg i.v. or midazolam 5 mg i.v., combined with pethidine (meperidine) 50–100 mg i.v.), the drowsy patient cannot co-operate or complain effectively, so the subtleties of colonoscopic technique may be ignored and there is no 'negative feedback' when loops form. The end result is that colonoscopy becomes a 'heavy' procedure with a potential for complications due to air distension and excessive force, whereas the total colonoscopy rate may be disappointing because of loops formed but not removed. Equally, some endoscopists who never employ sedation admit to only 70–80% success in performing total colonoscopy, presumably because some examinations were intolerable.

Most endoscopists use a balanced approach to sedation which will be affected by many factors including personal experience and the patient's attitude. A relaxed patient with a short colon having a limited examination rarely needs sedation, but a tense sick patient with a tortuous colon or severe diverticular disease requiring total colonoscopy needs some protection. Exceptional patients have such a morbid fear of colonoscopy, or such a low pain threshold, that it is justified to resort to light general anaesthesia if colonoscopy is particularly indicated. General anaesthesia is hazardous when combined with an inexperienced colonoscopist, who is able to use brutal technique because the anaesthetized patient cannot protest.

Nitrous oxide inhalation

We and others have recently described the use of a nitrous oxide/oxygen mixture as a useful 'half-way house' between no sedation and conventional intravenous sedation. The 50:50 nitrous oxide:oxygen mixture is self-administered by the patient, inhaling from a small cylinder fitted with a demand valve. Breathing the gas through a small sterile mouthpiece (Fig. 9.1) avoids the difficulties that can be experienced in getting a good fit with a face mask, and also the phobia that some patients feel for masks.

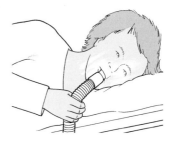

Fig. 9.1 Nitrous oxide/oxygen mixture is breathed through a mouthpiece.

The patient is shown how to inhale and pre-breathes for a minute or so as the endoscopist prepares to start the procedure, with the intention of achieving loading gas saturation of the body tissues. Thereafter it takes only 20–30s of gas breathing, when needed, to obtain a 'high' which makes short-lived pain significantly more tolerable. Nitrous oxide/oxygen inhalation should prove useful for some flexible sigmoidoscopies and is sufficient for motivated patients having total colonoscopy by a skilled endoscopist. Scared patients, prolonged or difficult examinations and examinations by inexpert endoscopists require conventional sedation.

Intravenous sedation

The ideal sedative for colonoscopy would last 5–10 min with a strong analgesic action but no respiratory depression or aftereffects. The nearest approach to the ideal at present is given by the combination of a benzodiazepine hypnotic such as midazolam (Versed 2.5–5 mg) or diazepam (Valium or Diazemuls 5–10 mg) either alone or with an opiate such as pethidine (meperidine 25–75 mg). The injection is given slowly over a period of at least 1 min, 'titrating' the dose to some extent by observing the patient's conscious state and ability to talk coherently—some patients merely become loquacious. Half dosage is used for older, sicker patients but the amount required is unpredictable; if in doubt it is safer to underdo the titration and give more later if necessary. The benzodiazepine contributes anxiolytic, sedational and amnesic effects whilst the opiate contributes analgesia and, in the case of pethidine, a useful sense of euphoria. In general, only a small dose of benzodiazepine should be given unless the patient is very anxious. For pathologically anxious or neurotic patients, premedication may occasionally be helpful before arriving in the endoscopy suite (giving, for instance, a beta-blocker (propranolol 40 mg or equivalent orally) or an intramuscular injection of pethidine (meperidine 75 mg)).

If increments of medication are needed during insertion it is usually best to use extra opiate rather than more benzodiazepine —which makes some patients even more restless and in any case has no pain-killing properties. Benzodiazepines and opiates potentiate each other, not only in effectiveness but also in side-effects such as depression of respiration and blood pressure, which can be sudden or gradual, and potentially serious. Pulse oximetry should therefore be routinely available and used in elderly, at-risk or heavily sedated (non-bronchitic) patients; if in doubt oxygen should be administered. Although it is increasingly suggested that pulse oximetry and low-dosage (2 litres/min) nasal oxygen should be used in *all* examinations where sedation is employed, we prefer to be selective, relying— in patients who are unsedated or only lightly medicated, comfortable and able to converse normally — on deliberately minimizing the overt technical complexity of the procedure and concentrating on its human aspects.

Benzodiazepines. Benzodiazepines have, as well as their anxiolytic effects, an additional mild smooth-muscle antispasmodic action. Diazepam (Valium) is poorly soluble in water and the injectable form is therefore carried in a glycol solution which can be painful and cause thrombophlebitis, especially if administered into small veins. If a hand vein is to be used, and also for paediatric practice, it is better either to use water-soluble midazolam (Versed) or diazepam in lipid emulsion (Diazemuls, where available), both of which are less irritant. Midazolam causes a greater degree of amnesia, which can be useful to cover a traumatic experience but unfortunately also 'wipes' any explanation of the findings, which must be repeated later on.

Opiates. Opiates, in addition to analgesic efficacy, can also variably induce a useful sense of euphoria. Pethidine may cause pain when administered through small veins, particularly in children, but this can largely be avoided by diluting the injection 1 : 10 in water. Some endoscopists prefer to give pethidine (meperidine) intramuscularly 1 h beforehand, which we do not favour. Pentazocine (Fortral) is a weaker analgesic, more hallucinogenic and seems to have little to recommend it. Fentanyl (Sublimaze) is a very short-lived opiate, but has the disadvantage of significant respiratory depressant effects without giving any sense of well-being.

Neurolept analgesia combinations. These combinations, usually haloperidol and droperidol, have been used by some, especially in France, but have the disadvantage of prolonged after-effects.

Propofol. Propofol (Diprivan), a short-lived intravenous emulsion anaesthetic agent, is widely used for colonoscopy in France and sporadically in other countries. It should ideally be administered by an anaesthetist because of the significant risk of marked respiratory depression but, with appropriate training and safeguards, has been employed by endoscopists alone. Its short duration of action, giving full recovery within about 30 min, is an advantage over excessive doses of conventional sedatives. On the other hand, the patient is rendered insensible and so unable to co-operate with changes of position or to give early warning of excessive pain. The routine use of propofol for all cases cannot, therefore, be commended.

Antagonists

Availability of antagonists to benzodiazepines (Anexate) and opiates (naloxone) provide an invaluable safety measure for occasions when inadvertent oversedation has occurred. Some endoscopists routinely give them (intravenously and/or intramuscularly) to speed up the recovery period, which suggests mainly that their routine dosage is excessive. We use Anexate extremely infrequently, but periodically administer naloxone intramuscularly on reaching the caecum in a patient who has requested or needed extra sedation. The patient is then conveniently awake by the time the examination is finished, without the risk of later 'rebound' re-sedation that is reported after intravenous naloxone wears off.

Antispasmodics

Either hyoscine *N*-butylbromide (Buscopan 20 mg) i.v. or Glucagon (0.5–1 mg) i.v. produce good colonic relaxation for at least 5–10 min and are helpful in improving the view during examination of a hypercontractile colon. The ocular side-effects of hyoscine may continue for several hours and the patient should not drive if vision is impaired, although cholinesterase-inhibitor eye drops will rapidly restore normality. Fears about anticholinergics initiating glaucoma are misplaced since patients previously diagnosed are completely protected by their eye drops, and those with undiagnosed chronic glaucoma are best served by precipitating an acute attack, which will cause the diagnosis to be made. Glucagon is more expensive, but has no ocular or prostatic side-effects.

The relatively short duration of action of intravenous antispasmodics leads some endoscopists to give them when the colonoscope is fully inserted; experienced endoscopists, sure of a rapid procedure, may give them at the start. There is an unproven suspicion that a bowel rendered more redundant and atonic by antispasmodics will be more difficult to examine; to the contrary, we find that the view is improved and insertion thereby speeded up after using hyoscine. Diazepam has a weak antispasmodic effect, relaxing most colons except for those which are 'irritable' or spastic; in the unsedated patient, therefore, antispasmodics may be particularly helpful—and can also be a useful placebo for those who cannot have routine sedation because they need to drive home, but expect an 'injection' to cover the procedure.

Patients with functional bowel disorder or diverticular disease may suffer from increased air retention after using antispasmodics, with the sudden onset of colic or abdominal discomfort an hour or more after the procedure when the pharmacological effects wear off.

Antibiotics

It is well proven from studies in which multiple blood cultures are taken during colonoscopy that transient bacteraemia occurs while the instrument is being inserted through the sigmoid colon. Both aerobic and anaerobic organisms can be released into the bloodstream at this time. Patients with ascites or on peritoneal dialysis have been reported to develop peritonitis following colonic instrumentation, presumably by transmural passage of bacteria as a result of local trauma. At-risk patients (including those with heart-valve replacements, cyanotic heart disease or previous endocarditis) and immunosuppressed or severely ill patients (especially immunocompromised infants) should have a suitable antibiotic combination administered beforehand so as to give therapeutic blood levels at the time of the procedure. The topic is more fully addressed in Chapter 3. Ampicillin 3 g orally 1 h beforehand (or 1 g in 2.5 ml 1% lignocaine i.m. just beforehand) *plus* another 0.5 g orally 6 h later and gentamicin 120 mg i.m. 1 h before (or intravenously just beforehand) is a possible adult regimen. Alternatively, a single intravenous dose of gentamicin (80 mg) and ampicillin (500 mg) before premedication has been advised. Vancomycin (20 mg/kg by slow i.v. infusion over the 60 min prior to the procedure) can be substituted for ampicillin in patients with a history of penicillin sensitivity. Children under 10 years of age receive half the adult dose of amoxycillin and gentamicin — 2 mg/kg body weight. In high-risk subjects it may be wise to continue antibiotics for up to 24–48 h.

Equipment

Colonoscopy room

The only special requisite for a colonoscopy room is good ventilation to overcome the evidence of occasional poor bowel preparation. In a few patients with particularly difficult and looping colons, it can be helpful to have access to X-ray facilities, particularly in teaching institutions. In the future, electronic imaging systems should become commercially available to show the endoscope configuration without X-rays. Until then most units perform colonoscopies in the ordinary endoscopy area, and either never use X-rays or arrange to have access to a mobile image intensifier or to an X-ray screening room on the rare occasions that it is needed.

Colonoscopes

Colonoscopes are engineered somewhat similarly to upper gastrointestinal endoscopes. They have a more flexible shaft, CO_2 insufflation and syringe-operated lens-washing facilities. The bending section of the colonoscope tip is also longer and so more gently curved, to avoid impaction in acute bends such as the splenic flexure. Ideally the colonoscope's control-section ergonomics will be modified (with a tracker ball or similar mechanism controlling power-steering facilities) to make one-handed steering and activation of the different buttons and switches easily possible, leaving the right hand free to manage the shaft. Present control mechanisms are almost unchanged from those of early gastrocameras and gastroscopes and are far from ideal for the more finicky steering required during colonoscopy.

Ignoring the slight variations between different makes of colonoscope, there are significant advantages in choosing the 'right colonoscope for the job' both at the stage of purchase and for particular patients. Long colonoscopes (165–180 cm) are able to reach the caecum even in redundant colons and are our preferred choice; the longer shaft needs careful handling and accessories take longer to insert. Intermediate-length instruments (130–140 cm) are considered by many to be a good compromise, and almost always reach the caecum. The 70 cm instruments used for flexible sigmoidoscopy have the advantage that the endoscopist knows from the onset that he is doing a quick procedure and is not tempted to go further and prolong it. However, flexible sigmoidoscopy can be performed with a longer instrument, so there is little need for a flexible sigmoidoscope in an endoscopy unit compared to its essential role in the office of a primary-care physician or a general clinic facility.

Paediatric colonoscopes, of intermediate length and smaller diameter (9–10 mm) are ideally available with either standard or 'floppy' shaft characteristics. They are invaluable for the examination of babies and children up to 2–3 years of age (see pp. 266–267) but also have a role to play in adult endoscopy. As well as allowing examination of strictures, anastomoses or stomas impassable with the full-sized colonoscope, they are often much easier to pass through areas of tethered postoperative adhesions or severe diverticular disease. Floppy paediatric instruments are particularly comfortable and easy to insert to the splenic flexure, tending to conform to the loops of the colon and to form a spontaneous 'alpha' loop which avoids difficulty in passing to the descending colon. The smaller diameter of the shaft is, however, less easy to torque or twist and is more easily damaged if used routinely for more extensive examination. For limited adult examinations, as for strictures or diverticular disease, a paediatric gastroscope can also be used (and has the bonus of an even shorter bending section, but the disadvantage of limited downward angling capability). Its very stiff shaft makes it less suitable for total colonoscopy in small children and babies than the paediatric colonoscope.

Video-colonoscopes, since they do not need to be held near the endoscopist's face, have both positional and hygienic advantages as well as allowing everyone to see and bringing all the benefits of high-resolution electronic-image handling. Nonetheless, a fibre-colonoscope used with a new generation 'video adaptor' or charged couple device (CCD) camera brings many of the same benefits.

Large channel size has particular advantages during colonoscopy. It permits aspiration of fibrous food residues or polyp fragments which would otherwise cause blockage and allows fluid aspiration whilst standard accessories (snare, biopsy forceps, etc.) are in place; dilatation balloons can be introduced with less trauma and larger accessories passed, such as the clipping device or the 'jumbo' forceps (for more certain diagnosis of malignancy or inflammatory disease). Larger or double-channel instruments usually have a marginally greater shaft diameter and consequent slightly stiffer handling characteristics. Doubtless, engineering skills will in future allow increased channel size without this small penalty, which is in any case of less concern during colonoscopy than in upper endoscopy.

Stiffness of the colonoscope shaft is generally an advantage to an expert but in the hands of an inexpert endoscopist can overstretch loops painfully and necessitate a routine of heavy sedation—which further removes any need for subtlety. Stiff or 'hard' colonoscopes are therefore not ideal for everyone. Floppier or 'soft' shaft instruments perhaps tend to loop more easily, but when they do will conform more easily to the colon and cause less stretch pain, and respond more easily to dexterity in handling. Selection of colonoscope shaft characteristics is therefore a matter of opinion. Ideally the anatomy of the individual patient would also be a factor; this is inapparent until the first examination, but a recommendation can sometimes be made for subsequent visits. Thus, a patient with a very redundant colon is best examined with a stiff instrument, whereas a floppier instrument will do better in a short colon with adhesions.

Few endoscopists have the luxury of having a variety of

instruments available. It is therefore important when buying a colonoscope to consider its likely major use, and in the individual patient to select one with regard to the clinical situation and the distance to be examined (and the tortuosity of the colon if a previous barium enema is available). The most experienced endoscopists are the least worried by changing instruments, but vary amazingly in their opinions as to what is the ideal — longer/shorter, more or less stiff—which suggests that there will never be such a thing as a single 'ideal' colonoscope. A physician who will want to be sure of being able to examine the proximal colon must either have a long instrument or have an intermediate-length instrument with a split overtube and/or fluoroscopy available. A busy unit needs at least two functional colonoscopes used alternately to permit adequate disinfection during a routine list; a third standard instrument should be available as a backup during any period of breakdown. A surgeon who is only interested in occasional and left-sided examinations or peroperative procedures will be satisfied with a single instrument of intermediate length. Ideally any endoscopist should also have access to a paediatric endoscope for special cases.

Accessories

All usual accessories such as biopsy forceps, snares, retrieval forceps or baskets, sclerotherapy needles, cytology brushes, washing catheters, dilating balloons, etc. are used down the colonoscope. Long- and intermediate-length accessories work equally well down shorter instruments, so it is sensible to order all accessories to suit the longest instrument in routine use. Other manufacturers' accessories also work down any particular instrument and, since some are better than others, it is worth taking advice when buying replacements.

   The only specialized accessory in colonoscopy is the stiffening tube, stiffener or split overtube, the use of which is described later (p. 246). Although not used by many endoscopists, and potentially hazardous if wrongly used, it is still very occasionally invaluable in avoiding recurrent loop formation of the sigmoid colon, for exchange of instruments or for retrieving multiple polyps.

Carbon dioxide

Most colonoscopes have CO_2 buttons, but few colonoscopists use CO_2 insufflation. This is because, with the exception of bowel preparation using mannitol (and other similar agents such as sorbitol, lactulose or lactitol), colonoscopic bowel preparation has been shown to leave no residual explosive gas in the colon as a polypectomy hazard. However, even for routine examinations, the use of CO_2 offers the striking advantage that it clears 100

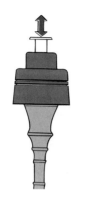

Fig. 9.2 A CO$_2$ button can replace the normal air button.

times faster than air (through the circulation, to the lungs and then breathed out). This means that after CO$_2$ insufflation the colon and small intestine are free of any gas in 15–20 min, whereas air distension can remain and cause abdominal discomfort for many hours, especially in patients with functional bowel symptoms. Colonoscopy with CO$_2$ insufflation can, therefore, be followed immediately by a DCBE or scanning, whereas residual air distension, especially if antispasmodics have been used, will increase the amount of barium needed to fill and then coat the colon and may degrade the quality of the examination. In the unlikely event of perforation or gas leak (pneumoperitoneum), air under pressure would add to the hazard whereas rapidly absorbed CO$_2$ and a well-prepared colon should markedly reduce it. Any patient with ileus, pseudo-obstruction, stricturing, severe colitis, diverticular disease or functional bowel disorder should benefit from the added safety and comfort of using CO$_2$ rather than air insufflation.

In some instruments it is now possible to fit a CO$_2$ insufflation button (Fig. 9.2) as a replacement in the usual air button position, which makes instrument handling easier than activating an alternatively sited CO$_2$ button. Cheaper low-pressure, metered-flow CO$_2$ delivery systems are also becoming available, which removes the previously valid objection that CO$_2$ was cumbersome to use and expensive to install.

Principles of colonoscopy

Embryological anatomy

The embryology of the colon is complex, especially in terms of mesenteries and attachments, which explains the extraordinarily variable configurations which can result during colonoscopy. The fetal intestine and colon lengthen into a U-shape on a longitudinal mesentery (Fig. 9.3a) but, as the whole embryo at that stage is only 1 cm long, become forced out into and rotate within (Fig. 9.3b) the umbilical hernia which is normal at this 5-week stage (Fig. 9.3c). The gut loop thus differentiates into the small and large intestine outside the abdominal cavity. By the third month of development the embryo is 4 cm in length and there is room within the peritoneal cavity for first the small and then the large intestine to be returned into the abdomen. This occurs in a fairly predictable manner, with the end result that the colon is rotated around so that the caecum lies in the right hypochondrium and the descending colon on the left of the abdomen (Fig. 9.4a). With further elongation of the colon, the caecum normally 'migrates' down to the right iliac fossa. At this stage, the mesentery of the transverse colon is free but then the mesenteries of the descending and ascending colon, pushed against the peritoneum of the posterior abdominal wall, fuse with it and are

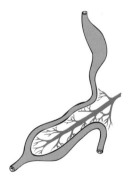 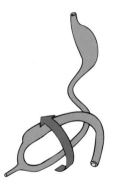 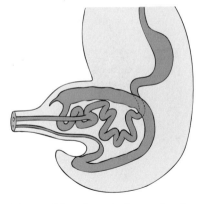

Fig. 9.3 (a) The fetal intestine and colon start on a longitudinal mesentery . . .

(b) . . . then rotate as the small intestine elongates . . .

(c) . . . and from 5 weeks (1 cm embryo) to 3 months (4 cm embryo) are in the umbilical hernia.

absorbed so that the ascending and descending colon become retroperitoneal (Fig. 9.4b).

In some cases *incomplete fusion* of the mesocolon and posterior wall occurs and a variable amount of the original mesocolon remains, resulting in variable mobility of the right and left colon. How often this incomplete fusion occurs is not clear from the literature, but a persistent descending mesocolon has been found in postmortem studies in 36% and an ascending mesocolon in 10% of subjects. The persistence of a descending mesocolon explains most of the strange configurations caused by the colonoscope in the left colon and splenic flexure (Fig. 9.5). Occasionally the caecum fails to descend and becomes fixed in the right hypochondrium (Fig. 9.6); in others, where a free meso-

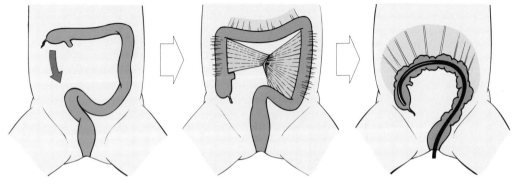

Fig. 9.4 (a) The embryonic colon extends on its mesentery at 3 months' gestation . . .

(b) . . . then partial fusion of the mesentery and peritoneum occurs at 5 months . . .

(c) . . . although sometimes the mesocolons persist.

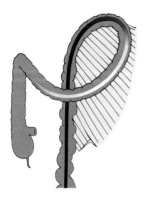

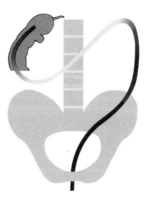

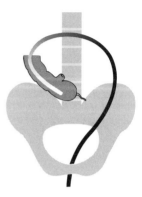

Fig. 9.5 Persistent descending mesocolon or mesentery.

Fig. 9.6 Inverted caecum.

Fig. 9.7 Mobile caecum.

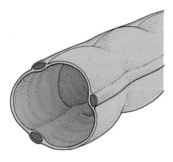

Fig. 9.8 The longitudinal muscle bundles (taeniae coli) bulge visibly into the colon.

colon persists, the caecum remains completely mobile (Fig. 9.7). Peroperative studies that we have undertaken show that colons in Oriental subjects are more predictably fixed than those in Western subjects.

The *musculature* surrounding the colon develops as three external longitudinal muscle bundles or taeniae coli and, within these, the circular muscles. Both muscle layers are sometimes visible to the endoscopist (Fig. 9.8), one or more of the taeniae as an inward longitudinal bulge and the circular musculature as fine reflective indenting in the mucosal surface. Haustral folds segment the interior of the colon; those that are prominent in the proximal colon sometimes create 'blind spots' whereas their muscular hypertrophy in diverticular disease can also create mechanical difficulties for the endoscopist.

Instrument characteristics

There are various basic points relevant to colonoscope handling that are worth highlighting before considering the anatomical variations and complexities that are encountered in practice.

Colonoscopy involves the insertion of a long flexible tube with a steerable tip through a long flexible cylinder which is elastic and can move around unpredictably. It is thus no surprise that the technique and its results are also unpredictable, multifactorial and dynamic—changing from moment to moment in a way that is often difficult to understand, let alone to simplify sufficiently to explain in print or to teach. Effectively, the endoscopist is like a puppeteer propelling a snake puppet by the tail, with control of its head, a view through its eyes, but scant idea of what is happening to its body because this is invisible within the abdomen.

Some of the problems of colonoscopy, and the tricks for overcoming them, relate primarily to the instrument characteristics. For instance the clinician used to rigid proctosigmoidoscopy is not used to the perverse tendency of the colonoscope to flex when it is pushed; he therefore tends to lose patience, use force and is surprised that insertion becomes increasingly difficult (and painful) as loops inevitably form.

1 *Straight is good* is therefore a cardinal principle in colonoscopy. A straight instrument will respond instantly to delicate shaft movements, whether in/out or rotational, with no force. If this responsive feeling is lost, because of looping, it can easily be regained by the simple expedient of pulling back—as one would need to do repeatedly if forced to *push* a flexible hosepipe (something which, in other circumstances, no sane person would think of doing).

2 *Pulling back is the most important move in colonoscopy.* Any fool can push, and most do — relentlessly. When pulling back, the shaft straightens so that it, the angling wires within it and the controls all become more responsive; conversely the colon shrinks or convolutes, reducing peritoneal and mesentery stretch and so making the patient more comfortable.

3 *Twisting the shaft only affects the tip when the shaft is straight* (Fig. 9.9). When a loop is present in the shaft, twisting forces applied will be lost within it (as well as moving the loop of colon). When the shaft is straight, twist becomes an excellent way to corkscrew or 'slalom' around bends. This is particularly useful if the angle to be traversed is acute or fixed, because simply trying to push around will encounter severe resistance (and so often result in looping rather than progress).

4 *Twist will have the most steering effect when the tip is angled*, and the same twist will have an opposite steering effect depending on whether the tip is up or down (Fig. 9.10).

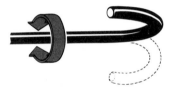

Fig. 9.9 Twist only affects the tip if the shaft is straight.

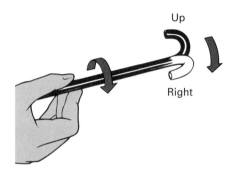

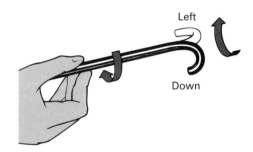

Fig. 9.10 With a clockwise shaft twist: (a) an up-angled tip moves to the right . . .

(b) . . . and a down-angled tip moves to the left.

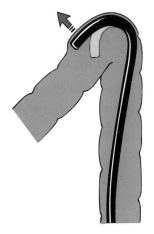

Fig. 9.11 The lateral control knob angulation has little effect if the tip is maximally up/down-angled.

Fig. 9.12 De-angulate at the splenic flexure to avoid impaction —the 'walking-stick handle' effect.

5 *Steering with the control knobs has least effect when the tip is already angled.* Try this outside the patient. When one control knob is fully angulated, applying the other one swivels the bending section a little but hardly affects the degree of angulation (Fig. 9.11). Vicious steering movements are therefore rarely helpful (but can damage the angling control wires).

6 *A fully angulated tip will not slide along the colon.* It is easy to forget, in the quest to get a view around bends, that overangling can be counterproductive (the 'walking-stick handle' phenomenon) (Fig. 9.12).

7 *An impacted tip cannot be steered.* Try it yourself. Hold the very tip of the bending section firmly and operate the angling control(s); the shaft will move because the tip cannot (Fig. 9.13). This is a limiting factor of flexible endoscopes, and is why the endoscopist is sometimes so impotent in fixed diverticular disease or a tight stricture.

8 *Twisting often increases or decreases a loop.* Loops formed by the colonoscope within the colon usually have a 3D spiral configuration, clockwise or anticlockwise. Try out on the table top the effect of twist. Clockwise twist applied to a clockwise spiral will tend to straighten it (or progress it forward if the tip is free to slide) (Fig. 9.14a). Anticlockwise twist of the same loop will do the opposite and make the spiral worse (or cause it to slide back if it is not fixed) (Fig. 9.14b). Applying the appropriate steady twisting force (torque) to the shaft can sometimes therefore be very helpful in either progressing, straightening or keeping it straight.

Instrument handling

The majority of skilled endoscopists favour, as we do, the 'single-handed' or 'one-man' approach, but there are still experts working successfully with the 'two-man' method, using an assistant to manipulate the shaft.

Single-handed colonoscopy. This depends on the endoscopist managing the colonoscope controls mostly or wholly with the left

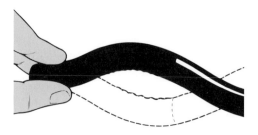

Fig. 9.13 If the tip is fixed it cannot be steered (the shaft moves instead).

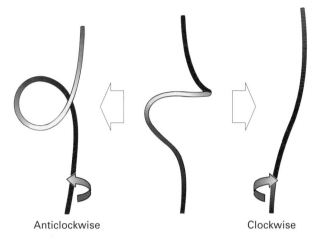

Anticlockwise   Clockwise

Fig. 9.14 A clockwise spiral is straightened by a *clock*wise twist. An *anti*clockwise twist worsens it.

hand, leaving the right hand free to hold the shaft (Fig. 9.15). The endoscopist should stand relaxed (see also p. 54), with the control section held in whatever position is comfortable and the shaft gripped 25–30 cm away from the anus (to avoid too fre-

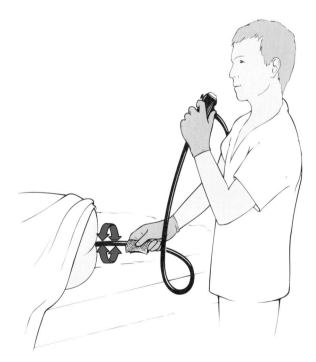

Fig. 9.15 Single-handed manoeuvring of the instrument shaft.

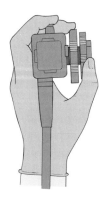

Fig. 9.16 The thumb can reach the lateral control knob if the hand is positioned appropriately.

quent changes of grip and jerky insertion which result from holding close to the anus, as many do).

For those with a reasonably large hand it is practicable for the left thumb to reach both the up/down and the lateral control knob (Fig. 9.16). Single-handed steering is made easier if the *first finger alone* operates the air/water or suction buttons and the second finger (forefinger) acts as *'helper'* to the thumb in managing the angling controls. In practice, the skilled single-hander mostly achieves lateral movement by shaft rotation transmitted to the up- or down-angulated tip rather than bothering with the lateral control knob. The result is to 'slalom' or twist around bends, particularly those in the distal colon, in a surprisingly fluent manner (providing the instrument can be kept reasonably straight).

Those with a small hand may be unable to reach the lateral control knob and may need, from time to time, to use the right hand for this purpose. This means briefly letting go of the instrument shaft whilst the angulation is made. Some endoscopists position the patient so that they can lean and trap the shaft transiently against the couch whilst the right hand is otherwise occupied. If the right hand is used too often the endoscopist is not using rotatory movements enough; if it is too long away from the shaft and working the lateral knob he is being indecisive — it takes at most a second or two to make an angling adjustment.

Shaft grip should at all times be with a paper towel or gauze square, for the combined reasons of hygiene and better grip. The most dexterous grip is, as when rolling a cigar, mainly between the thumb and two fingers (Fig. 9.17), rather than the more restricted and clumsy control which results from holding the shaft in the clenched fist. If you do not believe this, try rolling a pen maximally around in your fingers, and compare this with the half-rotation which is the most that can be accomplished in the fist—which is effectively a wrist movement.

Two-man colonoscopy. This allows the endoscopist to use the control body of the instrument in the way that it is, unfortunately for the colonoscopist, currently designed — namely with the left hand working the up/down control (and air/water/ suction buttons) and the right hand kept for the right/left angulation control knob. The assistant performs the role ascribed to the right hand of the single-handed endoscopist, pushing and pulling according to the spoken instructions of the endoscopist. A good assistant learns to feel the shaft to some extent and to apply some twist. More often, an assistant pushes with concealed gusto, causing unnecessary loops that are inapparent to the endoscopist.

It is perfectly possible to get the best of both worlds if the endoscopist takes over the shaft from the assistant from time to time, particularly when the shaft is being withdrawn, so getting a 'feel' of the situation and being able to make his own judge-

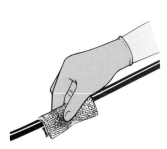

Fig. 9.17 The instrument shaft should be held delicately between the thumb and fingers.

ments. Unless the endoscopist/assistant team is well-honed and interactive the two-man approach to colonoscopy can be as illogical and clumsy as would be expected of two people attempting any intricate task, neither knowing fully what the other is doing.

Handling the colonoscope

Our rationale for preferring the *single-handed* approach to colonoscopy has been covered previously (pp. 212–214). With so many different instruments, techniques, hand sizes and degrees of dexterity, it is pointless to suggest that there is only one method of handling an endoscope, although the single-handed method seems to us the most logical and is favoured by most skilled colonoscopists. Others prefer an assistant to advance and withdraw the instrument, especially during the learning phase and difficult phases of insertion. The exact handling technique is unimportant if it is relaxed, gentle and effective. However, anyone who achieves less than 95% total colonoscopy (when indicated), hurts patients, needs to use heavy sedation or has complications during diagnostic colonoscopy needs to re-assess their technique.

The stance should be relaxed for what can be a prolonged examination and the endoscopist should also hold the colonoscope in a relaxed manner. Colonoscopy mostly requires fine and fluent movements, like those of a violin player, and similarly balanced position and handling are needed.

Hand control and finger skills are of paramount importance. For single-handed endoscopy, each hand is disciplined to fulfil only its appropriate tasks; the left hand holds the instrument in balance, manages the air/water/suction buttons and up/down control knob (see Fig. 9.15) with minor adjustments of left/right angling as well (see Fig. 9.16), while the right hand controls the shaft of the instrument with only occasional major alterations to the lateral control knob. Because the colon is a continuous series of short bends requiring multiple combinations of tip and shaft movement and frequent air/water and suction button activations, small delays and unco-ordinated movements rapidly summate to prolong the procedure unnecessarily. Handling efficiency can be considerably increased by the simple means of disciplining the fingers of the left hand (Fig. 9.18) so that (as detailed above) the left forefinger alone activates the air/water/suction buttons and only the left thumb and left middle finger control the up/down angling knob. By using just the two littlest (third and fourth) fingers to grip the control body, the middle finger assumes an invaluable role as 'helper' to the thumb in managing the angling controls; this role is especially important for major up or down angulations, for which purpose the middle finger steadies the control knob when the thumb needs to shift position.

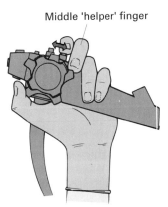

Middle 'helper' finger

Fig. 9.18 Single-handed control: the forefinger alone activates the air/water and suction knobs; the middle finger acts as 'helper' to the thumb for angulation.

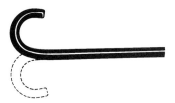

Fig. 9.19 A single-handed dexterity test: five full up/down angulations can be done in 20 s.

A table-top dexterity test which can be done to demonstrate the problems, or to check the efficiency of left-hand angling technique, is to time five full bending section retroflexions from maximally up to maximally down (with no help from the right hand); it can be done in around 20 s (Fig. 9.19). Adding full lateral angulation at each maximal up and maximal down position, skewing the tip first in one direction and then in the other, challenges the one-hand finger control of even the most dexterous. Such extreme movements are not often needed except for the occasional difficult polypectomy or awkward bend when the right hand is otherwise occupied, but the training exercise is useful in showing up limitations in finger skills.

Shaft handling must be equally dexterous. Whereas in gastroscopy the instrument runs a short and fixed course, so that looping and twisting of the shaft is of less relevance, in endoscopic retrograde cholangiopancreatography (ERCP) the need for the mechanical efficiency of a straight endoscope position is well recognized; it is just as important in colonoscopy, if inward push is to be transmitted to the tip and if the endoscope is to work to maximal efficiency. The mechanical construction of an endoscope, with its protective wire claddings and four angling wires, means that each shaft loop both increases the resistance of the instrument to twisting/torquing movements and decreases tip angulation by causing friction in the angulation wires. Shaft loops are also as counterproductive *outside* the patient as inside the abdomen. Thus the shaft should be made to run in an easy curve to the anus, without unnecessary bends, and any loops forming outside the patient should be derotated and straightened. This is best done by rotating the control body to transfer the loop to the umbilical, which can accommodate up to three to four loops without harm to its internal structures (Fig. 9.20). Where possible the shaft of the long colonoscope should be arranged on the table so as to make it easy to twist clockwise, since this is such a frequent action.

The right hand makes rotational twisting/torquing movements of the shaft and also feels whether the shaft moves easily (is straight) or there is resistance (due to looping). To feel and manipulate the shaft deftly, hold it in the fingers (see Fig. 9.17) as you would any other delicate instrument (and not in the fist like a hammer or an offensive weapon). Rolling the shaft between the fingers and thumb allows major steering rotations with minimal effort. Quick, almost reflex, logical responses and co-ordination between the right and left hands develop with practice; colonoscopy, from slow deliberate beginnings, thus becomes a rapid and fluent procedure.

Concentration is also vital. Whilst being relaxed in stance and instrument handling, obsessional attention to keeping the endoscopic view at all times is a key aspect of efficient and accurate colonoscopy. The endoscopist, if he is not to lose orientation

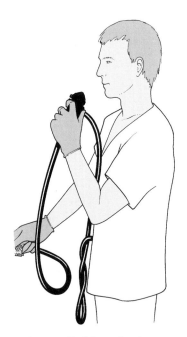

Fig. 9.20 Shaft loops forming *outside* the patient can be transferred to the umbilical by rotating the control body.

or miss diagnostic minutiae, must learn to be able to suppress normal social reflexes such as looking at the patient or endoscopy room staff when talking to them. It is perfectly possible to converse or give instructions without eye contact and often important to do so. Some acute bends or small polyps, for instance, may slip from view in the moment that the endoscopist looks away and then take a surprising time to find again. Intense concentration, on both mechanical and visual aspects of the procedure, makes colonoscopy quicker and more efficient. It takes all the endoscopist's faculties to assess the view, predict the correct action, keep a running mental log of decisions taken and their result, so as constantly to optimize the situation or to reverse it rapidly when necessary. Colonoscopy is an algorithm of small responses to ever-varying situations and it takes alertness, motivation and concentration to make the best of it.

Anus and rectum

Endoscopic anatomy

The anal canal, 3 cm long, is lined with sensitive squamous epithelium to the squamocolumnar junction or 'dentate line'. Sensory innervation, and so mucosal pain sensation, may in some subjects extend several centimetres higher into the distal rectum. Around the canal are the anal sphincters, normally in tonic contraction. The anus may be deformed, scarred or made sensitive by present or previous local pathology, including haemorrhoids or other conditions—and normal subjects may be sore from the effects of bowel preparation.

The rectum, although reaching only 15 cm proximal to the anal verge, may have a capacious 'ampulla' in its midpart as well as three or more prominent folds (valves of Houston) which create potential blind spots, in any of which the endoscopist can miss significant pathology. Digital examination, direct inspection and, where appropriate, a rigid proctoscope are needed for complete examination of the area. Prominent, somewhat tortuous veins are a normal feature of the rectal mucosa and should not be confused with the rare, markedly serpiginous veins of a haemangioma or the distended, tortuous ones in some cases of portal hypertension.

The rectum is extraperitoneal for its distal 10–12 cm, making this part relatively safe for therapeutic manoeuvres such as removal or destruction of sessile polyps; proximal to this it enters the abdominal cavity, invested in peritoneum.

Insertion

Pre-check the endoscope and equipment. All functions of the endoscope, light source and accessories should be thoroughly checked before insertion. In particular make sure that air (or CO_2) insufflation is fully operational, with no rinse water remaining in the air channel. The tip should bubble briskly when held underwater (if in doubt wrap a rubber glove around the tip and watch it inflate). It is very easy during the examination to think the colon is hypercontractile and difficult to inflate when in fact one of the connections is loose, the insufflation button misplaced or faulty, or the air outlet semi-obstructed, any of which will result in decreased pressure and so only partial function. Polishing the objective lens with a silicone stick or spectacle lens fluid helps to keep it clean during the examination.

Insertion through the anus should be gentle. The instrument tip is unavoidably blunt (the necessity for flat lenses means that it cannot be streamlined), so too fast or forcible an insertion may be quite uncomfortable for patients with tight sphincters or sore anal epithelium. The squamous epithelium of the anus and the sensory mechanisms of the anal sphincters are the most pain-sensitive areas in the colorectum, and digital examination or insertion of the endoscope should be done carefully. The patient is in the left lateral position, lying as comfortably as possible, and the endoscopist dons examination gloves. A clear water-soluble jelly (e.g. K-Y or local anaesthetic lubricating jelly) is best but some use oil or even silicone liquid, which is messier; additional lubrication may be needed from time to time during the procedure to minimize friction and so keep a good 'feel' of the shaft.

Many start with two gloves on the right hand and perform a digital examination with a generous amount of lubricant before inserting the instrument, both to check for pathology in this potentially 'blind' area and to prelubricate and relax the anal canal. Alternatively, a large blob of lubricant jelly can be squeezed out over the anal orifice and the instrument inserted directly through it (Fig. 9.21a), which saves a glove and a few

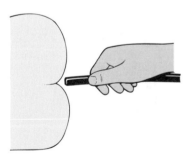

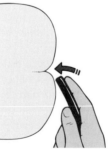

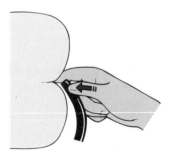

Fig. 9.21 Different methods of colonoscope insertion: (a) straight on through the jelly . . .

(b) . . . finger support of the bending section . . .

(c) . . . or the tip pushed in as the examining finger withdraws.

seconds; inflating air down the endoscope whilst pressing the tip into the anal canal gives direct vision and facilitates insertion. Sometimes the instrument tip will pass in more easily if pressed in obliquely, supported by the examiner's forefinger until the sphincter relaxes (Fig. 9.21b). Alternatively, the examiner can use his thumb to push the tip inward along the line of his examining forefinger as this withdraws from the anal canal (Fig. 9.21c). The tendency of the bending section to flex can be avoided by starting with it straight, fixing the control knob brakes and pressing in gently.

Particularly tight or tonic sphincters may take some time to relax; asking the patient to 'bear down' is said to help this. Allowing an extra 15–20 s, if necessary, for sphincter relaxation is a humane start to proceedings, especially for a patient with anorectal pathology or anismus; the sphincters of colitis patients are noticeably more tonic than normal, presumably because of the longstanding need to keep control.

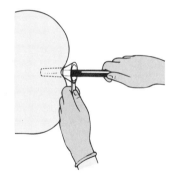

Fig. 9.22 Video-proctoscopy.

Video-proctoscopy

If a rigid proctoscope is used the patient can be shown the appearances by the simple expedient of inserting the video-endoscope tip up the proctoscope once the insertion trocar is removed. The colonoscope simultaneously provides a convenient source of illumination and an excellent close-up view. The endoscopist can perform video-proctoscopy (Fig. 9.22) entirely from the monitor view, with the opportunity of taking tape or videoprints — which in many cases of 'unexplained bleeding' persuasively show the patient and referring doctor the likely (haemorrhoidal) origin.

Rectal insertion

After the scope has been inserted into the rectum there is usually little to see except a 'red-out' because the rectal mucosa is pressed against the lens. At this point, the following steps should be performed in sequence:

1 *Insufflate air* to distend the rectum.

2 *Pull back* and angulate or rotate slightly to find the lumen (this is the first of many times during the examination when withdrawal, inspection and cerebration bring success more quickly than following instinct and pushing blindly).

3 *Rotate the view so that any fluid lies inferiorly.* The suction port of the colonoscope tip lies just below the bottom right-hand corner of the image (Fig. 9.23) and should be selectively placed in the fluid before activating the suction button. To do this co-ordination will be required between forcible shaft rotation with the right hand and synchronous compensatory up or down angulation with the left hand so as to keep the view. During examina-

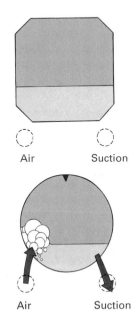

Air   Suction

Air   Suction

Fig. 9.23 The suction/instrumentation port opens below and to the right of the view; the air port opens below and left.

tion a skilled single-handed endoscopist often uses twist to steer or 'corkscrew' the tip; the capacious rectum is the ideal place in which to practise this; the need to suction fluid efficiently is a good reason to do so.

4 *Aspirate fluid or residue* to avoid any chance of anorectal leakage during the rest of the examination, when instrument pressure, in/out movements and air insufflation often combine to give the patient a distressing illusion of being incontinent.

5 *Push in*, finally, only when an adequate view has been obtained, and only as fast as a reasonable view can be obtained.

6 *Corkscrew or 'slalom' round the first few bends*, using up or down angulation and shaft-twist alone to achieve most lateral movements, rather than unnecessarily using the lateral angulation control. This is an economic way of steering in at this stage and demonstrates the efficacy of finger twist when the shaft is straight—which it inevitably is in the rectosigmoid region.

Retroversion can be important since the rectum, often being very capacious, can be surprisingly difficult to examine completely. Care is needed to combine angling and twist movements sufficiently to see behind the major folds or valves. In a capacious rectum the most distal part is a potential blind spot but the generous size of the rectal ampulla will make tip retroflexion easy. Look around to choose the widest part, angulate both control knobs fully and push gently inward to invert the tip towards the anal verge (Fig. 9.24). Retroversion is not always possible in a small or narrowed rectum, but in a narrow rectum the wide-angled (140°, nearly 'fish-eye') lens of the endoscope should see everything without risk of blind spots.

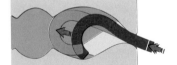

Fig. 9.24 Angulate both knobs and *push in* to retrovert.

Sigmoid and descending colon

Endoscopic anatomy

The distal colon, needing to cope with formed stools, has a thick circular musculature which results in a tubular appearance (Fig. 9.25) broken by the ridged indentations of the haustral folds. The three external taeniae coli or longitudinal muscle bundles are only seen to indent if the sigmoid or descending colon are unusually capacious. From the internal view, extracolonic structures, probably muscle tissue, are occasionally seen as a blue-grey discoloration through the colonic wall (less obviously than the spleen or liver more proximally); vascular pulsations of the adjacent left iliac artery are frequently visible in the mid- or proximal sigmoid.

The sigmoid is 40–70 cm long when stretched by the instrument during insertion, although it will crumple down to only 30–35 cm once the instrument is straightened fully — which is why careful inspection is important during insertion if lesions are not to be missed during the withdrawal phase. The sigmoid

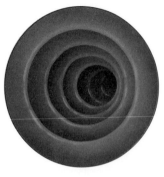

Fig. 9.25 The distal colon is usually circular.

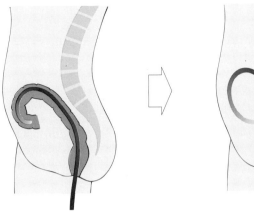

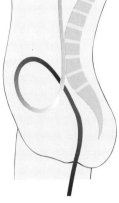

Fig. 9.26 (a) The sigmoid colon loops anteriorly . . .

(b) . . . then passes up into the left paravertebral gutter.

colon mesentery is inserted in a V-shape across the pelvic brim, but is very variable in both insertion and length, and also quite frequently modified by adhesions from previous inflammatory disease or surgery. In elderly subjects the sigmoid colon anatomy is often narrowed and deformed internally by the thickened circular muscle rings of hypertrophic diverticular disease, and sometimes also fixed externally by pericolic post-inflammatory processes. The redundant and prolapsing mucosal folds overlying the muscular rings in diverticulosis often appear reddened from traumatization and sometimes focally inflamed as well (Plate 9.1). After hysterectomy the distal sigmoid colon can also be angulated and fixed anteriorly onto the area previously occupied by the uterus.

The 3D anatomy of the distal colon is relevant to understanding both the spiral loops that can form and the basis of the rotatory movements and tricks with which they can be managed. The inserted colonoscope may stretch the bowel to the limits of its attachments or the confines of the abdominal cavity. The shape of the pelvis, with curved sacral hollow and the forward-projecting sacral promontory, cause the colonoscope to pass anteriorly (Fig. 9.26a) so that the shaft can often be felt looped onto the anterior abdominal wall before it passes posteriorly again to the descending colon in the left paravertebral gutter (Fig. 9.26b). The result is that an anteroposterior loop occurs during passage of the sigmoid colon and, since the descending colon is usually laterally placed, it forms a clockwise spiral loop (Fig. 9.27); the importance of this will be discussed later (see pp. 235–6). When the sigmoid loop runs anteriorly against the abdominal wall it is possible partially to reduce or modify the sigmoid looping of the colonoscope by pressing against the left lower abdomen with the hand (Fig. 9.28).

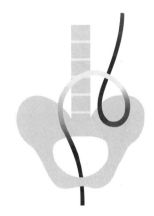

Fig. 9.27 Sigmoid loop—anterior view (clockwise spiral).

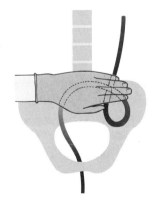

Fig. 9.28 Hand pressure restricts the sigmoid spiral loop.

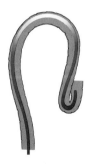

Fig. 9.29 Fixed (iatrogenic) hairpin bend at the sigmoid–descending junction.

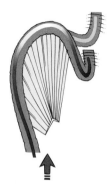

Fig. 9.30 The length of mesentery and the extent of retroperitoneal fixation determine the acuteness of the sigmoid–descending junction.

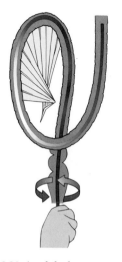

Fig. 9.31 An alpha loop—a beneficial iatrogenic volvulus.

The descending colon is normally bound down retroperitoneally and ideally runs in a fixed straight line which is easy to pass with the colonoscope, except that there is usually an acute bend at the junction with the sigmoid colon (Fig. 9.29). This junction is only a theoretical landmark to the radiologist but, once the sigmoid colon is deformed upwards and outwards by the inserted colonoscope shaft, becomes a very real challenge to the endoscopist. The acuteness of the sigmoid–descending angle depends on anatomical factors, including how far down in the pelvis the descending colon is fixed, and also on colonoscopic insertion technique. A really acute hairpin bend results when the sigmoid colon is long or elastic enough to make a large loop and the retroperitoneal fixation of the descending colon happens also to be low in the pelvis (Fig. 9.30). Sometimes, when the sigmoid colon is long an alpha loop occurs, which avoids any angulation at the sigmoid–descending junction. The 'alpha' is the fluoroscopic description of the spiral loop of sigmoid colon twisted around on its mesentery or sigmoid mesocolon in what is, in effect, a partial iatrogenic volvulus (Fig. 9.31). Formation of the loop depends on the anatomical fact that the base of the sigmoid mesocolon on its short inverted 'V' at the pelvic brim allows easy rotation (Fig. 9.31).

Mesenteric variations from the norm occur in at least 15% of subjects because of partial or complete failure of retroperitoneal fixation of the descending colon *in utero* (see p. 209). The result is persistence of varying degrees of descending mesocolon, which in turn has a considerable effect on what shapes the colonoscope can push the colon into during insertion; the descending colon can, for instance, run up the midline (Fig. 9.32) or allow a 'reversed alpha' loop to form (Fig. 9.33). Surgeons are well aware that there is great patient-to-patient variation in how easily the colon can be mobilized and delivered outside the abdominal cavity; occasionally the whole colon can be lifted out without dissection. A mobile colon which is 'easy' for the surgeon is, however, often extremely unpredictable and difficult for the endoscopist.

Insertion—principles for sigmoidoscopy and colonoscopy

The objective is to insert the endoscope gently, but in a reasonably short time, because it is the push and mesenteric (or peritoneal) stretch of the insertion phase that is uncomfortable or painful for the patient. Full inspection should be on the return journey—although better views of some areas are obtained on the way in when the colon is stretched; any small polyps seen should therefore be destroyed during the insertion phase, as they can easily be missed in the shortened colon on the way back. The paradox of flexible endoscopy is that aggression and attempts at speed are often self-defeating because of a combination of factors: the tendency of the instrument tip to get bent up in folds, of its shaft to flex into counterproductive loops and of the colon to be squashed into impossibly tight configurations. If the object of the examination is a limited view up the sigmoid these factors are often less important, but if the intention is to reach the caecum it is fundamental to understand the principles for efficient insertion and how to avoid or remove the loops that can form.

In nine patients out of 10 (the exceptions being those with colons fixed by adhesions or impossibly long and loopy or, worst of all, a combination of both) colonoscopy can be made a virtually painless, even enjoyable, experience. The sigmoid colon is an elastic tube (Fig. 9.34). Inflated it becomes long and tortuous; deflated it is significantly shorter. When stretched by a colonoscope the bowel forms loops and acute bends (Fig. 9.35) but if shortened down by the same colonoscope it can be telescoped into a few convoluted centimetres (Fig. 9.36) (rather like pushing a coat- or shirt-sleeve up to expose the arm). The following are simple principles for comfortable and safe insertion.

1 *Suction air frequently and fluid infrequently.* Whenever fully distended colon is seen or if the patient feels discomfort it takes only a second or two to suction off excess air until the colon outline starts to wrinkle and collapse, making it shorter and also easier to manipulate. In contrast, after having evacuated fluid from the rectum, only aspirate fluid during the rest of the insertion phase when absolutely necessary to keep a view, and only do so when there is enough air present and a good enough view to suction accurately (sucking blind when already immersed is

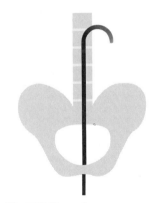

Fig. 9.32 The endoscope may push a fully mobile distal colon up the midline.

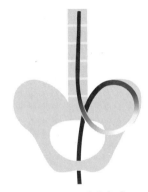

Fig. 9.33 A reversed alpha loop due to a persistent descending mesocolon.

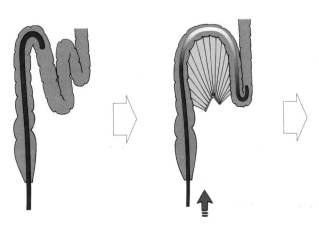

Fig. 9.34 The sigmoid colon is an elastic tube . . .

Fig. 9.35 . . . pushing loops it . . .

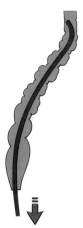

Fig. 9.36 . . . but pulling back shortens and straightens the colon.

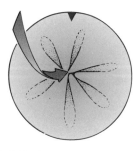

Fig. 9.37 Aim at the convergence of folds.

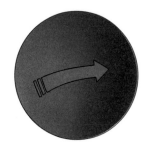

Fig. 9.38 Aim at the darkest area.

usually rather ineffectual). During insertion there will be numerous local 'sumps' or pools of residual fluid; aspirating each one wastes a lot of time, loses the view and requires reinflation. It is usually possible to inflate a little and steer in over the fluid level rather than plunging into it and having to suction. Even solid stool can often be successfully passed, deliberately angling the tip to slide along the mucosa for a few centimetres rather than impacting against a bolus, which can coat the lens irrevocably. Any residue can easily be suctioned or removed from view by changes of patient position on the way back when a perfect view is important.

2 *Insufflate as little as possible.* Gentle air insufflation is needed throughout the examination, except when there is an excellent view. The policy is 'as much as necessary, as little as possible'; it is essential to see, but counterproductive and uncomfortable to overinflate. Remember that bubbles are caused by insufflating under water, which can usually be avoided by the simple means of angling above it. If fluid preparation and bile salts do result in excessive bubbles, these can be dispersed instantly by injecting an antifoam preparation solution containing particulate silicone down the instrument channel.

3 *Use all visual clues.* A perfect view is not needed for progress; but the correct direction or axis of the colonic lumen should be ascertained *before* pushing in. The lumen when deflated or in spasm is at the centre of converging folds (Fig. 9.37).With only a partial or close-up view of the mucosal surface, there are usually sufficient clues to detect the luminal direction. Aim towards the darkest area, worst illuminated because it is furthest from the instrument and nearest the lumen (Fig. 9.38). The convex arcs formed by visible wrinkling of the circular muscles (Plate 9.2), the haustral folds or the highlights reflected from the mucosa over them, all indicate the centre of the arc as the correct direction in which to angle (Fig. 9.39). The slight bulge of the underly-

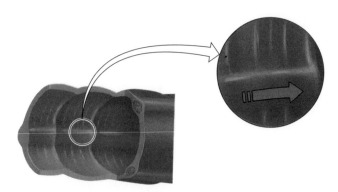

Fig. 9.39 Aim at the centre of the arc formed by folds, muscle fibres or reflected highlights.

ing longitudinal muscle bundles (taeniae coli) is another, occasionally useful, clue. The expert can make his steering decisions on evidence which would be inadequate for the beginner. On the other hand, each time the expert is 'lost' for more than 5–10 s he pulls back quickly to regain the view and re-orientate, whereas the beginner can flounder around blindly for a minute or more in each difficult spot and is surprised that the overall examination takes so long.

4 *Steer carefully and cautiously.* Steering movements should be early, slow and exact (rather than jerky and erratic). A slow start to each angulation movement allows it to be terminated at once, within a few degrees of travel, if it proves to be moving the tip in the wrong direction. A rapid steering movement in the wrong direction can simply lose the view altogether, quite unnecessarily, and then tends to be corrected by another large movement so that the effect is to flail around—often hopelessly, certainly inelegantly. Each individual movement should be slow and purposive and every action during insertion should be thought out and executed in response to the view, or whatever visual clues there are to suggest the correct luminal direction.

5 *If there is no view, pull back at once.* If lost at any point in the examination, keep the control knobs still or let them go entirely, insufflate and then gently withdraw the instrument until the mucosa and its vascular pattern slips slowly past the lens in a proximal direction (Fig. 9.40); follow the direction of slippage by angling the controls or twisting the shaft and the lumen of the colon will come back into view. Thrashing around blindly with the instrument rarely works; *pulling back* must do, for the bending section self-straightens if left free to do so.

6 *Rehearse steering actions before bends while there is a good view.* Unlike the stomach, where there is usually sufficient room to see what is happening during steering manoeuvres, colonic bends are unforgivingly tight and it is very easy to become unsighted and uncertain when angling around them. Stop before any acute bend and try out, whilst stationary and still able to see, the best steering movements to use within it.

7 *Use the lateral angling knob as little as possible.* There are a limited number of possible tip-steering movements for the single-handed endoscopist:

(a) the easiest is up/down thumb control (left hand);

(b) the next easiest is clockwise/anticlockwise twist (right hand);

(c) the least convenient is left/right angling (by the thumb on the lateral knob or taking the right hand off the shaft to activate the lateral control knob).

Thus, when steering, first angle up or down as appropriate; next, rather than using the right/left control knob, try rotating the instrument shaft clockwise or anticlockwise with the right hand. Because the tip is already slightly angled this rotation should

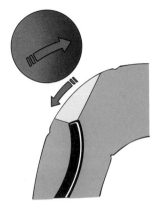

Fig. 9.40 Pull back when lost—the mucosa slides away in the direction of the lumen.

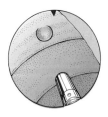

Fig. 9.41 (a) If a lesion is badly placed for the suction/instrumentation channel . . .

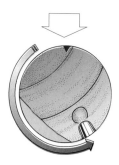

(b) . . . rotate the straightened shaft to target it optimally.

corkscrew it around laterally (see Fig. 9.10), precisely and quickly, and will often make use of the lateral control knob unnecessary.

8 *Use twist and torque.* With the single-handed method, twisting the shaft becomes second nature and a most essential part of the colonoscopist's range of tricks and manoeuvres. It should be appreciated, however, that there are three different twisting effects:

(a) *twisting with the shaft and tip straight* rolls the instrument around on its axis. This can be useful to re-orientate the biopsy forceps, injection needle or polypectomy snare into the ideal quadrant to target a particular lesion, or to place the suction channel precisely over a fluid pool to be aspirated (Fig. 9.41). When approaching a bend, twisting may adjust the axis of the instrument so that up/down angulation alone will steer around the bend. Appreciating the 'free and easy' feel and responsiveness of a really straight colonoscope to twist and push/pull movements is an essential part of skilled colonoscopy;

(b) *twisting with the shaft straight but the tip angulated* deviates the tip very rapidly according to the direction of twist and angulation. Thus with the tip angled up, twisting clockwise moves it right (see Fig. 9.10); with the tip down, the same clockwise twist will move it left (droop or cock your wrist and then rotate the forearm one way or the other to simulate this). Such corkscrewing movements are particularly effective when the colon is fixed, as by adhesions or diverticular disease, or when the tip is already acutely angulated in a sharp bend;

(c) *twisting with a loop in the shaft will alter the position of the loop,* and often its size and configuration as well. Because the course of most sigmoid colon loops is spiral (usually a clockwise spiral due to shaft passage anteriorly from the pelvis and curving laterally and posteriorly into the descending colon (see Fig. 9.27)), twist is particularly effective in this region. Since the colonoscope is free to move within the colon, but the colon itself is fixed at the rectum and retroperitoneally in the descending region (as well as being constrained by the anterior and lateral abdominal wall), a clockwise twist will also usually shorten (pleat/accordion) the mobile sigmoid over the shaft, whilst the tip moves forward up the fixed descending colon. Other spiral loops (large alpha, large N, reversed splenic or 'gamma' loops) need to be first reduced in size by pulling back before they can be successfully twisted about and straightened in the confined space of the abdominal cavity.

9 *Torque is the application of continued twist* whilst inserting or withdrawing the instrument. Clockwise torque is a major help in keeping the colonoscope shaft straight in the sigmoid colon whilst advancing up the descending colon, but also in controlling the sigmoid (and other potential loops) during the later phases of insertion. Whether to torque/twist clockwise or anticlockwise is an empirical decision according to results, but with conventional mesenteric anatomy clockwise is the more likely to help. Remember that if torque is being applied in one direction (e.g. clockwise) to affect a loop, any attempt to use corkscrewing or twist steering movements in the opposite direction will be counterproductive.

10 *Push little and slowly, pull often and fast.* The challenge to the endoscopist is to progress the instrument tip without losing the view or causing the shaft to flex unnecessarily. For both reasons pushing movements should start slowly, giving time for simultaneous twist or steering movements and also allowing the endoscope to slide in (rather than just buckle and loop, as tends to happen with a rapid push). By contrast, withdrawal movements needed to straighten out loops in the shaft and colon must be vigorous to be fully effective. The commonest mistake of the less experienced endoscopist is to be overcautious in pulling back, compared to the expert who will start withdrawal movements very quickly and only slow down when the tip starts to slip back excessively, the shaft feels straighter and more responsive or the 'catapult' feel of pulling against the hooked tip becomes apparent.

11 *Be aware of the 'feel' of the straight endoscope.* For much of the insertion the colonoscope should feel as free and responsive in the fingers as a gastroscope does. The endoscopist should expect to feel the same precise and easy responsiveness to shaft movement or twist that a pool or snooker player gets from his cue. If this 'free and easy' feeling is lost, a loop has been formed and should be removed as soon as possible, for the sake of the patient's comfort and easier insertion.

12 *'Set up' bends so that steering around them is easy.* During ERCP, orientation of the endoscope tip into the midline axis is an essential preliminary to easy cannulation; similarly in upper gastrointestinal endoscopy, when passing around the greater curve to the gastric antrum and pylorus, the instrument is made to run in the midline (see Figs 4.21 and 6.14). Similarly, the colonoscopist should, whenever possible, adjust the instrument so that an acute bend can be passed with its axis upwards or downwards (for easy thumb steering), as well as optimizing mechanical efficiency by having the colonoscope shaft straight (for better push) and the bending section not overangled (to help it slide around). A good 'racing line' is fundamental to ski and car racing and, at infinitely slower speed, is just as applicable to atraumatic flexible endoscopy.

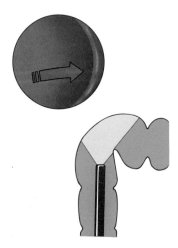 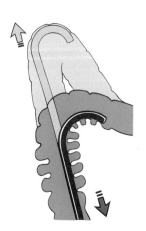

Fig. 9.42 Endoscopic view of an acute bend, with a bright fold on the angle, and the 'aerial' view.

Fig. 9.43 Pulling back flattens out an acute bend and improves the view.

Sigmoid colon 'slalom' or corkscrewing technique

Single-handed manoeuvring is particularly useful in the multiple bends of the sigmoid, where co-ordination with an assistant can be difficult. Each of the succession of serpentine bends requires a conscious steering decision. The quicker and more accurately each decision is made, the faster the whole examination will be. It is easier to judge direction around a bend from afar, so the tip should not be rushed into it. First observe the bend carefully from a distance; it will be seen as a bright semi-lunar fold of mucosa against the shadowed background (Fig. 9.42). Having decided on the direction to be taken, try out in mini-movement rehearsal (a few millimetres or degrees of movement are enough) the best combination of angling and rotation needed to steer around correctly when subsequently pushing through the bend, often close-up and relatively blind. If finger rotation of the shaft is used much of the sigmoid can be traversed with little or no use of the lateral angling knob, the angled tip corkscrewing first one way and then the other round the succession of bends.

Acute and mobile bends

Having angled in the correct direction, if the view is poor gently pull back the angled/hooked tip, which should simultaneously reduce the angle, shorten the bowel distally, straighten it out proximally and disimpact the tip to improve the view (Fig. 9.43). If all fails, de-angle, pull back below the bend again and re-check its direction more carefully; the colon can rotate on its attachments and the nature of bends may change during manoeuvring, any rotation being visible in close-up as a rotation of the visible vessel pattern (Fig. 9.44; Plate 9.3); watching the direction towards which the vessels rotate indicates in which direction to follow a mobile bend.

Hook and withdraw frequently

As soon as an acute bend is passed and a luminal view is regained, the instrument should be withdrawn again to shorten the loop that forceful insertion will inevitably have caused. Trying to pull back repeatedly and as much as feasible (bearing in mind the small possibility of damage) after every major bend is at the basis of colonoscopy. 'Hook and withdraw' is the concept; the practicality is that steering around an acute bend automatically produces a 'hooked' tip, so the bend is the best landmark for trying withdrawal. Pulling back, especially having just pushed in, is instinctively unnatural to most endoscopists, and yet one of the most important points of technique. However much of a struggle has been involved in rounding a bend, as soon as the tip is well past it, the instrument is withdrawn until catapult-like shaft resistance is felt and the tip is beginning to slide back, indicating that the shaft is as straight as possible.

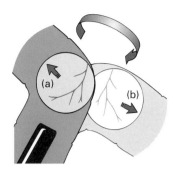

Fig. 9.44 Rotation of the vessel pattern (from (a) to (b)) indicates the rotation of the colon, so the endoscopist needs to change the steering direction.

Corkscrew during withdrawal

As the endoscope straightens out the tip will start to respond to shaft twist but also, if there is any spiral element, it will often advance slightly without any need to push. At any major bend try first pulling back fairly forcibly and then applying twist one way or the other. When this works it makes the most of the 3D configuration of the colon and minimizes the need to push and so form unnecessary loops. The classic expression of this pull-and-twist approach (deflating also helps) is at the sigmoid–descending junction, where the anatomy often favours clockwise twist both to corkscrew round into the descending colon and to hold the sigmoid straight. The result is a most satisfying feeling for the endoscopist of 'getting something for nothing', quite apart from avoiding pain for the patient.

Check the inserted shaft distance from time to time

As well as the responsive 'feel' of the straightened shaft, the appropriate depth of insertion for the probable anatomical location is a valuable cross-check. The straightened endoscope at the sigmoid–descending junction should be at 40–45 cm; any greater distance means that a significant sigmoid loop remains, which will make direct insertion into the descending colon more difficult than necessary. Similarly, the straight endoscope at the splenic flexure is at around 50 cm only, and the caecal pole should be at 70–80 cm.

Avoid overangulation

At all times manoeuvre the instrument until the best reasonable view of the bend or lumen ahead is obtained with the minimum of angulation. Overangling into a 'walking-stick handle' position (see Fig. 9.12) inevitably means that it is going to be difficult to persuade the tip to slide around that particular bend. Taking a few seconds at any bend, even a minute or so at a major bend, to optimize the view but minimize angulation pays dividends in avoiding the need to push forcefully and the tendency to re-loop the shaft.

If necessary push hard—but then withdraw again

As an absolutely last resort, if it is quite certain that the instrument is pointing in the correct direction but attempts at angling and twisting and simultaneous gentle pull or push have not given a luminal view, it *is* permissible simply to push blind for a few centimetres around a bend. Providing the tip is pointing correctly, it should slip gradually over the mucosa with the 'slide by' appearance of the mucosal vascular pattern traversing the field of view. Continue to push if 'slide by' continues smoothly; stop if the mucosa blanches (indicating excessive local pressure) or if the patient experiences pain (indicating undue strain on the bowel or mesentery).

Similarly, if repeated attempts at a more subtle approach have failed but the direction is certain, it may be better to warn the patient and push in calculatedly than to struggle on indefinitely or to abandon the procedure when clinical indications for it are strong. It should not be necessary to push strongly and uncomfortably like this *for more than 20–30 s at the most*; the instrument can then be straightened back rapidly, taking the strain off the colon and its attachments and making the patient comfortable.

How does an 'expert' make insertion look so easy?

Much of sigmoidoscopy (and colonoscopy) is a matter of patience—'two steps forward and one step back'. Impatience or relentless pushing tend to result in loops, pain and a slower examination in the end. The more experienced colonoscopist, being more careful and rational, and using less air, ends up with fewer acutely angled bends. He also steers accurately in spite of the more restricted view of an only partially inflated and shorter bowel. He is more fluent because he chooses the right combination of movements to move the tip in the desired direction, with simultaneous twist, push or pull as necessary to straighten the bowel or advance the tip, without losing control or sense of luminal direction. He slows down, or even pulls back, before an acute bend to maintain a view at all times. Whilst he does nothing fundamentally different from the beginner, there are fewer mistakes, little waste of time and effort, and the colonoscope seems magically to snake up the colon.

In the learning phase the two commonest reasons for becoming 'stuck', particularly in the sigmoid colon, are either that the instrument has become looped and jammed in a bend (it should be withdrawn as far as possible both to straighten it out and get a proper view) or simply that, having manoeuvred into the right position, the endoscopist has not the courage of experience to 'slide by' through the difficult area. Warn the patient of stretch pain and then push hard for a few seconds to get around the bend—before pulling back to straighten it out again.

Be prepared to abandon

A caveat is called for. Not *every* sigmoid colon can be safely intubated. Operative or peridiverticular adhesions may fix the pelvic colon so as to make the attempt impossible or dangerous. If there is difficulty, if the instrument tip feels fixed and cannot be moved by angling or twisting and the patient complains of pain during attempts at insertion, there is a danger of perforation and the attempt should be abandoned. Sometimes a different endoscope (e.g. paediatric) or another endoscopist may succeed, but only a very experienced colonoscopist with very good clinical reasons should risk the patient and instrument under these circumstances; usually the most experienced are the most prepared to stop.

Adhesions and diverticular disease

Adhesions, as after hysterectomy, cause angulation and difficulty but rarely result in failure because of the ability of the colon to straighten over the instrument. Even in severe diverticular disease, where there are the difficulties of a narrowed lumen, pericolic adhesions and problems in choosing the correct direction (Fig. 9.45a), once the instrument has been laboriously inched through the area, the 'splinting' effect of the abnormally rigid sigmoid usually facilitates the rest of the examination. In the presence of diverticular disease the secret is extreme patience, with care in visualization and steering, combined with greater than usual use of withdrawal, rotatory or corkscrewing movements. It helps to realize that a close-up view of a diverticulum means that the tip must be deflected to a right angle (by withdrawal and angulation or twist) to find the lumen (Fig. 9.45b). Using a thinner and more flexible paediatric colonoscope or gastroscope may make an apparently impassable narrow, fixed or angulated sigmoid colon relatively easy to examine — which sometimes also saves the patient from surgery.

In some patients with very hypertrophic circular musculature

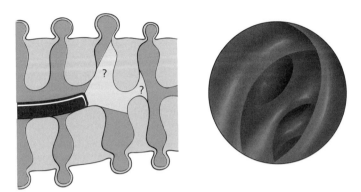

Fig. 9.45 (a) Choosing the correct path can be difficult in diverticular disease . . .

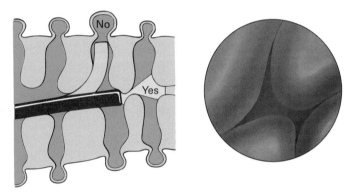

(b) . . . a circular view is a *diverticulum*—the lumen will be at 90° and is often squashed.

in diverticular disease, and redundant mucosal folds as well, it can be very difficult to obtain an adequate view. An occasionally useful trick is to distend the segment with water; the water jet has the combined advantages of being non-compressible, remaining in the dependent sigmoid colon (rather than the tendency of air to rise and distend the proximal colon) and holding the mucosal folds away from the lens to keep at least a partial view.

Sigmoid–descending junction

All colonoscopists occasionally, and the inexperienced frequently, have trouble in passing into the descending colon because, having rounded the sigmoid with panache, they probably have stretched up a large sigmoid spiral N-loop (Fig. 9.46) and created iatrogenic difficulty. An endoscopist who has been more careful, using less air and frequent withdrawals should

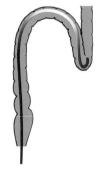

Fig. 9.46 An N-loop stretching up the sigmoid colon.

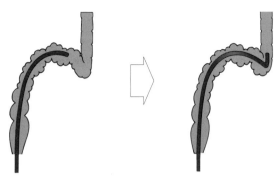

Fig. 9.47 (a) Pull back and deflate to keep the sigmoid short . . .

(b) . . . which may allow direct passage to the descending colon.

be rewarded by a straighter or even direct passage from the sigmoid to descending colon (Fig. 9.47). On the other hand a large spiral alpha loop may be formed during insertion, intentionally or unintentionally, but nonetheless resulting in easy passage (see p. 237). So much depends on the anatomy of the particular patient that anything can happen and the colonoscopist may need all his skills and some luck to pass this region reasonably quickly and without undue pain. The sigmoid–descending colon junction is often the most difficult part of colonoscopy and the greatest challenge to the endoscopist.

Although the endoscopist may not be certain when he has reached the proximal sigmoid, the appearance of an acute bend at approximately 40–70 cm is suggestive evidence, particularly (in the left lateral position) if it is water-filled. The sigmoid–descending junction can be so acute as to appear at first to be a blind ending, especially if the bowel is overinflated. In a capacious colon there may be a longitudinal fold pointing towards the correct direction of the lumen, caused by the muscle bulk of a taenia coli (Fig. 9.48 & Plate 9.4); follow the longitudinal fold closely to pass the bend.

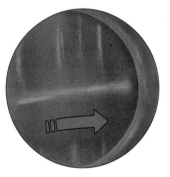

Fig. 9.48 At acute bends a longitudinal bulge (taenia coli) shows the axis to follow.

'Direct passage' to the descending colon

It can prove difficult to wriggle the tip around the sigmoid–descending bend, particularly when it has been made acute by a large N-loop. As soon as the tip is even partially round these steps should be followed:

1 *Pull back* the shaft to reduce the loop, which creates a more favourable angle of approach to the junction and also optimizes the instrument mechanics.

2 *Apply abdominal pressure*, the assistant pushing on the left lower abdomen so as to compress the loop or reduce the abdominal space within which it can form.

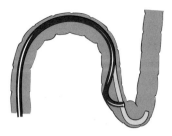

Fig. 9.49 'Pre-steer' before pushing into an acute bend.

3 *Deflate the colon* (without losing the view) to shorten it and make it as pliable as possible and help to relax the flap-like inner angle of the sigmoid–descending bend.

4 *'Pre-steer'* into the bend, the tip being steered at the mucosa just before the inner angle (Fig. 9.49), so that on pushing in the pre-steering causes the tip to slip past the angle to point straight at the lumen of the descending colon.

5 *Try shaft twist* in case the configuration allows corkscrewing force to be applied to the tip, which may have the very satisfying effect of swinging it around the bend with no inward push pressure required.

6 *Changing the patient to the right lateral position* can improve visualization of the sigmoid–descending junction (air rises, water falls) and may sometimes also cause the distal descending colon to drop down into a more favourable configuration for passage.

7 *Use of force to 'push through' the loop* should be the last resort. Having warned the patient to expect discomfort, a few seconds of careful 'persuasive pressure' may slide the instrument tip successfully around the bend and then allow straightening again.

'Clockwise twist and withdrawal' manoeuvre

Once the tip is successfully hooked into the descending colon the colonoscope must be straightened to allow direct upwards passage of the shaft too. Pulling back is effective in doing this because the tip is now retroperitoneal and relatively fixed (Fig. 9.50a). An inevitable, but unwanted, consequence of pulling

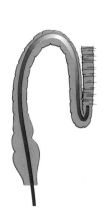

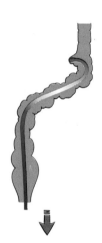

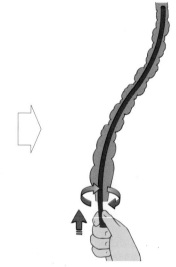

Fig. 9.50 (a) The tip is hooked into the retroperitoneal descending colon, then pulled back . . .

(b) . . . and when the endoscope is maximally straightened the tip is re-directed . . .

(c) . . . and the endoscope pushed in, with clockwise twist, into the descending colon.

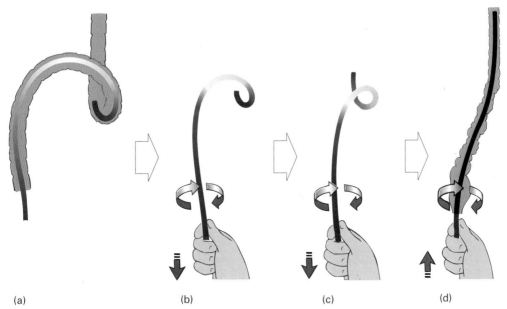

(a)   (b)   (c)   (d)

Fig. 9.51 (a) An N-loop with the tip at the sigmoid–descending junction . . . (b) . . . twist clockwise and withdraw . . . (c) . . . keep twisting and find the lumen of the descending colon . . . (d) . . . then push in (still twisting to avoid re-looping).

back is that the hooked tip will impact into the mucosa. A complex simultaneous movement is needed, combining withdrawal with tip steering towards the lumen of the descending colon (Fig. 9.50b). A wrong move at this point will lose the critical retroperitoneal fixation and the instrument will fall back into the sigmoid. Careful interpretation of the close-up view, minimal insufflation, twist, delicate steering movements and patience are all needed to pass in without re-looping (Fig. 9.50c), which results from excessive push or tip impaction. The importance of using clockwise torque rotation to prevent re-looping of the straightened instrument is such that this method of direct passage has been called by Shinya the 'right twist (clockwise) withdrawal' manoeuvre. The 3D looping of the sigmoid colon, with both left/right and anteroposterior components creating a clockwise spiral is illustrated (Fig. 9.51) to show why twisting is so important at this stage.

'N' or spiral sigmoid looping

Some degree of looping of the endoscope in the sigmoid is unavoidable.The usual N-loop in the sigmoid colon can be anything from a minor deviation (which may, however, be fixed and not straightenable) following hysterectomy or previous diverticulitis, to a huge loop reaching towards the diaphragm in some patients with a redundant or megacolon. The exact shape will vary from moment to moment according to the constraints of the abdomen, the mesenteries and the activities of the endoscopist propelling or twisting the colonoscope. Although based on its typical anteroposterior fluoroscopic appearance, the loop is conventionally described as an N-loop; it is actually a 3D spiral of which the N-type is mainly rotated to occupy the left side of the abdomen, whilst the alpha-type is rotated more to the right side. Most N-loops can eventually be straightened out completely by including a degree of forcible twisting (usually clockwise) to assist in undoing the spiral element. For shorter loops it is worth attempting this during passage through the sigmoid colon, or certainly when the sigmoid–descending junction is reached, so as to attempt direct or 'straight scope' passage to the descending colon, as described above.

With a longer colon, complete removal of the N-loop may be difficult until the instrument tip has reached nearly to (or around) the splenic flexure, so as to give adequate purchase at the bending section, for forcible withdrawal. With some colons that seem to have no acute bends to angle around, it may even be necessary to fix both control knobs in maximum angulation, simply wedging the tip against the colon wall to get a hold and allow straightening without slippage. However, as for direct passage, manual pressure by the assistant in the left lower abdomen will often help by reducing or minimizing the size of the loop (see Fig. 9.28), acting as a buffer to transmit some of the inward push on the shaft laterally towards the descending colon. If the assistant can actually feel the loop, the objective is to reduce it back towards the pelvis (i.e. with downward, as well as inward, pressure). Although it is worth the endoscopist trying one or two withdrawal movements to shorten the N-loop, especially near the apex of the sigmoid colon but also at any obvious fold or bend which allows 'hooking', often there is little to be done until the sigmoid junction is reached and an attempt can be made at the 'clockwise twist and withdrawal' manoeuvre, described above.

The troublesome N-loop

Most of the difficulties experienced later in the examination whilst passing the proximal colon (splenic flexure, transverse colon and hepatic flexure) also stem from recurrent or persistent N-looping in the sigmoid. This removes the motive power of the endoscopist's inward push unless the loop can be avoided, removed or at least minimized. It is for this reason that repeated straightening, clockwise shaft twist and assistant hand pressure over the sigmoid colon can still be important when inserting through the proximal colon. N-looping is also the major cause of pain during colonoscopy.

Pain in the sigmoid

Remember that if the patient experiences excessive pain there is a potential danger of damage to the bowel or mesentery. In the longest colons there may be a sufficient length of sigmoid colon and mesentery to let the instrument loop below the sigmoid–descending junction and to pass relatively easily into the descending colon without the acute hairpin bend usually formed when an N-loop is present (Fig. 9.52). Having to use force or cause pain is inelegant and to be avoided if possible. However, it may be preferable for the patient to suffer briefly and get the instrument into the descending colon quickly and successfully rather than to struggle on and on with repeated failed attempts at gentle passage, particularly as the analgesic effects of i.v. pethidine diminish considerably by about 5 min after administration. Before using force, and at any stage during colonoscopy when pushing in may cause pain due to looping, the patient is warned beforehand (e.g. 'this will hurt for a few seconds, but there is no danger'). Inward push should also be applied gradually, avoiding any sudden shoves and should be limited to a tolerable time—no more than 20–30 s. Looping pain stops at once when the instrument is withdrawn slightly. There is no excuse for long continued periods of pain, even in those miserable examinations when recurrent looping cannot be avoided.

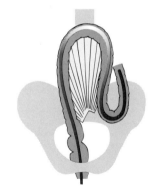

Fig. 9.52 A very long sigmoid may allow the scope to loop enough to avoid a hairpin bend.

The alpha loop and manoeuvre

When the colonoscope is passed through the sigmoid colon it can form spontaneously into the configuration known as an alpha loop (Fig. 9.53). From the endoscopist's point of view, the formation of an alpha loop is a blessing, as there is no acute bend between the sigmoid and descending colon and the splenic flexure can always be reached. If, during insertion, no particularly acute flexure is encountered in the sigmoid colon and the instrument appears to be sliding in a long way without problems or acute angulations, it can be suspected that an alpha loop is being formed. If so (especially if confirmed on fluoroscopy or the imager) it is better to spend a little time and care passing to the proximal descending colon or splenic flexure at 90 cm (sometimes even around the splenic flexure into the transverse colon) before trying any withdrawal/straightening manoeuvre. Straightening half-way round an alpha loop can cause the alpha configuration to flop across and form back into the more difficult N-loop.

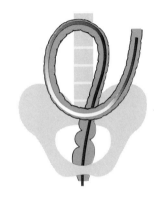

Fig. 9.53 An alpha loop.

The alpha manoeuvre is the intentional formation of an alpha loop. This was originally always performed using fluoroscopy and was an important dodge in the 1970s when first colonoscopes would only angulate 90° or less, making it sometimes

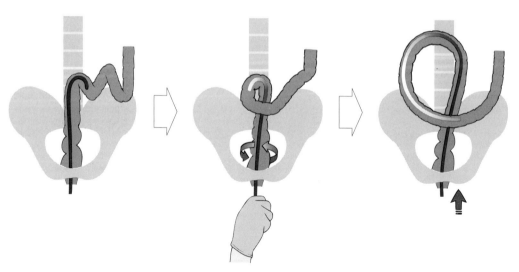

Fig. 9.54 (a) At the first sigmoid colon bend, 15–20 cm from the anus . . .

(b) . . . rotate the angled tip counterclockwise . . .

(c) . . . and push in to make an alpha loop.

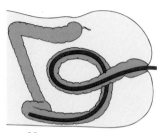

90cm

Fig. 9.55 In an alpha loop the scope runs through the fluid-filled descending colon to the splenic flexure at 90 cm (posterior view).

impossible to steer around into the descending colon. If the colon is known to be long or feels long and mobile during normal insertion into the distal sigmoid colon, it is worth trying to make an alpha loop so as to avoid the greater problems of an N-loop. The principle is to twist the sigmoid colon around into a partial volvulus (see Fig. 9.31), which is easy to demonstrate but difficult to explain. As soon as the instrument is felt to be angling upwards into the distal sigmoid colon at around 15–20 cm from the anus (Fig. 9.54a), start to rotate the shaft firmly counterclockwise at every opportunity, so that the angled tip swings anteriorly across the pelvic brim to point towards the caecum, pulling the sigmoid colon across with it (Fig. 9.54b). Continue the insertion through the sigmoid with as much counterclockwise twist as possible at all stages and avoid clockwise twist (so that the loop does not swing back to the 'N'-position). Equally, do not withdraw or attempt to straighten the shaft (even if the patient has mild stretching pain) but push (Fig. 9.54c) and steer carefully until the tip has passed through the fluid-filled descending colon to the splenic flexure, reached at 90 cm (Fig. 9.55).

It is *not* always possible to achieve the alpha manoeuvre. Endoscopists who claim 'always' to do so are shown, when they demonstrate their technique under fluoroscopy, equally often to form an unrecognized N-loop, which they pass with elan (and extra sedation because of the pain). A short or fixed sigmoid mesocolon probably prevents the formation of an alpha loop;

thus patients with diverticular disease or any other cause of peri-colic adhesions are not suitable for the manoeuvre, and are most unlikely to form a spontaneous alpha loop.

Straightening an alpha loop

Any loop puts some stress and limitation on tip angulation due to friction in the control wires, as well as often being uncomfortable for the patient, so it is logical to remove the alpha loop at some stage. Opinions differ concerning the correct time to do so. With current very flexible and full-angling instruments, it is occasionally better to attempt to pass straight on into the proximal transverse colon with the alpha loop in position rather than to straighten it at the splenic flexure and then have difficulty with re-looping.

Most colonoscopists prefer to straighten out the alpha loop as soon as the upper descending colon is safely reached and to pass the splenic flexure with a straightened instrument. However, every colonoscopist has also experienced the chagrin of struggling to reach the descending colon and the frustration of seeing the tip slide back out of the descending colon when an attempt is made, too early, to withdraw and straighten the shaft. A reasonable compromise is to pass the tip up to, but not necessarily around, the splenic flexure at about 90 cm and then to take care that it does not slip back excessively during removal of the alpha loop. If fluoroscopy is used the whole alpha loop cannot be seen in one fluoroscopic field and the best plan is to centre the view over the point where the looped shaft crosses itself. If the instrument is seen to be slipping back too far down the descending colon, it is quickly advanced again and the tip hooked or wedged around the splenic flexure for extra support before repeating the straightening manoeuvre.

The alpha loop is straightened by combined withdrawal and clockwise derotation. Slightly withdrawing the shaft initially reduces the size of the loop and makes derotation easier, but the tip can start to slide down the descending colon; derotation alone will undo the alpha volvulus of the sigmoid into the 'N' position, but does not reduce the size of the loop. The two actions must be combined by simultaneously pulling back and twisting the whole instrument (Fig. 9.56). Strong clockwise twist during straightening will tend to push the tip up towards the splenic flexure and any tendency of the tip to slip back can usually be stopped by applying more twist and less pull. Twisting forces are not harmful to the colonoscope.

Again there is a caveat. Derotation should be easy and atraumatic; if straightening the loop proves difficult or the patient has more than the slightest discomfort the situation should be reassessed. Adhesions can make derotation difficult and occasionally impossible. Do not use force. The sigmoid loop that has

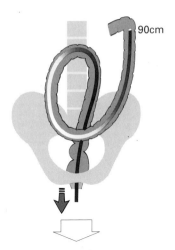

Fig. 9.56 (a) An alpha loop . . .

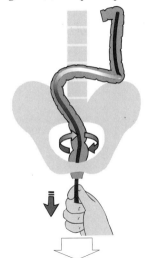

(b) . . . derotates with clockwise twist and withdrawal . . .

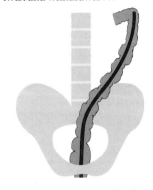

(c) . . . to straighten completely.

formed may not be a true alpha loop but a 'reversed alpha', which can form when there is persistent descending mesocolon and freely mobile left colon (see Fig. 9.33). This reversed loop may need *counter*clockwise derotation during straightening and, in the absence of imaging, the endoscopist must judge this by *feel* (and results).

Loops in the external shaft and umbilical

Having rotated the colonoscope 180° or more in the process of straightening an alpha loop, and probably having made previous clockwise twisting movements as well, it is likely that there will be a resultant loop in the shaft external to the patient. Because of the negative effect that this has on instrument handling, it is my practice to rotate the control body to transfer this loop to the umbilical (see Fig. 9.20) and keep the external shaft straight at all times. Several loops can be accommodated in the umbilical without harm, but sometimes it may be necessary to unplug the instrument from the light source and unravel the umbilical. The alternative for the dexterous, and if the instrument is straight, is to derotate the external shaft loop whilst steering the tip into the lumen so that the colonoscope rotates on its axis within the colon; however, if the shaft is not straight the instrument tends to slip back in the process.

Descending colon

The conventional descending colon is normally traversed in a few seconds as a 20 cm long 'straight'. For the gravitational reasons described above, when the patient is in the left lateral position, there is characteristically a horizontal fluid level within it (Fig. 9.57). Often there is sufficient air interface above the descending colon fluid (or blood in emergency cases) so that the tip can be steered above it. If fluid makes steering difficult, it may be quicker, rather than wasting time suctioning and re-inflating, to turn the patient onto the right side to fill the descending colon with air. Apart from this positional trick, and the frequent use of clockwise twist or hand pressure to minimize sigmoid colon re-looping, no particular skills or manoeuvres are needed in the average descending colon. Sometimes the descending colon is far from straight and the endoscopist, having struggled through a number of bends and fluid-filled sumps believes the tip to have reached the proximal colon when it is in fact only at the splenic flexure.

Distal colon mobility and 'reversed' looping

In the absence of the normal fixation of the descending colon, all normal control and sense of anatomy can disappear; at the most

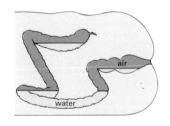

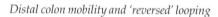

Fig. 9.57 Fluid levels in the left lateral position.

extreme, the colonoscope may run through the 'sigmoid' and 'descending' distal colon straight up the midline (see Fig. 9.32), resulting inevitably in a 'reversed splenic flexure' and consequent mechanical problems later in the examination.

The endoscopist is alerted to the probability that there is partial fixation, with a descending mesocolon allowing the descending colon to deviate medially when *counterclockwise* rotation seems to help insertion at the sigmoid–descending junction. This indicates that an unconventional counterclockwise spiral loop or 'reversed alpha' has been able to be formed by the instrument (see Fig. 9.33), with the corollary that other oddities may occur during insertion. If possible, the endoscopist tries to use this counterclockwise twist and the springiness of the colonoscope shaft to push the mobile descending colon outwards against the lateral margin of the abdominal cavity. This regains the conventional configuration so that the instrument runs medially (rather than in reverse) around the splenic flexure, and is able to adopt the favourable question-mark shape to reach the caecum. Such apparently mysterious manipulations are understandable to anyone who has done colonoscopy under fluoroscopic control or used the electromagnetic imager; they can also be achieved, unknowingly, by an experienced endoscopist without these aids by the simple expedient of responding to the 'feel' of the endoscope, and empirically using whichever twisting movement (in this case counterclockwise) makes the instrument insert most easily.

Splenic flexure and transverse colon

Endoscopic anatomy

The descending colon, after running up the paravertebral gutter, bends medially and anteriorly around the splenic flexure. The splenic flexure is situated beneath the left costal margin, and so is inaccessible to hand pressure. Its position is variably fixed according to the degree of mobility of the fold of peritoneum called the phrenicocolic ligament, which attaches it to the diaphragmatic surface (Fig. 9.58). In some subjects the splenic flexure is relatively tethered up into the left hypochondrium, in others it is relatively free and can be pulled down towards the pelvis (Fig. 9.59). A lax phrenicocolic ligament, a common feature of redundant colons, makes control of the transverse colon difficult by depriving the endoscopist of any fixed point or fulcrum with which to exert leverage during withdrawal manoeuvres (the cantilever or 'balance beam' effect). The configuration of the splenic flexure is also affected by the patient's position, principally because of the effects on it of the transverse colon, sagging down in the left lateral position but pulling on it in a right lateral position (see Fig. 9.66).

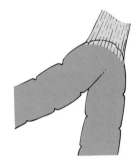

Fig. 9.58 The phrenicocolic ligament.

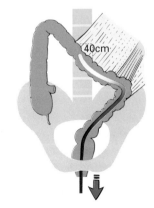

Fig. 9.59 The splenic flexure can pull back to 40 cm if there is a free phrenicocolic ligament.

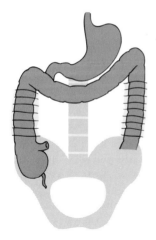

Fig. 9.60 The transverse colon is anterior, over the duodenum and pancreas; the descending and ascending colon are fixed retroperitoneally.

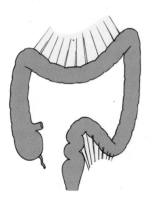

Fig. 9.61 Colon mesenteries—the transverse and sigmoid mesocolons.

The *transverse colon*, which lies anteriorly just beneath the abdominal wall, is held forward by the vertebral bodies, the duodenum and pancreas and relates to the left and right lobes of the liver (Fig. 9.60). It is enveloped in a double fold of peritoneum called the transverse mesocolon (Fig. 9.61) which originates from the posterior wall of the abdomen and hangs down posterior to the stomach, varying considerably in length. In a barium enema study, the transverse colon of 62% of females drooped down to into the pelvis, compared to only 26% of males. This longer transverse loop largely accounts for the 10–20 cm greater mean colon length found in women despite their smaller stature (total colon length was 80–180 cm) and probably also contributes to our experience that 70% of difficult colonoscopies are in females (previous hysterectomy making only a small contribution). The depth of the looped transverse colon also affects the angle at which the endoscope approaches the hepatic flexure, in the same way that the size of the sigmoid colon loop causes an acute sigmoid–descending bend. Because the transverse mesocolon (Fig. 9.62a) is broad-based it does not usually allow a gamma loop to form (Fig. 9.62b). From an anatomical and endoscopic viewpoint, the hepatic flexure is a nearly 180° hairpin bend, similar in many respects to the bend at the sigmoid–descending junction but more constant in its fixation and more voluminous.

The characteristic triangular configuration of the transverse colon (Fig. 9.63 and Plate 9.5) depends on the relative thinness of the circular muscles compared to the longitudinal muscle bundles of the taeniae coli (Fig. 9.64). In some patients (such as those with longstanding colitis but also some normals) the circular musculature is thicker and the transverse colon can be tubular. Both at the mid-transverse flexure and at the hepatic flexure a true 'face-on' view may be obtained of the haustral folds, which present a characteristic knife-edge appearance (Fig.

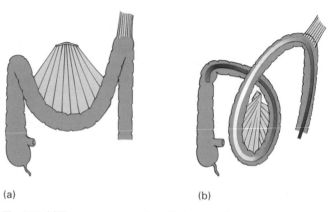

(a)   (b)

Fig. 9.62 (a) Transverse mesocolon. (b) A gamma loop.

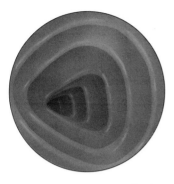

Fig. 9.63 The transverse colon is usually triangular.

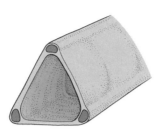

Fig. 9.64 The triangular configuration is due to the taeniae coli.

9.65); it is therefore easy to confuse the mid-transverse flexure with the hepatic flexure. The mid-transverse bend should be less voluminous, show no blue liver patch and may show transmitted cardiac or aortic pulsation; it can also be distinguished by imaging, local palpation of the anterior abdominal wall or transillumination (if the room is darkened).

Insertion

The splenic flexure represents the 'half-time' point during colonoscopy and is an excellent moment at which to ensure that the instrument is properly straightened to 50 cm from the anus and under control before tackling the proximal colon. The commonest reason for experiencing problems in the proximal colon is because the colonoscope has been inadequately straightened at the splenic flexure; persistence of loops make the rest of the procedure progressively more difficult or impossible. If the splenic flexure is passed with straight shaft configuration at 50 cm using the above rules, the rest of a total colonoscopy insertion should usually be finished within a minute or two. Anyone who frequently finds the proximal colon or hepatic flexure difficult to traverse should apply the '50 cm rule' at the splenic flexure, and is likely to find most of the problem solved.

Passage of the splenic flexure is usually obvious when the instrument has passed around the apex of the splenic flexure, because it emerges from fluid into the air-filled, often triangular, transverse colon (see Fig. 9.63 & Plate 9.5). However, whilst the flexible and angled tip section of the colonoscope passes around without effort, the stiffer segment at 10–15 cm at the leading part of the shaft does not follow so easily. This problem is accentuated in the left lateral position, because drooping of the transverse colon causes the splenic flexure to be acutely angled (Fig.

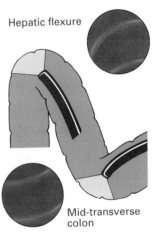

Hepatic flexure

Mid-transverse colon

Fig. 9.65 Similar 'knife-like' haustra are seen at the mid-transverse colon and hepatic flexure.

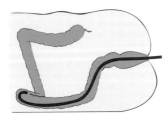 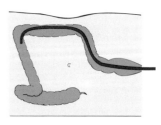

Fig. 9.66 (a) In the left lateral position the transverse colon flops down making the splenic flexure acute . . .

(b) . . . whereas in the right lateral position gravity rounds off the splenic flexure, making it easy to pass.

9.66a) compared to its configuration when opened out by gravity in the right lateral position (Fig. 9.66b).

To pass the splenic flexure, without force or re-looping, follow these rules:

1 *Ensure that the colonoscope is truly straight* and therefore mechanically efficient. Pull back with the tip hooked around the flexure until the instrument is 40–50 cm from the anus, which both straightens any sigmoid loop and pulls down and rounds off the flexure. Note that splenic avulsions or capsular tears have been reported, so be gentle.

2 *Avoid overangling the tip.* Full angulation of a colonoscope can result in the bending section effectively impacting in the splenic flexure, preventing further insertion (the 'walking-stick handle' effect). Having obtained a view of the transverse colon and pulled back, consciously de-angulate a little so that the instrument runs around the outside of the bend (see Fig. 9.12), even if this means worsening the view somewhat — but avoid the tip impacting in the haustral folds.

3 *Deflate the colon* slightly to shorten the flexure and make it malleable.

4 *Apply assistant hand pressure* over the sigmoid colon. Any resistance encountered at the splenic flexure is likely to result in stretching upwards of the sigmoid colon into an N- or alpha loop, which dissipates more and more of the inward force applied to the shaft as the loop increases (Fig. 9.67). It is immediately obvious to the single-handed endoscopist that such a loop is forming, because the 1:1 relationship between insertion and tip progress is lost—in other words, the shaft is being pushed in but the tip moves little or not at all. Pull back again to re-straighten the shaft if this occurs.

5 *Use clockwise torque on the shaft.* As explained above, the clockwise spiral course of the sigmoid colon from the pelvis to its point of fixation in the descending colon means that applying clockwise torque to the colonoscope shaft tends to counteract any looping tendency in the sigmoid colon whilst pushing in

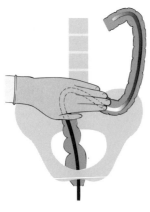

Fig. 9.67 Control sigmoid looping by hand pressure to help pass the splenic flexure.

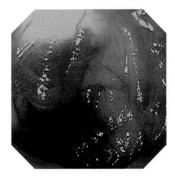

Plate 9.1 Traumatized redundant mucosal folds in diverticular disease, which may show focal inflammation on biopsy.

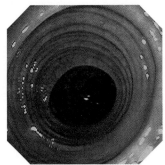

Plate 9.2 Normal colon showing circular muscle rings and reflected highlights, which help to indicate lumen direction.

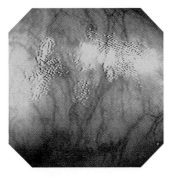

Plate 9.3 Normal submucosal vessel pattern in the colon; the reflected highlights show up the transparent mucosal surface, including the crypt openings or 'pit pattern'.

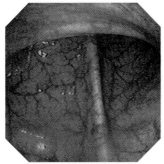

Plate 9.4 A prominent longitudinal muscle bundle or taenia coli indicates luminal direction (upwards).

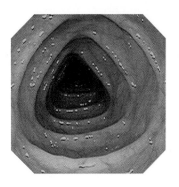

Plate 9.5 Triangular appearance of colon (due to the three taeniae coli) characteristic of the transverse, but sometimes seen in the descending.

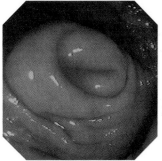

Plate 9.6 Appendix orifice — usually a crescentic slit but sometimes a whorl of folds.

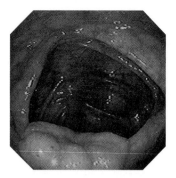

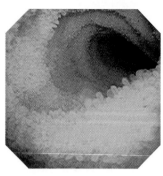

Plate 9.7 The ileocaecal valve bulge on the first large circumferential fold back from the caecal pole.

Plate 9.8 Terminal ileum – under water view causing the ileal villi to stand out prominently.

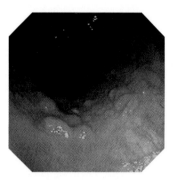

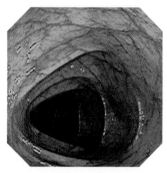

Plate 9.9 Peyer's patch in the terminal ileum – a normal finding in children and young adults.

Plate 9.10 Bluish coloration due to adjacent extra-colonic structures – here the liver against the transverse colon.

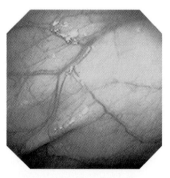

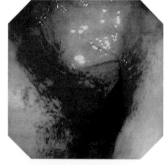

Plate 9.11 Vessel pattern in close-up – note the pairing of arterioles and venules.

Plate 9.12 Mucosal traumatization in the splenic flexure region – due to transmitted instrument pressure passing the looped-up sigmoid colon.

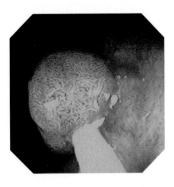

Plate 9.13 Shiny submucosal lipoma – soft, cystic and indentable with biopsy forceps (the 'cushion sign'): do *not* attempt snare polypectomy.

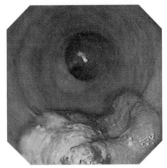

Plate 9.14 Close-up of a tubulo-villous adenoma showing the typical 'cerebral' or 'sulcal' appearance of the surface.

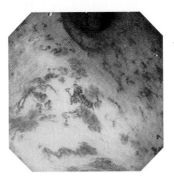

Plate 9.15 Rectal telangiectasia after irradiation therapy (DXT).

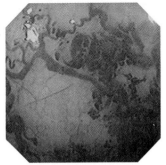

Plate 9.16 Serpiginous vessels of a colonic haemangioma – often a purely endoscopic diagnosis. The abnormality can be extensive.

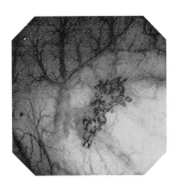

Plate 9.17 A 3 mm angiodysplasia, bright red because it is highly perfused. Look for others, and treat the most dependant first – in case of bleeding.

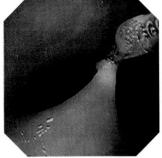

Plate 10.1 'Mount Fuji effect' during hot biopsy, showing safe *limited* electrocoagulation of a 2 mm polyp base, tented up with the forceps.

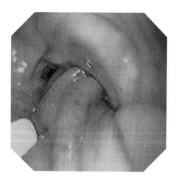

Plate 10.2 Pre-injection with adrenaline of the basal stalk of a large polyp before polypectomy – as a safety measure.

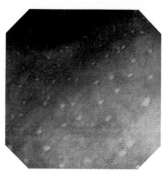

Plate 10.3 'Melanosis coli' with lipofuscin pigmentation showing up usually invisible lymphoid follicles.

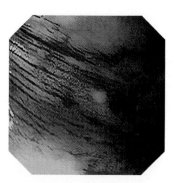

Plate 10.4 Dye-spray (dilute ink or 0.1% indigo carmine) shows fine mucosal detail – here 1 mm micro-adenomas in an adenomatous polyposis child.

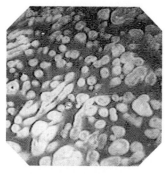

Plate 10.5 Post-inflammatory (pseudo-) polyps, here accentuated by dye spray, occur after severe colitis of any kind and have *no* cancer potential.

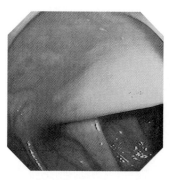

Plate 10.6 'Tattoo' of intramucosal india ink visible 5 years after marking a malignant polyp site.

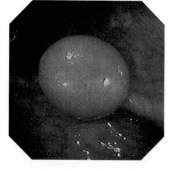

Plate 10.7 'Appendix stump' at the caecal pole after appendicectomy – snaring it can cause perforation!

(Fig. 9.68). Clockwise torque will only be effective on the shaft if the colonoscope has previously been straightened, if the descending colon is normally fixed and if any sigmoid loop is small. (Because the tip is angulated, applying clockwise shaft torque inevitably loses or affects the luminal view into the transverse colon, and readjustment of the angling controls may be needed).

6 *Finally, push in, but slowly.* Obviously the instrument tip will not advance around the splenic flexure without inward push, so as well as clockwise twist, continued gentle inward pressure is needed (aggressive pushing simply reforms the sigmoid loop). Firm, but nearly isometric, inward pressure on the shaft causing a gradual millimetre-by-millimetre slippage of the tip into the transverse colon is all that is needed for success. Whilst pushing in it may be possible to deflate again, or it may be necessary to make compensatory movements of the steering controls. A combination of these various manoeuvres, together or in sequence, whilst using the control knobs to 'squirm' the bending section, or the suction button to aspirate a little more, may help the tip and the stiffer shaft behind it to slide around the splenic flexure.

7 *If it does not work, pull back and start again.* If the tip is not progressing but, from the amount of shaft being inserted, it is obvious that a sigmoid loop is reforming, pull back, run through all the above actions again before pushing in once more. It may take two or three attempts to achieve success.

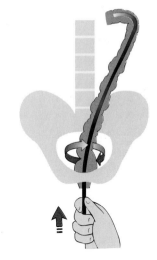

Fig. 9.68 Twist the shaft clockwise while advancing to keep the sigmoid straight.

Position change

If it *still* does not work, change position. As pointed out earlier, the left lateral position used by most endoscopists has the undesirable effect of causing the transverse colon to flop down (see Fig. 9.66a) and make the splenic flexure acutely angled. Turning the patient to the right lateral position has the opposite effect, the transverse colon sags to the right side and, together with gravity, pulls the splenic flexure into a smooth curve without any apparent 'flexure' at all (see Fig. 9.66b). Even having the patient turn supine has a significant gravitational effect and, since this is an easier move to make, is worth trying before a fully-fledged right lateral move.

The first angulation encountered by the instrument on passing round the splenic flexure, after a change to the right lateral position, is usually the mid-transverse colon or even the dependent and fluid-filled hepatic flexure. Change of position is almost invariably and immediately effective in passing the splenic flexure, but it does take a few seconds to achieve, and the patient has to be returned to the left lateral position to inflate and visualize the proximal colon properly and to reach the caecum. It is also cumbersome if the patient is obese, disabled or oversedated.

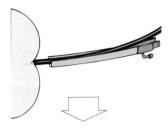

Fig. 9.69 (a) Insert the split overtube onto the colonoscope shaft . . .

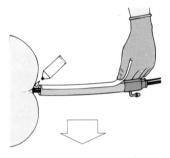

(b) . . . seal the slit with sticky tape and lubricate . . .

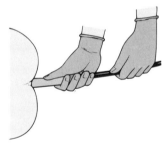

(c) . . . and slide the overtube in; keep the endoscope stationary with the other hand.

We therefore change position if 'stuck' at the splenic flexure for over 60 s or so, allowing several attempts at direct passage, first in the left lateral position, then the supine, before full rotation to the right. The ability to perform postural changes easily is an additional reason for reducing routine sedation (or avoiding it altogether when possible).

Position changing should be a simple routine. Except for heavily sedated or otherwise immobile patients, position change can be quick and effortless. It helps to have a routine. Mine (CBW) involves changing to hold the instrument control body in the right hand, the endoscopist's left hand lifts the patient's lowest foot off the couch, the shaft is slid through to the other side and the patient can then turn over. Providing the shaft is kept away from the patient's heel (and perhaps rotated a little as the body rotates) there is nothing to go wrong and the whole manoeuvre takes at most 20–30 s.

The stiffening or 'overtube'

If all this fails (perhaps one case in 500–600 in our hands) use of a stiffening overtube, sometimes called a 'splinting device', is almost guaranteed to hold the sigmoid colon straight and allow easy passage into the proximal colon. An overtube can only be inserted when the sigmoid colon has been completely straightened and the tip of the instrument is in the proximal–descending colon or splenic flexure.

The original, extremely stiff wire-reinforced overtubes had disadvantages which have discouraged most endoscopists from using them routinely; the tube must be on the instrument before starting (or the endoscope completely withdrawn before it can be put on) and insertion can be traumatic and requires fluoroscopy. The principle of a soft-plastic split overtube overcomes all of these disadvantages, especially new atraumatic versions made of frictionless and very flexible plastic material (Gortex, Olympus). The split overtube is softened in hot water and placed over the shaft of the colonoscope after this has been straightened to 50 cm at the splenic flexure (Fig. 9.69a). The overtube split is sealed with adhesive tape and lubricated with jelly (Fig. 9.69b), then inserted (without fluoroscopy) as far into or through the shortened sigmoid colon as proves easy and comfortable for the patient (Fig. 9.69c).

Resistance to insertion of an overtube means impaction against a fold, loop or flexure and discomfort means the same—both are indications that further insertion or use of force could be dangerous (the same rules apply even when fluoroscopy is used). The tube is 45 cm long to accommodate long colons, but 'successful' insertion is usually only to around 30–40 cm, the handle of the overtube then being held by the assistant and the shaft of the colonoscope pushed in through it (Fig. 9.70). As soon as the colonoscope has been passed in satisfactorily (or at once if the overtube cannot be inserted successfully) it takes only a few seconds to remove the split overtube again, strip off the tape and to return to normal handling of the instrument.

As well as its use for stiffening a looping sigmoid colon, the overtube can be invaluable for exchanging colonoscopes or removing multiple polypectomy specimens.

The 'reversed' splenic flexure

In about one patient in 20, if imaging is available, the instrument tip will be seen to pass *laterally* rather than medially around the splenic flexure, because the descending colon has moved centrally on a mesocolon (Fig. 9.71) (see p. 209). This is of more than academic interest because, having passed laterally round the flexure and displaced the descending colon medially, the advancing instrument forces the transverse colon down into a deep loop. The instrument is then mechanically under stress and difficult to steer, and the hepatic flexure is approached from below at a disadvantageous angle which makes it difficult to reach the caecum and virtually impossible to steer into the ileocaecal valve. Even when the instrument tip can be hooked onto the hepatic flexure, the sheer bulkiness of the reversed loop configuration at the splenic flexure actively holds down the transverse loop and stops it being straightened and lifted up into the ideal 'question-mark' shape.

Derotation of a reversed splenic flexure loop will avoid these problems later in the examination. This can be done by twisting the shaft strongly *counter*clockwise (rather than the usual clockwise twist), usually after withdrawing the tip to the splenic flexure; the subsequent examination is so much quicker, and also more comfortable for the patient, that the time spent is worthwhile. Counterclockwise derotation makes the tip pivot around the phrenicocolic suspensory ligament and swing medially (Fig. 9.72a). After that, by maintaining counterclockwise torque while pushing in, the instrument can be made to pass across the transverse colon in the usual configuration, forcing the descending colon back laterally against the abdominal wall (Fig. 9.72b).

Although this counterclockwise straightening manoeuvre is most easily performed under imaging, it is also quite feasible without fluoroscopy, using these guidelines and a little imagination whenever atypical looping is suspected in the proximal colon. A reversed splenic flexure/mobile descending colon is the most frequent reason for an unexpectedly difficult adult or paediatric colonoscopy. It happens more commonly in children due to the relative elasticity of the attachments of the colon in childhood. Sometimes the best solution, if the problem is suspected but imaging is not available and attempts at counterclockwise

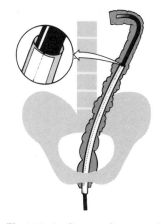

Fig. 9.70 A split overtube inserted to 30–40 cm prevents looping of the sigmoid.

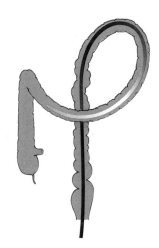

Fig. 9.71 A 'reversed' splenic flexure will result in a deep transverse loop.

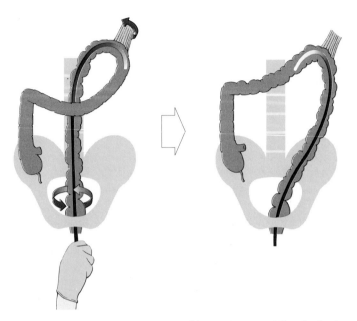

Fig. 9.72 (a) Counterclockwise rotation . . .

(b) . . . swings a mobile colon back to a normal position.

derotation have failed, is simply to get a move on, push harder than usual (if necessary with extra sedation) and to stop as soon as a reasonable view of the right colon has been obtained. If a reversed splenic loop is present, for the reasons given above, it is rare to be able to enter the ileum without successful derotation, because the looped and stressed instrument will not angulate sufficiently. If ileoscopy is essential and a reversed loop is present it is likely to be necessary to pull the instrument out to 50 cm at the splenic flexure, attempt counterclockwise derotation and pass in again; simply trying to angulate the tip forcibly without doing so is likely to stress the bending section, but not to succeed.

Transverse colon

Insertion through the transverse colon should present little problem if the sigmoid colon does not bow up into an N-loop and so reduce the transmitted pressure, but in the mid-transverse colon there is often a surprisingly sharp bend where the colonoscope tip can push downwards into the pelvis. A drooping transverse colon, frequently found in females and those with long colons, inevitably results in greater friction resistance to passage; the force required then results in sigmoid looping as well. This combination can be a major obstacle to those who have not learned to shorten and control colonic loops.

In a voluminous transverse colon the antimesenteric taeniae coli may infold into the colon, acting as a useful pointer to the correct longitudinal axis to follow — rather like the white line down the centre of a road (Fig. 9.73 & Plate 9.4). Appreciating this is particularly helpful at acute angulations, where a taenia coli can be followed blindly to push round the bend and see the lumen beyond (Fig. 9.74).

Having passed the mid-point of the transverse, it may be slow and difficult to 'climb the hill' up the proximal limb of the looped transverse colon (Fig. 9.75a). The most important manoeuvre is to pull back repeatedly. The tip, being hooked around the transverse loop, lifts up and flattens the transverse (Fig. 9.75b) and the tip often advances as the shaft is withdrawn—the phenomenon of 'paradoxical movement'. Substantial and repeated in-and-out movements (like playing a trombone) may be needed, the instrument advancing little by little towards the hepatic flexure. Hand pressure can be helpful, whether over the sigmoid colon during inward push or in the left hypochondrium to lift up the transverse loop. Deflation of the colon, torquing movements and even change of position (usually to the left lateral position, sometimes to the supine, right lateral or even prone positions) can all also help. When the tip is established in the proximal transverse colon counterclockwise torque often helps it to advance towards the hepatic flexure; this useful phenomenon results from flattening out of the *counterclockwise* spiral formed by the shaft running anteriorly and medially around the splenic flexure from the descending colon to the transverse colon.

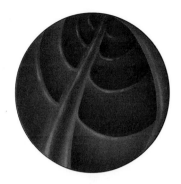

Fig. 9.73 The longitudinal bulge of a taenia coli shows the axis of the colon.

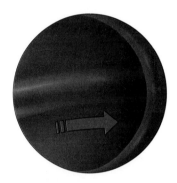

Fig. 9.74 Follow the longitudinal bulge (taenia coli) round an acute bend.

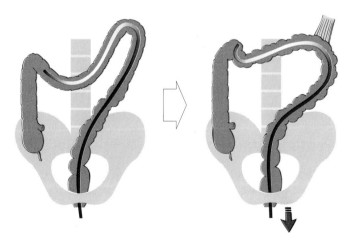

Fig. 9.75 (a) If passage up the proximal transverse is difficult . . . (b) . . . pull back to lift and shorten.

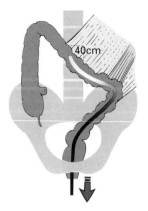

Fig. 9.76 (a) If the phrenicocolic ligament is lax, withdrawal manoeuvres are ineffective . . .

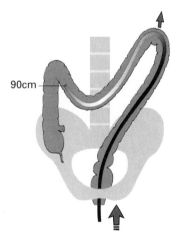

(b) . . . and pushing in simply reforms the loop.

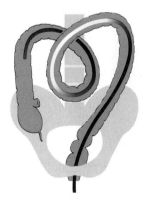

Fig. 9.77 A gamma loop in a redundant transverse colon.

Effect of a mobile splenic flexure

During these 'lift' manoeuvres, the fulcrum or cantilever effect (sometimes called 'balance beam' effect) of the phrenicocolic ligament fixing the splenic flexure is crucial. In some patients this attachment is lax, allowing the splenic flexure to be pulled back to 40 cm (rather than the usual 50 cm) (Fig. 9.76a); the colon is then found to be hypermobile and unresponsive to any of the normally effective withdrawal or twisting movements (Fig. 9.76b). When this occurs the use of force is ineffectual, but deflation, hand pressure, posturing (usually to the right lateral position) and gentle perseverance will eventually coax the tip up to the hepatic flexure.

Gamma looping of the transverse colon

In occasional patients with a very redundant transverse colon, the formation of a spontaneous gamma loop can be seen (Fig. 9.77); this is rarely removable because the instrument falls back when withdrawn. If it is removed, this is by combined withdrawal and strong clockwise twist to lift up the transverse colon into a more conventional position. It is usually impossible to enter the ileocaecal valve with a gamma loop in position, since friction stops the instrument tip angulating sufficiently.

Hand pressure

Since the major mechanical problem of colonoscopy is to stop the flexible shaft of the scope looping within the confines of the abdominal cavity, and to encourage it by any means to proceed straight onto the caecum in an easy curve (the 'question-mark' configuration), it is scarcely surprising that external hand pressure is valuable. The rationale for pressure in the lower left abdomen over the looping sigmoid colon has been described (see Fig. 9.67). The tendency of the sigmoid to re-loop at all stages of the examination has also been mentioned. Because of this tendency, hand pressure over the sigmoid colon is a good bet whenever the instrument is looping, and its application has therefore been called '*non-specific*' hand pressure.

Other loops also cause problems which can be reduced by appropriate hand pressure, notably the drooping of the transverse colon into a deepening loop which results in 'paradoxical movement' so that the tip slips back more and more as the instrument shaft is pushed in. Pulling back when this occurs reverses the slippage, so that the tip approaches the hepatic flexure again and aspiration collapses the colon and brings it nearer still. At this point changing the assistant's hand pressure empirically to the left hypochondrial region to lift the loop and the tip across the abdomen towards the hepatic flexure, or in the mid-abdomen to counteract the sagging transverse colon, can be the final critical additive action to reach the flexure (Fig. 9.78). When such hand pressure fails to help, in the transverse colon or elsewhere, it is well worth the endoscopist optimizing both the view and the position of the instrument (by push, pull, rotation, deflation, angulation, etc.) and then either the endoscopist or assistant palpating the patient's abdomen with the other hand to attempt to push the tip further in. This manoeuvre has been called '*specific*' hand pressure. At any time in the proximal colon that a few extra centimetres of insertion are needed, but cannot be achieved, try abdominal hand pressure, first 'non-specific' (in the left lower abdomen) but, if this fails, 'specifically' according to the results of local palpation.

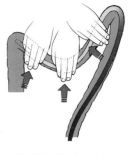

Fig. 9.78 'Specific' hand pressure may elevate the transverse colon.

Hepatic flexure

One of the most frustrating problems for the colonoscopist is to be able to see the hepatic flexure but not be able to reach it . If the flexure is only 2–3 cm away in spite of a reasonably straight colonoscope (around 70–80 cm), hand pressure and clockwise torque, there is a sequence of actions which should ensure rapid passage around the hepatic flexure:

1 *Assess from a distance* the correct direction around the flexure for, after the tip reaches into it, it will be so close to the opposing mucosa that it is very difficult to steer except by a predetermined plan. At all costs avoid impacting the tip forcibly against the opposing wall or it will catch in the haustral folds and there will be no view at all.

2 *Aspirate air carefully* from the inflated hepatic flexure, to collapse it towards, but not actually onto, the tip as it moves around (Fig. 9.79).

3 *Steer the tip blindly in the previously determined direction* around the arc of the flexure. Since the hepatic flexure is very acute, it takes some confidence to angulate nearly 180° around in the same direction without seeing well (Fig. 9.80). Use both angling control knobs simultaneously to achieve full angulation; adding clockwise twist may be helpful.

4 *Withdraw the instrument* substantially for up 30–50 cm to lift up the transverse colon and straighten out the colonoscope (Fig. 9.81a,b) for passage into the ascending colon.

5 *Aspirate air again* once the ascending colon is seen, in order to shorten the colon and drop the colonoscope down towards the caecum (Fig. 9.81c).

In practice, a combination of these manoeuvres is used simultaneously, so that aspiration brings the hepatic flexure towards the tip until the inner fold of the flexure can be passed, the colonoscope is withdrawn (either by manipulation of the shaft or by the endoscopist pulling the colonoscope out, using both hands on the control body simultaneously working both angling

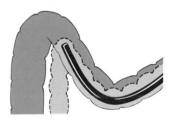

Fig. 9.79 Aspirate to shrink the hepatic flexure towards the scope.

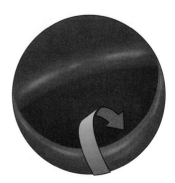

Fig. 9.80 Suction toward, then angle acutely (180°) around the acute hepatic flexure.

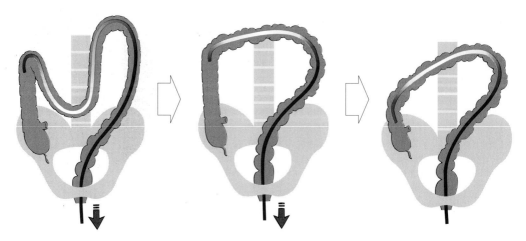

Fig. 9.81 (a) When around the hepatic flexure and viewing the ascending colon . . .

(b) . . . pull back to straighten . . .

(c) . . . and aspirate to collapse the colon and pass towards the caecum.

controls) whilst the tip is steered maximally around until it can be sucked down into the ascending colon. A parallel has already been drawn between the 'hook, withdraw and clockwise twist' situation in the transverse loop and hepatic flexure and the 'right twist and withdrawal' method of shortening the sigmoid N-loop at the sigmoid–descending colon angle; the same instrument manoeuvres apply to both, except that they must be exaggerated at the hepatic flexure because of its larger dimensions.

When things do not go according to plan, other tricks which help coax the colonoscope tip into and around the hepatic flexure, apart from pressing in the left hypochondrium to lift the transverse colon, are to get the patient to inspire deeply (to lower the diaphragm and thus the hepatic flexure too), to use the split overtube to control the sigmoid colon or to change position (to supine, prone or sometimes even right lateral positions) if the usual left lateral position has been ineffective. Using brute force rarely pays off, since the combined sigmoid and transverse colon loops can take up most of the length of the colonoscope shaft. With the instrument really straightened at the hepatic flexure, only about 70 cm of the shaft should remain in the patient; this is one of the situations where a distance check helps to ensure a straight colonoscope and to result in easy and painless insertion.

A final, embarrassing, point is that if things are not working out at the hepatic flexure after applying the various tips, the colonoscope may actually still be in the *splenic* flexure. In a redundant colon it is possible to be over-optimistic and hopelessly lost.

Ascending colon and ileocaecal region

Endoscopic anatomy

The ascending colon is posteriorly placed at its origin from the hepatic flexure, but then runs anteriorly so that where it joins the caecum it is just under the anterior abdominal wall and is accessible to finger palpation or transillumination. In 90% of subjects, the ascending colon and caecum are predictably fixed retroperitoneally but the remainder may be mobile on a persistent mesocolon, with correspondingly variable positions.

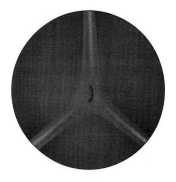

Fig. 9.82 Appendix orifice.

At the pole of the caecum the three taeniae coli fuse down into the appendix (Fig. 9.82); between the taeniae coli and the marked caecal haustra there can be cavernous outpouchings which are difficult to examine. The appendix orifice is normally an unimpressive slit (Plate 9.6), which is often crescentic because the appendix is folded around the caecum. Only rarely is the appendix orifice tubular, and it may be unobvious in a local whirl of mucosal folds. The operated appendix usually looks no different unless it has been invaginated into a stump, when it can sometimes resemble a polyp (take care — by all means take a biopsy but do not attempt polypectomy!).

The ileocaecal valve is situated on the medial part of the prominent ileocaecal fold which encircles the caecum about 5 cm from its pole. Unfortunately for the endoscopist, the orifice of the valve is often a slit on the invisible 'caecal' aspect of the ileocaecal fold. The most the endoscopist normally sees is the slight bulge (Plate 9.7) of the upper lip — much as the mouth would look if seen by an endoscope emerging from the nose. It is therefore rare to see the orifice directly without specific close-up manoeuvres.

Insertion

On seeing the ascending colon from around the hepatic flexure the temptation is to push in, but this usually results in the transverse loop re-forming and the tip sliding back. The secret is to *deflate*; the resulting collapse of the capacious hepatic flexure and ascending colon will drop the tip downwards towards the caecum (see Fig. 9.81c); it also lowers the position of the hepatic flexure relative to the splenic flexure and with this mechanical advantage, pushing inwards should become effective. Make short aspirations and steer carefully down the centre of the deflating lumen, then push the last few centimetres into the caecum. If it proves difficult to reach the last few centimetres to the caecal pole, change the patient's position to prone (even a partial position change may help) or, if that does not work, to supine. Once in the caecum, the bowel can be reinflated to get a view.

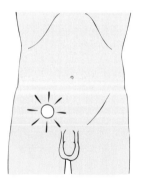

Fig. 9.83 Transillumination deep in the iliac fossa suggests the caecum.

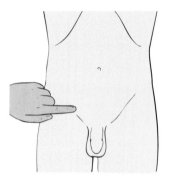

Fig. 9.84 Finger pressure in the right iliac fossa indents the caecum.

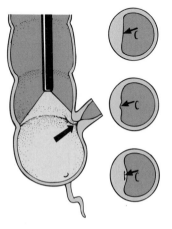

Fig. 9.85 The ileocaecal valve is a bulge on the ileocaecal fold and can be a single bulge, double bulge or 'volcano'.

The caecum can be voluminous and its pronounced haustral infoldings and tendency to spasm may make it confusing to examine. In particular, it is possible to be mistaken about whether the pole has actually been reached. One catch is that the ileocaecal valve fold, the major circumferential fold at the junction of the ascending colon and the caecum — on which is situated the give-way bulge of the valve — has a tendency to be in tonic spasm. The fold in spasm can easily be mistaken by the unwary for either the appendix orifice or the ileocaecal valve. Insufflating and pushing in with the instrument tip and/or using extra intravenous antispasmodic medication will reveal the cavernous caecal pole beyond.

The endoscopist should therefore be very careful about assuming that true *'total colonoscopy'* has been performed. The appendix orifice or ileocaecal valve should be identified as landmarks, with or without imaging; also use right iliac fossa transillumination (Fig. 9.83) or finger palpation indenting the caecal region (Fig. 9.84) to confirm location of the tip. At the same time the colonoscope should, after withdrawal, be at 70–80 cm. The caecal pole is often difficult to examine, is not always completely clean and is sometimes in tonic spasm; a 'too good to be true' appearance may therefore actually be only the ascending colon or even the hepatic flexure. Inability to locate the ileocaecal valve opening and noting that the shaft distance on withdrawal is only at 60–70 cm should warn of this possibility.

Entering the ileocaecal valve

First find the valve. Pull back about 8–10 cm from the caecal pole and look for the first prominent circular haustral fold, around 5 cm back from the pole; somewhere on this 'ileocaecal' fold will be the tell-tale thickening or bulge of the valve. A common mistake is to look for the valve when the endoscope tip is in the caecal pole, rather than pulling back to the mid-ascending colon to get a proper overall view from a distance. Looking at this ileocaecal fold, with the caecum moderately inflated, one part of it should be seen to be less perfectly concave than the rest. It may be simply flattened out, bulge in (especially on deflation, when it often bulges more obviously and may bubble or issue ileal contents), show a characteristic 'buttock-like' double bulge or, less commonly, have obvious protuberant lips or a 'volcano' appearance (Fig. 9.85 & Plate 9.7). It is rather uncommon to see the actual slit orifice or pouting lips of the valve straight on, because the opening is normally on the caecal side of the ileocaecal fold. The best the endoscopist can usually achieve is a partial, close-up and tangential view, and only often after careful manoeuvring. Change of patient position may be helpful if the initial view is poor or disadvantageous for tip entry.

Consider pre-inserting the biopsy forceps to the instrument

tip, especially if an ileal biopsy may be required. The forceps will insert easily when the endoscope is straight in the ascending colon, but may not do so at all (or only with undesirable force) when the tip is angulated into the ileum. It is particularly aggravating to have to withdraw back out of the ileum to insert the forceps if it has been a struggle to get in—and the forceps can in any case be helpful in this, as described below.

After these preliminaries there are three ways to enter the ileo-caecal valve.

Direct entry with the instrument tip. To do this there is a sequence of actions to follow so as to angle in towards the valve and enter it:

1 *Rehearse at a distance* (about 10 cm back from the caecal pole) the easiest movements, preferably combining shaft twist and down-angulation to point the tip towards the valve (Fig. 9.86a). If possible rotate the endoscope so that the valve lies in the downward (6 o'clock) position relative to the tip, because this allows entry with an easy downwards angulation movement (lateral or oblique movements are awkward single-handedly) and because the tip air outlet is situated below the lens, but needs to enter the valve first in order to open up the ileum on insufflation.

2 *Pass the colonoscope tip in* over the ileocaecal valve fold in the region of the valvular bulge and angle in towards the valve (Fig. 9.86b). Overshoot a little, so that the action of angling directs the tip into the opening, not short of it.

3 *Deflate the caecum partially* to make the valve supple (Fig. 9.86c).

4 *Pull back the scope, angling downwards* until the tip catches in the soft lips of the valve, resulting in a 'red-out' of transilluminated tissue (Fig. 9.86c), typically with the tell-tale granular appearance of the villus surface in close-up (as opposed to the pale shine of colonic mucosa).

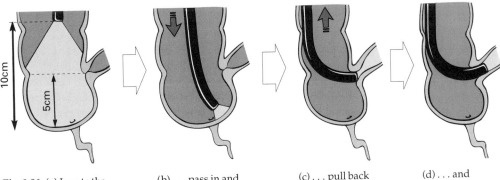

Fig. 9.86 (a) Locate the ileocaecal valve (preferably at 6 o'clock)...

(b)... pass in and angulate and deflate slightly...

(c)... pull back until the 'red-out' is seen...

(d)... and insufflate to open the valve.

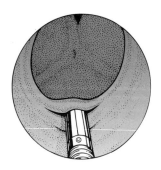

Fig. 9.87 The biopsy forceps can be used to locate, and then pass into, the ileocaecal valve.

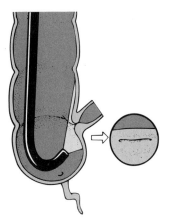

Fig. 9.88 A slit-like valve may only be visible in retroversion.

5 *On seeing the 'red-out', freeze all movement,* insufflate air to open the lips (Fig. 9.86d) and wait — gently twisting or angling the scope a few millimetres if necessary until the direction of the ileal lumen becomes apparent; if considerable angulation has been used to enter the valve *de*-angulation may be needed to straighten things out and let the tip slide in.

6 *Multiple attempts may be needed* for success in locating the valve and entering the ileum, if necessary rotating to slightly different parts of the ileocaecal fold, hooking over it and pulling back to pass the area repeatedly. On each successive attempt try to learn from the problems of the previous one, fining down tip movements to a centimetre or two and a few degrees either way. Change of position may also help.

Using the biopsy forceps as guidewire. If only a distant, partial or uncertain view can be obtained of the ileal bulge or opening, it is usually possible to use the biopsy forceps to locate and then pass into the opening of the valve (Fig. 9.87), either to obtain a blind biopsy or to act as an 'anchor'. The forceps fix the position of the tip relative to the valve and facilitate endoscope passage through it on the guidewire principle. Even if entry into the ileum is not intended, the opened forceps can be used to hook back the bulge of the upper lip of the valve to visualize the ileal opening and make identification certain; suggestive bulges or flattenings can be identified misleadingly on more distal folds.

Entry into the ileum in retroflexion. The retroversion approach is particularly useful when the ileocaecal valve is slit-like and invisible from above (Fig. 9.88). Retroverting the tip to visualize and then enter the valve from below (Fig. 9.89a) can also occasionally be successful if direct approaches to enter the valve have failed, especially if the caecum is capacious and the colonoscope is straight and responsive. Very acute angulation of the colonoscope tip is needed, with maximum up/down and lateral angulation, and often some twist of the shaft as well. Fairly forceful inward push may be needed to impact low enough in the caecal pole to visualize the valve; with some video-endoscopes the extra length of the bending section may preclude this. Once the valve is located, pull back to impact the tip within it (Fig. 9.89b), then insufflate to open the lips and de-angulate and pull back further to enter the ileum, with or without use of the forceps (Fig. 9.89c).

Problems in finding or entering the ileocaecal valve. This can occur for a number of reasons. The endoscope may be in the hepatic flexure, not the caecum. Even if the tip is in the right place, the chosen 'bulge' on the ileocaecal valve may not be correct; some valve openings are entirely flat and slit-like, effectively invisible on the reverse side of the fold. Aiming the lens at the centre of the

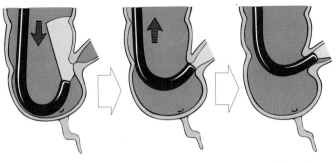

Fig. 9.89 (a) If necessary retroflex to see the valve . . .

(b) . . . pull back to impact . . .

(c) . . . and insufflate and de-angulate to enter the ileum.

endoscope tip exactly at the slit may mean that the rest of the tip impacts against the upper lip and cannot pass in (Fig. 9.90), which is why overshooting the opening slightly will let the angled tip edge in successfully even though the initial view is less good.

Those cases of inflammatory disease where the colonoscopist wants to see the terminal ileum are those where the valve is most likely to be narrowed and, although a limited view may be possible and biopsies taken, the valve may be impassable.

Terminal ileum

The terminal ileum surface characteristics are variable; it looks granular or matt in air, but under water small finger-like villi are seen projecting (Plate 9.8). It is often studded with raised lym-

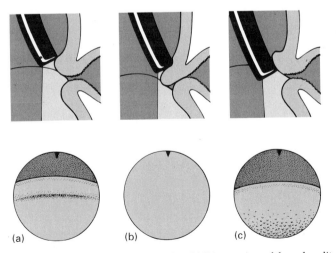

(a) (b) (c)

Fig. 9.90 Entering the ileocaecal valve. (a) Distant view of the valve slit. (b) Pushing in directly impacts against upper lip. (c) Overshooting the valve a little lets the tip angle-in successfully.

phoid follicles resembling small polyps or aggregated into plaque-like Peyer's patches (Plate 9.9). Sometimes the ileum is surprisingly colon-like with a pale shiny surface and visible submucosal vascular pattern. After colon resection the difference between colon and ileum may be imperceptible because of villus atrophy. Using the dye spray technique (1:4 dilution of washable blue ink, 0.1% indigo carmine or 5% methylene blue) to highlight the surface detail will rapidly discriminate between the granular or 'sandpaper' appearance of the ileal mucosa and the small circumferential grooves of the colonic surface, which give a 'fingerprint' effect.

The ileum is soft, peristaltic and collapsible compared to the colon, and should be handled more like the duodenum. Greater distances can be travelled by gentle steering and deflation — so that the intestine collapses over the colonoscope — than will be achieved by force, which simply stretches it. At each acute bend it is best to deflate a little, hook round, pull back and then steer gently (if necessary almost blindly) around and inwards before pulling back again to re-find the view — the 'two steps forward and one step back' approach which applies throughout colonoscopy. Once the colonoscope tip is in the ileum, it can often be passed for up to 30–50 cm with care and patience, although this length of intestine may be folded on to only about 20 cm of instrument. Air distension in the small intestine should be kept to a minimum since it is particularly uncomfortable and slow to clear after examination — another reason for routinely using CO_2.

Examination of the colon

Better views are obtained during withdrawal than on insertion and the more painstaking examination is usually performed on the way out. However, in many areas, especially around bends, a different and sometimes better view is obtained on insertion. For this reason when a perfect view is obtained of a polyp or other lesion during insertion (especially a small one) it is better to deal with it at once (snare, biopsy or video print) rather than have the humbling experience of not being able to find it again on the way out and thereby to waste time. A convincing example of the difference between insertion and withdrawal is in the number of diverticular orifices seen in travelling around bends, compared with the few seen on coming out with the colon straightened.

The view is better on the way back because the colonoscope is in the centre of the lumen and is straight. However, the colon has been shortened during the insertion, and during withdrawal the most convoluted parts, such as the transverse and sigmoid colon, can spring off the tip at such speed that it is difficult to ensure a complete view. At sharp bends or marked haustrations there may, therefore, be blind spots during a single withdrawal;

careful scanning and twisting movements should be used in an attempt to survey all parts of each haustral fold or bend, and some may need to be re-examined several times. At a flexure the outside of the bend may be seen on the first pass, but the colonoscope often has to be reinserted and hooked to get a selective view of the other side. Acute bends, including the hepatic and splenic flexures, the sigmoid–descending colon junction and the capacious parts of the caecum and rectum are potential blind spots where the endoscopist needs to take particular care to avoid 'misses' (Fig. 9.91).

Changes of position can also help to improve the completeness of inspection. The splenic flexure and descending colon are rapidly filled with air and emptied of fluid by asking the patient to rotate towards the right lateral position. In patients where accuracy is particularly important, such as those with increased risk of polyps or possible bleeding points, it is our policy to rotate them to the right oblique position for inspection of the left colon, then back to the left lateral position again for a better view of the sigmoid colon and rectum.

The single-handed technique (the endoscopist managing both controls and shaft) comes into its own during inspection on withdrawal. The endoscopist has precise control and the corkscrewing movements he makes by twisting the shaft are the quickest way of scanning a bend or haustral fold so that he can reflexly re-examine a problem area several times. With an assistant, difficulties of communication and co-ordination make it more difficult to be thorough and accurate.

As well as being obsessional the endoscopist must be honest, reporting not only what he sees but also when his view has been imperfect due to technical difficulty or bad bowel preparation. Even during an ideal examination, the endoscopist probably misses 5% of the mucosal surface and in a problematic examination he may miss up to 20–30% (although he is unlikely to miss large protuberant lesions).

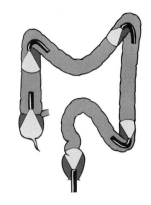

Fig. 9.91 Potential blind spots for colonoscopic visualization.

Localization

One of the endoscopist's most serious problems, especially during flexible sigmoidoscopy or limited colonoscopy, but even during supposed 'total' colonoscopy, is uncertainty of localization. This can be misleading in judging where the instrument has reached, and therefore which manoeuvres to employ; and catastrophic if the surgeon is given wrong information on which to plan a resection.

Distance of insertion of the instrument is sometimes used by inexperienced colonoscopists to express the position of the instrument or of lesions found ('the colonoscope was inserted to 90 cm', 'a polyp was seen at 30 cm', etc.). The elasticity of the colon makes this information meaningless; at 70 cm the instru-

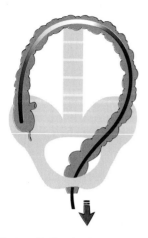

Fig. 9.92 Pulling back the scope shortens the colon.

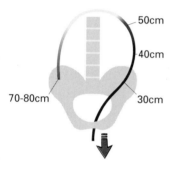

50cm

40cm

70–80cm

30cm

Fig. 9.93 If the scope is in the caecum at 70–80 cm, other anatomical sites are predictable by measurement.

ment may be in the sigmoid colon or in the caecum. On withdrawal, however, providing no adhesions are present and the mesenteric fixations are normal, the colon will shorten and straighten predictably (Fig. 9.92) so that measurement gives approximate localization. On withdrawal, the caecum should be at 80 cm, the transverse colon at 60 cm, the splenic flexure at 50 cm, the descending colon at 40 cm and the sigmoid colon at 30 cm (Fig. 9.93). The last two figures depend, of course, on the sigmoid colon being straightened. It is sometimes difficult to convince enthusiasts for rigid proctosigmoidoscopy that at 25 cm their instrument may still be in the rectum, whereas the flexible colonoscope (on withdrawal) may be in the proximal sigmoid colon. Equally, it is sometimes possible for the colonoscope to be withdrawn to 55–60 cm when the tip is in the caecum.

In a personal series, anatomical location during limited colonoscopy (when judged by withdrawal distance) was wrong in almost half the cases when checked on fluoroscopy. In 25%, a persistent loop (alpha or N) caused the endoscopist to judge the tip location to be at the splenic flexure when actually at the sigmoid–descending colon junction. In 20%, a mobile splenic flexure pulled down to 40 cm from the anus, causing the endoscopist wrongly to judge the instrument to be at the sigmoid–descending colon junction (see Fig. 9.59).

The internal appearances of the colon have already been described, but they too can be misleading. In the sigmoid and descending colon the haustra and the colonic outline are generally circular (see Fig. 9.25), whereas the longitudinal muscle straps or taeniae coli cause the characteristic triangular cross-section often seen in the transverse colon (see Fig. 9.63); the descending colon, however, may look triangular or the transverse colon circular in outline.

Fluid levels can be surprisingly useful clues to localization, especially after oral lavage. Just as the radiologist rotates the patient into the right lateral or left lateral position to fill the dependent parts of the colon with barium (Fig. 9.94), the endoscopist (with the patient in the usual left lateral position) knows that the instrument tip is in the descending colon when it enters fluid, and is in the transverse colon when it leaves the fluid for

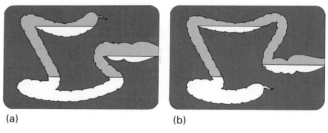

(a)

(b)

Fig. 9.94 Barium enema in (a) the left lateral position and (b) the right lateral position.

the triangular and air-filled lumen of the transverse colon (see Fig. 9.57).

Visible evidence of extracolonic viscera normally occurs at the hepatic flexure where there is seen to be a bluish indentation from the liver (Plate 9.10), but a similar appearance may sometimes occur at the splenic flexure or descending colon. The combination of an acute bend with sharp haustra and blue coloration is thus characteristic of the hepatic flexure and is a useful, but not infallible, endoscopic landmark. Pulsation of adjacent arteries are seen in the sigmoid colon (left iliac) and transverse colon (aorta) and sometimes in the ascending colon (right iliac).

The ileocaecal valve is, in the final analysis, the only definite anatomical landmark in the colon, but it has been stressed already that it is not always easy to find and mistaken identification is possible unless the ileum is entered or the orifice visualized.

Transillumination of the abdominal wall by instruments with bright enough illumination (not all video-endoscopes have this facility) can be very helpful if other imaging modalities are not available, but in obese patients may necessitate a darkened room. It should be remembered that the descending colon is so far posterior that no light is usually visible and that the surface marking of the splenic and hepatic flexures is by transillumination through the rib cage posteriorly. Light in the right iliac fossa is suggestive, but not conclusive, that the instrument is in the caecum; similar appearances can be produced if the tip stretches and transilluminates the sigmoid or mid-transverse colon.

Finger indentation, palpation or ballotting can be effective, particularly in the ascending colon or caecum, where close apposition to the abdominal wall should make the impression of a palpating finger easily visible to the endoscopist, unless the patient is fat. If in doubt indent in several places and beware the possibility of transmitted forces giving, literally, misleading impressions.

Reporting of localization of the instrument tip or lesions found in the colon should therefore be made by the endoscopist in broad anatomical terms (e.g. 'the polyp was seen on withdrawing the instrument at 30 cm in the proximal sigmoid colon'), or even omit the measurement altogether so that there is no chance of confusion in the mind of someone unfamiliar with the shortening of the colon possible during flexible endoscopy. Inaccurate localization can occur even when fluoroscopy is employed and the endoscopist usually needs to rely on a combination of assessments — distance inserted, distance after withdrawal and straightening of the shaft, appearances and visualization of palpating fingers or transillumination. Knowing the pitfalls and being careful should make localization reasonably accurate, but even experienced endoscopists can mistake the sigmoid colon for the splenic flexure, or the splenic flexure for the hepatic flexure, which can be a serious error if localizing a lesion before surgery.

Normal appearances

The form and internal anatomy of the colon have been considered earlier. The colonic mucosa normally shows a generalized fine, ramifying vascular pattern which can often be seen to be composed of parallel pairs of vessels comprising a venule (larger, bluer) and an arteriole (Plate 9.11). The veins become particularly prominent in the rectum, notably so in the anal canal if a proctoscope is used to impede venous return, and distend the haemorrhoidal plexus. The vessel pattern in the colon depends on the transparency of the normal colonic epithelium, since the vessels seen are in the submucosa. If the epithelial capillaries are dilated (as may occur after bowel preparation) the vascular pattern may be partly obscured. If hyperaemia is marked (as in inflammatory bowel disease) there is no visible pattern. If the epithelial layer is thickened (as in the 'atrophy' of inactive chronic inflammatory disease) the mucosa appears pale and featureless even though biopsies may be essentially normal. The most convincing demonstration of how poorly the endoscopist normally sees the epithelial surface is to spray dye (25% dilution of washable blue ink or 0.2% indigo carmine) onto the colonic mucosa. Small irregularities and lymphoid follicles stand out and there is a fine interconnecting pattern of circumferential 'innominate grooves' on the surface into which the dye sinks, providing there is no excess of mucus on the surface.

There is a considerable size range of normal submucosal vessels; even if they seem unusually prominent they should not be thought of as abnormal, and they are not likely to be haemangiomatous, unless the vessels are tortuous or serpentine. It is not surprising that there can be areas of mucosal trauma (Plate 9.12) during insertion of the colonoscope, and red or even haemorrhagic patches may sometimes be seen on withdrawal, especially in the sigmoid or where the looped sigmoid colon has impinged on the upper descending colon; sometimes it may be wise to take biopsies to ensure that these appearances are not evidence of inflammatory change.

Abnormal appearances

It is not the purpose of this book to cover more than the most obvious points of endoscopic pathology. Fortunately for the endoscopist, nearly all colonic abnormalities are either mucosal, with characteristic discoloration, or project into the lumen so that they are easy to see and excise or biopsy. Submucosal lesions which may be very difficult to diagnose include secondary carcinoma, endometriosis, a few large-vessel haemangiomas and carcinoma in chronic ulcerative colitis. The endoscopist has a poor appreciation of colonic contour due to the nearly fish-eye lens and flat illumination of modern endoscopes. He may also see nothing, or remarkably little compared to the radiologist, of extracolonic communications such as tracks or fistulae. Any experienced endoscopist has also, through bitter experience, learnt humility in visual interpretation and takes care to provide appropriate specimens for pathological opinion as well.

Polyps

The normal colonic mucosa is pale, so that submucosal abnormalities projecting into the lumen such as hamartomatous polyps, lipomas (Plate 9.13) or gas cysts may be pale. The very smallest polyps (of whatever histology) are also pale; those of 1–3 mm diameter may be transparent and invisible except on light reflex or by the dye spray technique. In polyps 4–6 mm in diameter, there may be little difference in appearance between a normal mucosal excrescence and a metaplastic, adenomatous or any other type of polyp, although small adenomas are more often red and frequently have a matt-looking or even 'sulcal' surface in close-up view (Plate 9.14). The combination of high-resolution or zoom endoscopes with vital straining (methylene blue) or surface enhancement by dye spraying (indigo carmine) stands in future to give the endoscopist nearly microscopic views, but the clinical impact that this will have is uncertain. Adenomatous polyps over about 7–8 mm in diameter, being vascular, have a characteristic red colour which makes them easy to see. Even the smallest polyps are easy to pick out if the patient has been a purgative taker, since the dusky appearance of melanosis coli (often most marked in the right colon) does not stain either polyps, which stand out like pale islands, or the ileocaecal valve.

Flat, sessile, villous adenomas are also usually pale, soft and shiny, but these are rare above the rectum except in the caecum. Apart from lipomas or shiny, worm-like inflammatory polyps, which sometimes have a cap of white slough, all other polyps are best removed. Macroscopic differentiation is inaccurate and there is no sure way of anticipating which polyp will prove histologically to be malignant. A malignant polyp may be obviously irregular, may bleed easily from surface ulceration or be paler and is usually firmer than usual to palpation with the biopsy forceps. Such signs of possible malignancy in a stalked polyp warn the endoscopist to electrocoagulate the base thoroughly, to obtain a histological opinion on the stalk and to localize and tattoo the polyp carefully in case subsequent surgery is indicated. Carcinomas are usually very obvious (Plate 9.14). They are larger and have a more extensive irregular base; carcinomatous ulcers are uncommon in the colon but look like malignant gastric ulcers. Conditions which can mimic malignancy are granulation tissue masses at an anastomosis, larger granulation tissue polyps in chronic ulcerative colitis, and (rarely) the acute stage of an ischaemic process. Biopsy evidence should always be obtained, bearing in mind that the pathologist may only be able to report 'dysplastic tissue' since there may not be diagnostic evidence of invasive malignancy in the small pieces presented to him, which is why either a large-forceps biopsy or snare-loop specimen should be taken whenever possible. Even with standard forceps, a surprisingly large specimen can be taken by the 'avulsion' or 'push biopsy' approach; the instrument is then withdrawn with the forceps at the tip so as not to shear off parts of the tissue by pulling it back through the biopsy channel.

Inflammatory bowel disease

The degree of mucosal abnormality in different forms of inflammatory bowel disease can vary enormously. The mucosa can even appear normal with an intact vascular pattern or show the most minute haziness of vascular pattern, slight reddening or tendency to friability, and yet the pathologist may find very significant abnormality on the biopsies. The endoscopist is, therefore, wise not to rely too much on his eyes and must have an extremely low threshold for suspecting abnormality and taking biopsies, particularly if there is diarrhoea or any clinical suspicion of inflammatory disease.

Colonoscopic biopsies unfortunately rarely yield diagnostic granulomas in Crohn's disease, whereas the appearance of multiple, small, flat or volcano-like 'aphthoid' ulcers set in a normal vascular pattern are characteristic. The differential diagnosis of the various specific and non-specific inflammatory disorders may not be easy; infective conditions, ulcerative, ischaemic, irradiation (Plate 9.15) and even Crohn's colitis can look amazingly similar in the acute stage but biopsies will usually differentiate them. Collagenous colitis, a rare cause of unexplained diarrhoea due to an extensive 'plate' of collagen deposition of unknown aetiology just under the epithelial surface, shows normal mucosa visually and the diagnosis can only be made histologically. The ulcer from a previous rectal biopsy or a solitary ulcer of the rectum can look endoscopically identical to a Crohn's ulcer, while tuberculous ulcers are similar but more heaped up, and amoebic ulcers more friable. Ulceration can also occur in chronic ulcerative colitis and ischaemic disease but against a background of inflamed mucosa. The endoscopic appearances must be taken together with the clinical context and histological opinion. In the severe or chronic stage it is often impossible for either endoscopist or pathologist to be categoric in differential diagnosis.

Unexplained rectal bleeding, anaemia or occult blood loss

Blood loss is a common reason for undertaking colonoscopy. Although colonoscopy gives an impressive yield of radiologically missed cancers and polyps, 50–60% of patients will show no obvious abnormality, which raises the spectre of whether anything has been missed. Haemorrhoids can be seen with the colonoscope (by retroversion in the rectum if necessary), but a proctoscope should be used for a proper view and the endoscope tip can be inserted within it to show the patient or take prints at video-proctoscopy. Haemangiomas (Plate 9.16) are rare, but they can assume any appearance from massive and obvious submucosal discoloration with huge serpentine vessels to telangiectases or minute solitary naevi, which could easily be missed in folds or bends. Angiodysplasias (Plate 9.17) mainly occur in the caecum or ascending colon, but also in the small intestine or very rarely in the distal bowel; they have variable appearances and are always bright red, but they can be small vascular plaques, spidery telangiectases or even a 1–2 mm dot lesion; they may be solitary or numerous.

Special circumstances

Pain mapping

Functional bowel disturbance in the apparently normal colon can take many forms, and 'spastic colon' pain may present with equally variable referred-pain radiation patterns—to the right or left loin, back or even into the thighs. An occasionally useful and very simple colonoscopic procedure is to map the pain experienced during distension at different sites in the colon produced by inflating a small balloon taped alongside the tip of the colonoscope (Fig. 9.95). A child's balloon, finger-cot or the cut-off finger of a rubber glove is bound with fine thread at the end of a small-bore flexible tube (include a short length of rigid tube inside the end to stop it collapsing during binding). The bound neck of the balloon is taped to the junction of the shaft and bending section—

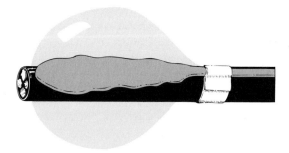

Fig. 9.95 Balloon for pain mapping taped behind the colonoscope tip.

placing the balloon at the tip can obscure the view—and two or three additional tapes secure it along the shaft. With a three-way tap and a 50 ml Luer-fitting syringe it is easy to inflate and deflate the balloon in representative sites during withdrawal of the colonoscope.

The balloon should not be inflated above 200 ml volume in the proximal colon and 100 ml distally, or mucosal stretch damage will occur. Because of the variability in colon size, quantification of the volume inflated to the pain experienced in different patients is unpredictable, but some patients with irritable bowel syndrome/spastic colon are notably hypersensitive to even 12–25 ml distension in the sigmoid colon. At each inflation site ask the patient about the quality and site of any pain experienced, and use this to map out referred-pain radiation sites and their correlation with the patient's 'usual' symptoms.

Colostomies, ileostomies and fistulae

Providing that a finger can be inserted into the stoma, a standard or paediatric colonoscope will also pass into a colostomy or ileostomy without trouble. The first few centimetres through the abdominal wall are sometimes difficult to negotiate and also to examine, partly because of the continual escape of insufflated air. It is quite normal for the stoma to change to an unhealthy-looking cyanotic colour and even for there to be a little local bleeding, but no harm ensues.

Through an ileostomy, the distal 20 cm of ileum are easily examined but further insertion depends on whether adhesions have formed. As in the sigmoid colon, the secret of passage through the small intestine is to pull the instrument back repeatedly as each bend is reached, which convolutes the intestine onto the instrument and straightens out the next short segment; thus even though only 30–40 cm of instrument can be inserted, as much as 50–100 cm of intestine may be seen. Since the sigmoid colon will usually have been removed in a colostomy patient, examination of the proximal colon is usually very easy; if there is a loop colostomy both sides can be examined providing they have been suitably prepared.

Limited examination of an ileal conduit or continent (Kock's) ileostomy is also possible providing that an acutely angling endoscope is available; a paediatric gastroscope or colonoscope is ideal. Pelvic ileoanal pouches are easy to examine with a standard instrument. Cholangioscopes have also been used to examine fistulous tracts and doubtless further endoscopic/radiological frontiers will be broached in the future.

Paediatric colonoscopy

Neonatal examinations are best performed with a thinner (1 cm), and preferably extra-flexible, paediatric colonoscope; but from the age of 2 years upwards adult colonoscopes can be used if necessary. The infant anus will accept an adult finger and so will take an endoscope of the same size, but the sphincter first requires gentle dilatation over a minute or two, using any small smooth tube (such as a nasogastric tube or a ballpoint pen cover). The main advantage of a purpose-built paediatric colonoscope is more the extra flexibility or 'softness' of its shaft than its small diameter, because it is easy with stiffer adult colonoscopes to overstretch the mobile and elastic loops of a child's colon. It is a mistake to use a paediatric gastroscope, which is thinner but much stiffer. An adult 13–15 mm colonoscope, although useable, is nonetheless too clumsy to be ideal in the colon of a small child—and stunting from disease means that age alone is a poor guide. The steering difficulties and looping problems that can ensure if a purpose-built smaller instrument is not available are reminiscent of driving a large articulated truck through small alleyways—uncomfortable for all concerned.

Bowel preparation in children is usually very effective. Pleasant-tasting oral solutions such as senna syrup or magnesium citrate are best tolerated. A saline enema will cleanse most of the colon of a baby. Children of any age can be colonoscoped without general anaesthesia providing that generous premedication is used (except for neonates, who may sometimes be more safely examined with no sedation at all). A suitable oral sedative premedication (such as antihistamine or pethidine) can be useful so that a particularly anxious child is relaxed before the procedure. A small dose of i.v. benzodiazepine (Diazemuls 2–5 mg or midazolam 1–3 mg) is usually combined with a larger dose of pethidine (meperidine) 25–50 mg i.v., slowly titrated according to response and body weight. When the child is somnolent and tolerates digital examination easily, the rest of the colonoscopy will be equally well tolerated.

Peroperative colonoscopy

Peroperative colonoscopy is normally only justified if attempts at colonoscopy have failed in a patient with known polyps, where the small intestine is to be examined in a patient with continued blood loss, or where the colon proximal to a constricting neoplasm is to be inspected to exclude synchronous lesions.

For non-obstructed patients, oral lavage or full colonoscopy bowel preparation must have been used, as most standard preoperative preparation regimens leave solid faecal residue. If the bowel has been completely obstructed, it is possible to perform on-table lavage through a temporary caecostomy tube or through a purse-string colotomy proximal to the obstructing lesion. During peroperative colonoscopy, overinsufflation of air can fill the small intestine and leave the surgeon with an unmanageable tangle of distended loops. This can be avoided if the endoscopist uses CO_2 insufflation instead of air, or if the surgeon places a clamp on the terminal ileum and the endoscopist aspirates carefully on withdrawal.

To examine the small intestine at laparotomy (see Chapter 11 for a fuller account), the long colonoscope can be used either per orally by the usual route or through an intestinal incision; 70 cm of instrument is required to reach either the ligament of Treitz per orally or the caecum per anally. It helps for the surgeon either to mobilize or manually support the fixed part of the duodenum (see Fig. 11.3) if the colonoscope is passed orally. The small intestine must be very gently handled on the endoscope to avoid local trauma or postoperative problems. A very flexible single channel endoscope (colonoscope or 'push enteroscope') is used to minimize stretching and it is also important to insufflate as little as possible. Clamps are sequentially placed on each segment of small intestine after it has been evacuated. The surgeon inspects the transilluminated intestine from outside (with the room lights turned off) whilst the endoscopist inspects the inside. The surgeon marks any lesion to be resected with a stitch whilst the endoscopist can perform conventional snare polypectomies as appropriate. A major source of confusion tends to be the artefactual submucosal haemorrhages which occur from handling the small intestine.

Hazards and complications

Colonoscopy is certainly more hazardous than barium studies (one perforation per 1700 colonoscopic examinations in published series against one perforation per 25 000 barium enemas), however these figures are likely to be pessimistic in view of the generally excellent safety record of modern colonoscopes, also bearing in mind the high mortality rate after intraperitoneal barium leakage. Nonetheless, inexpert or occasional endoscopists can perforate the colon, which makes it all the more important to certify for endoscopic skills and ensure that the potential for endoscopic cancer prevention is not besmirched by unnecessary morbidity or mortality.

Instrument or shaft tip perforations. Perforations reported in the past were usually due to inexperience and the use of excessive force when pushing in or pulling out. In a pathologically fixed, severely ulcerated or necrotic colon, however, forces may be hazardous that would be safe in a normal colon. Either the tip of the instrument or a loop formed by its shaft can perforate. When surgery is performed soon after colonoscopy, small tears have been seen in the antemesenteric serosal aspect of the colon as well as haematomas in the mesentery. In several reported cases the spleen has been avulsed during overaggressive straightening manoeuvres with the tip hooked around the splenic flexure.

Air pressure perforations. Perforations have also occurred from air pressure, including 'blow-outs' of diverticula; and unexplained pneumoperitoneum or ileocaecal perforation has followed colonoscopy limited to the sigmoid colon. Instruments with single-button control of both air and water can produce dangerously high air pressures if the tip is impacted in a diverticulum or if insufflation is continued for excessively long periods, as for instance when trying to distend and pass a stricture. Use of CO_2 insufflation effectively removes any chance of these serious sequelae since it is so rapidly absorbed. Great care and light finger pressure on the air button are indicated in the presence of diverticular disease. Diverticula are thin walled and have also been perforated with biopsy forceps or by the instrument tip; it is surprisingly easy to confuse a large diverticular orifice with the bowel lumen.

Hypotensive episodes. Hypotensive episodes and cardiac or respiratory arrest can be provoked by the combination of oversedation and intense vagal stimulus from instrumentation. Hypoxia can occur in elderly patients who are oversedated or suffer a vasovagal reaction during colonoscopy. These hazards too should be a thing of the past now that pulse oximetry is widely available. Except in occasional patients with chronic airways disease who might be disadvantaged, it may be wise to administer oxygen prophylactically to elderly, ill or heavily sedated patients.

Prophylactic antibiotics. Prophylactic antibiotics can be important in certain groups of patients, as has already been mentioned (p. 34) (for those with heart valve replacements, immunosuppressed or immunodepressed patients, especially babies, or those with ascites or peritoneal dialysis fluid). Gram-negative septicaemia can result from instrumentation (especially in neonates or the elderly) and unexplained pyrexia or collapse should be investigated with blood cultures and managed appropriately.

Electrosurgery and snare polypectomy. These contribute additional specific hazards (see Chapter 10).

Safety during colonoscopy lies in being aware of possible complications and in avoiding pain (or oversedation which masks the pain response, as well as contributing pharmacological side-effects). Before starting a colonoscopy it is impossible to know if there are adhesions, whether the bowel is easily distensible and whether its mesenteries are free-floating or fixed; pain is the only warning that the bowel or its attachments are being unreasonably strained and the endoscopist must respect any protest from the patient. A mild groan in a sedated patient may be equivalent to a scream of pain without sedation. Total colonoscopy is not always technically possible, even for the experts. If there is a history of abdominal surgery or sepsis, or if the instrument feels fixed and the patient is in pain, the correct course is usually to stop. The experienced endoscopist learns to take his time, to be obsessional in steering correctly and to be prepared to withdraw from any difficult situation, and if necessary to try again. Too often the beginner has a relentless 'crash and dash' approach, and may be insensitive to the patient's pain because he causes it so often.

Despite the potential hazards, skilled colonoscopy is amazingly safe; it is certainly justified by its clinical yield and the high morbidity of colonic surgery (which would often be the alternative).

Instrument trouble-shooting

Colonoscopy can be difficult enough without adding problems in instrument performance. Ideally the functions of all instrument controls should have been checked before the examination, because they can be difficult to spot or tedious to remedy during it.

Vision

Check the illumination and clarity of view beforehand. Is the light source functioning properly and the brightness control turned up? Is the view crisp or is there debris on the lens or light-bundle lenses which may need washing, polishing or even gentle scratching off? Colonic mucus and debris can be solidified by the protein-denaturing effects of strong antiseptics such as glutaraldehyde. Use a hand-lens to inspect the tip optics closely and to help with local cleaning.

Air

If there is no insufflation from the tip, check the light source—is the air pump switched on, are the umbilical and water-bottle connections pushed in fully and the water bottle screwed on? Is the rubber O-ring in place on the water-bottle connection? Is the air/water button in good condition and seated properly and the CO_2 button in position (where relevant), since it will otherwise allow air leakage? As already mentioned, proper air insufflation is difficult to assess by bubbling under water, but very obvious when blowing up a rubber glove or balloon placed over the tip. It is easy to miss the fact that there is inadequate air flow during an examination, which then becomes technically difficult and the colon apparently 'hypercontractile' because it collapses continually and inflates with difficulty. A great deal of wasted time can be avoided by noticing this defect before starting, or by withdrawing the scope at an early stage to check and rectify the problem.

Organic debris and mucus is the usual cause of poor insufflation, since this tends to reflux under the positive pressure within the colon back up the air channel when it is not in active use (and therefore at atmospheric pressure). A particular culprit is the small, angled air (or air plus water) nozzle at the tip of the instrument. A single plug or an accretion of layers of proteinaceous material can solidify within this nozzle, especially after glutaraldehyde exposure. Paradoxically, the units with the greatest 'air-blockage' problems are often those with the highest cleaning standards, where full antisepsis is rigorously employed. The problem can be minimized by careful water-flushing of the air channel for at least 30–40 s immediately after each examination. Preferably, this should be achieved with a single-channel flushing device, since any adaptor which flushes both the air and water channels simultaneously will simply by-pass an absolute or partial blockage in one channel without this being apparent. Using enzyme detergents is also very effective in the cleaning process, including domestic non-foaming versions for endoscope washing machines.

If a complete or partial blockage has occurred in the air channel of an instrument with a separate CO_2 button, the quickest remedy is to try forcing first air, and if this fails water, by syringe down the CO_2 channel—remembering to press the CO_2 button at the same time. The CO_2 system connects directly with the air channel and so gives convenient access to it for flushing purposes. Water is preferable for forced perfusion since it is non-compressible and a smaller (5–10 ml) syringe gives greatest pressure. Some manufacturers have special 'flush buttons' which allow direct pressure syringing after replacing the usual air/water button. A messy alternative is to activate the regular air button, put a finger over the water-bottle port on the umbilical to avoid leakage and then to syringe through the air-input channel at the end of the umbilical using a suitable syringe attachment, such as a micropipette tip cut to size.

The angled metal air nozzle at the instrument tip is often the logical place for a direct attack on a blockage problem. First try probing its slit-like opening, or even water-injecting this using a fine-gauge intravenous needle. If this proves ineffective it is possible, as a last resort, to remove the air nozzle altogether. Although it may be more diplomatic to have this done by the manufacturer's service department, or at least by skilled technicians, removal, cleaning and reinsertion are actually an easy matter. A small jeweller's screwdriver is necessary and the covering layer of soft silicone sealant must be prised off, but under this will be found a simple slotted grub-screw which can be unscrewed for a turn or two, releasing the air nozzle The channel or nozzle are ram-rodded with a fine wire (such as the stilet of an ERCP cannula) or can be syringe perfused until all debris is removed, rapidly solving the problem.

If the air channel cannot be unblocked during the process of an examination, a simple dodge is to empty the water bottle, then to activate the water button to achieve air insufflation (use the water syringe attachment if lens washing is needed).

To check that the air pump itself is working properly (the lamp must be ignited in some light sources before the air pump will operate), insert any syringe into the rubber air-output tube and the syringe plunger will rapidly blow out, demonstrating high pressure.

Water

Failure of the water system is relatively unusual, because mucus or debris do not reflux back up the filled water system as easily as up the empty air channel. None-the-less, particles of the rubber O-ring or other matter can become lodged in the water system. They should be quickly cleared by water-syringing with a micropipette tip into the small hose that normally lies under-water within the water bottle—remembering to press the water button simultaneously to allow flow.

Suction

Particulate debris can also block the suction channel. If in the shaft, this can be dislodged by water-syringing through the biopsy port. Removing the suction button and covering the opening on the control head with a finger is a quick way of improving suction pressure and can result in rapid clearance of the whole system (as when sucking polyp specimens). Applying the sucker tube directly to the suction-channel opening can also be effective in clearing particulate debris. As a final resort the whole suction system can be cleared by retrograde-syringing using a 50 ml bladder syringe to wash through tubing attached to the suction port on the umbilical. Push the suction button and also cover the biopsy port during this procedure to avoid unpleasant (refluxed) surprises.

Further reading

General sources

Cotton PB, Tytgat GNJ, Williams CB, eds. *Annuals of Gastrointestinal Endoscopy.*London: Current Science, 1988–96.

Hunt RH, Waye JD. *Colonoscopy: Techniques, Clinical Practice and Colour Atlas.* London: Chapman and Hall, 1981.

Raskin JB, Nord HJ, eds. *Colonoscopy: Principles and Techniques.* Tokyo: Igaku-Shoin, 1995.

Sakai Y. *Practical Fiberoptic Colonoscopy*. Tokyo: Igaku-Shoin, 1981.

Shinya H. *Colonoscopy: Diagnosis and Treatment of Colonic Diseases*. Tokyo: Igaku-Shoin, 1982.

Sivak MV Jr, ed. *Gastroenterologic Endoscopy*, 2nd edn. Philadelphia: WB Saunders, 1995.

Bowel preparation

Cohen SM, Wexner SD, Binderow SR *et al.* Prospective, randomised, endoscopic-blinded trial comparing precolonoscopy bowel cleansing methods. *Dis Colon Rectum* 1994;**37**:689–96.

Davis GR, Santa-Ana CA. Development of a lavage solution with minimal water and electrolyte absorption and secretion. *Gastroenterology* 1979;**78**:991–5.

Hickson DEG, Cox JGC, Taylor RG, Bennett JR. Enema or Picolax as preparation for flexible sigmoidoscopy? *Postgrad Med J* 1990;**66**:210–11.

Marshall JB, Pineda JJ, Barthel JS, King PD. Prospective, randomised trial comparing sodium phosphate solution with polyethylene glycol-electrolyte lavage for colonoscopy preparation. *Gastrointest Endosc* 1993;**39**:631–4.

Rösch T, Classen M. Fractional cleansing of the large bowel with Golytely for colonoscopic preparation: a controlled trial. *Endoscopy* 1987;**19**:198–200.

Techniques and indications

Arigbabu AO, Badejo OA, Akinola DO. Colonoscopy in the emergency treatment of colonic volvulus in Nigeria. *Dis Colon Rectum* 1985;**28**:795–8.

Harned RK, Consigny PM, Cooper NB, Williams SM, Woltzen AJ. Barium enema examination following biopsy of the rectum or colon. *Radiology* 1982;**145**:11–16.

Hixson LJ, Fennerty MB, Sampliner RE, Garewal HS. Prospective blinded trial of colonoscopic miss-rate of large colorectal polyps. *Gastrointest Endosc* 1991;**37**:125–7.

Jensen DM, Machicado GA. Diagnosis and treatment of severe hematochezia. The role of urgent colonoscopy after purge. *Gastroenterology* 1988;**95**:1569–74.

Kalvaria L, Kottler RE, Marks IN. The role of colonoscopy in the diagnosis of tuberculosis. *J Clin Gastroenterol* 1988;**10**(5):516–23.

Kingham JGC, Levison DA, Ball JA, Dawson AM. Microscopic colitis—a cause of chronic watery diarrhoea. *Br Med J* 1982;**285**:1601–4.

Koltun WA, Coller JA. Incarceration of colonoscope in an inguinal hernia 'pulley' technique of removal. *Dis Colon Rectum* 1991;**34**:191–3.

Kozarek RA. Hydrostatic balloon dilation of gastrointestinal stenoses: a national survey. *Gastrointest Endosc* 1986;**32**:15–19.

Kozarek RA, Botoman VA, Patterson DJ. Prospective evaluation of a small caliber upper endoscope for colonoscopy after unsuccessful standard examination. *Gastrointest Endosc* 1989;**35**:333–5.

Rauh SM, Coller JA, Schoetz DJ. Fluoroscopy in colonoscopy. Who is using it and why? *Am Surg* 1989;**55**:669–74.

Rossini FP, Ferrari A, Spandre M *et al.* Emergency colonoscopy. *World J Surg* 1989;**13**:190–2.

Swarbrick ET, Bat L, Hegarty JE, Dawson AM, Williams CB. Site of pain from the irritable bowel. *Lancet* 1980;**443**:446.

Waye JD. The differential diagnosis of inflammatory and infectious colitis. In: Sivak MV Jr, ed. *Gastroenterologic Endoscopy*. Philadelphia: WB Saunders, 1987:881–99.

Waye JD, Bashkoff E. Total colonoscopy: is it always possible. *Gastrointest Endosc* 1991;**37**:152–4.

Waye JD, Yessayan SA, Lewis BS, Fabry TL. The technique of abdominal pressure in total colonoscopy. *Gastrointest Endosc* 1991;**37**:147–51.

Webb WA. Colonoscoping the 'difficult colon'. *Am Surg* 1991;**57**:178–82.

Williams CB, Baillie J, Gillies DF, Borislow D, Cotton PB. Teaching gastrointestinal endoscopy by computer simulation: a prototype for colonoscopy and ERCP. *Gastrointest Endosc* 1990;**36**:49–54.

Williams CB, Guy C, Gillies DF, Saunders BP. Electronic three-dimensional imaging of intestinal endoscopy. *Lancet* 1993;**341**:724–5.

Wyllie R, Kay MH. Colonoscopy and therapeutic intervention in infants and children. In: Gastrointestinal Endoscopy Clinics of North America, Vol. 4(0) (series ed. Sivak MV). Philadelphia: WB Saunders, 1994:143–60.

Sedation, hazards and complications

Bigard MA, Gaucher P, Lasalle C. Fatal colonic explosion during colonoscopic polypectomy. *Gastroenterology* 1979;**77**:1307–10.

Bond JH, Levitt MD. Colonic gas explosion: is a fire extinguisher necessary? *Gastroenterology* 1979;**77**:1349–50.

Church JA, Stanton PD, Kenny GNC, Anderson JR. Propofol for sedation during endoscopy: assessment of a computer-controlled infusion system. *Gastrointest Endosc* 1991;**37**:175–9.

Fleischer D. Monitoring the patient receiving conscious sedation for gastrointestinal endoscopy: issues and guidelines. *Gastrointest Endosc* 1989;**35**:262–5.

Habr-Gama A, Waye JD. Complications and hazards of gastrointestinal endoscopy. *World J Surg* 1989;**13**:193–201.

Hart R, Classen M. Complications of diagnostic gastrointestinal endoscopy. *Endoscopy* 1990;**22**:229–33.

Hussein AMJ, Bartram CI, Williams CB. Carbon dioxide insufflation for more comfortable colonoscopy. *Gastrointest Endosc* 1984;**30**:68–70.

Kavin RM, Sinicrope F, Esker AH. Management of perforation of the colon at colonoscopy. *Am J Gastroenterol* 1992;**87**:161–7.

Kozarek RA, Earnest DL, Silverstein ME, Smith RG. Air-pressure induced colon injury during diagnostic colonoscopy. *Gastroenterology* 1980;**78**:7–14.

Macrae FA, Tan KG, Williams CB. Towards safer colonoscopy: a report on the complications of 5000 diagnostic or therapeutic colonoscopies. *Gut* 1981;**24**:376–83.

Phaosawasdi P, Cooley K, Wheeler J, Rice P. Carbon dioxide insufflated colonoscopy — an ignored superior technique. *Gastrointest Endosc* 1986;**32**(5):330–3.

Rockey DC, Weber JR, Wright TL, Wall SD. Splenic injury following colonoscopy. *Gastrointest Endosc* 1990;**36**:306–9.

Saunders BP, Fukumoto M, Halligan S *et al.* Patient-administered nitrous oxide/oxygen inhalation provides effective sedation and analgesia for colonoscopy. *Gastrointest Endosc* 1994;**40**:418–21.

Schembre D, Bjorkman DJ. Review article: endoscopy-related infections. *Aliment Pharmacol Ther* 1993;**7**:347–55.

Stevenson GW, Wilson JA, Wilkinson J, Norman G, Goodacre RL. Pain following colonoscopy: elimination with carbon dioxide. *Gastrointest Endosc* 1992;**38**:564–7.

Colonoscopic Polypectomy and Therapeutic Procedures

10

Equipment

The equipment requirements for endoscopic polypectomy are few, and in many ways the fewer the better. It is preferable to be completely familiar with one electrosurgical unit and only a few accessories, since from this familiarity it becomes easy to recognize when polypectomy is going right and when it is not.

Electrosurgical units

Any isolated-circuit electrosurgical unit can be used for polypectomy. For flexible endoscopy the unit is used only at low power settings (typically 15–50 W, usually equivalent to dial settings around 2.5–4 for 'coag' current) and should preferably have an automatic warning system in the circuitry in case a connection is faulty or the patient plate is not in contact. Most electrosurgical units have separate 'cut' and 'coagulate' circuits, which can often be blended to choice. As will be explained below, in electro-surgery the type of current is much less important than the amount of power produced. High settings (high power) of co-agulating current provide satisfactory cutting characteristics, whereas in units whose output is not rated directly in watts the 'cut' power output is much greater than 'coag' power at the same setting. The difference in current type used for polypectomy is therefore often illusory, and use of pure coagulating current alone is considered by most expert endoscopists to be safer and more predictable.

Lasers and argon beam electrocoagulators

The higher power needed for tissue destruction of sessile tumours, or no-touch coagulation of vascular anomalies, is best supplied by laser (usually neodymium-yttrium aluminium garnet (Nd-YAG)) or the cheaper alternative of the argon gas coagulator. The latter uses the electrical conductivity of argon gas passed down a catheter and high-power electrosurgical current to produce a local plasma arc.

Snare loops

Several makes of snare loop are available. For anyone doing a limited number of polypectomies it is advisable to be familiar with one snare only, although some endoscopists prefer to use a

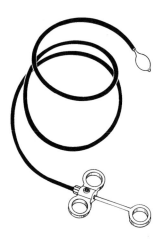

Fig. 10.1 Use one commercial snare type for familiarity.

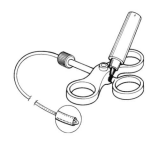

Fig. 10.2 Mark the handle when the loop is fully closed.

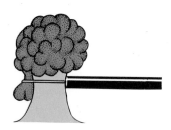

Fig. 10.3 Polyp tissue can be trapped in the snare, reducing its efficiency.

standard larger snare (for up to 3 cm polyps), a mini-snare (for smaller polyps) and specialist spiked or stiffer snares for sessile polyps (Fig. 10.1). Various configurations of snare loop or variations of handle are available, but are mainly a matter of personal preference. With any snare there are several points that should be checked *before* starting polypectomy:

1 *Mark the snare handle* with a pencil or indelible pen at the point that the snare is just closed to the tip of the outer sheath (Fig. 10.2). This is arguably the single most important safety factor in polypectomy. It allows the assistant to stop snare closure before the wire closes too far into the tube and there is danger of a smaller stalk being cut off by 'cheese-wiring' mechanically without adequate electrocoagulation; it also warns if the stalk is larger than apparent or head tissue has become entrapped (Fig. 10.3).

2 *A smooth 'feel'* is essential for safety; the snare handle and wire should open and close very easily so that the endoscopist (or assistant) has an accurate idea of what is happening when the snare loop is out of view behind the polyp or its stalk. A snare inner wire that has been bent and no longer moves freely within its plastic outer sheath is hazardous and should be discarded because this prevents any proper feeling of snare loop against polyp tissue.

3 *Snare wire thickness* greatly affects the speed of electrocoagulation. Most loops are made of relatively thick wire so that there is little risk of cheese-wiring unintentionally and there is a larger contact area which favours good local coagulation rather than electrocutting. Some disposable snares have thin wire loops and need a lower current setting or considerable care in closure to avoid cutting too rapidly, before full coagulation of stalk vessels. Be careful if using a new snare type.

4 *Squeeze pressure.* A 15 mm closure of the loop into the snare outer tube (Fig. 10.4a) is also very important when snaring large polyps. This ensures that the loop will squeeze the stalk tightly even if the plastic outer sheath crumples slightly under pressure, a particular problem with large stalks (see p. 281). If squeeze pressure is inadequate (Fig. 10.4b) the final cut may have to rely entirely on using high-power electrical cutting and may not coagulate the central stalk vessels enough, with potentially disastrous (bleeding) consequences. If the loop closes too far (Fig. 10.4c) cheese-wiring can occur before electrocoagulation is applied. This can also result in bleeding.

Other devices

Hot biopsy forceps. These are found by many to be a good compromise way of destroying small polyps up to 5 mm in diameter and even for electrocoagulating telangiectases or angiodysplasia (see p. 299).

A polyp-retrieval Dormia basket or grasping forceps. This is sometimes useful, but the snare loop itself is usually adequate for picking up the severed polyp and saves time in changing accessories.

A long sclerotherapy needle. This may be invaluable for adrenaline injection, whether to elevate a sessile polyp, to prevent or arrest polypectomy bleeding or to tattoo a polypectomy site for subsequent re-identification.

A washing or dye-spray cannula. This should be available to allow visualization of very small polyps (diagnosis or exclusion of familial adenomatous polyposis) or to demonstrate the margin of larger sessile ones.

Clipping or nylon-loop placement devices. These have an occasional place, either to deal with post-polypectomy bleeding or to prevent it. The metal clips available are too short-jawed to be useful for the thick stalks most at risk, and the nylon loop is difficult to place over a larger head, but either can be placed on the residual stalk where there is increased risk of delayed post-polypectomy bleeding—as in patients with a bleeding diathesis or on anticoagulants or antiplatelet medication.

Principles of polyp electrosurgery

The reason for using electrosurgical or diathermy currents in polypectomy is to cause *heat*, with resultant coagulation of blood vessels — especially the large ones. Coincidentally, the cooked tissue becomes easier to transect with the snare wire, but this is of secondary importance. Heat is generated in tissue by the passage of electricity (electrons), the flow of which causes collisions between intracellular ions and release of heat energy in the process (Fig. 10.5). The use of a high-frequency or 'radiofrequency' electric current, alternating in direction at up to a million times per second (10^6 c/s, 1000 kc/s or 10 Hz) (Fig. 10.6), is important because at such frequencies there is no time for muscle and nerve membrane depolarization before the current alternates again; therefore there is no 'shock' due to massive muscle contraction or afferent nerve impulse. Electrosurgical current is not felt by the patient and there is equally no danger to cardiac muscle.

Cardiac pacemakers are also unaffected at the relatively low power used for endoscopic electrosurgery, an additional safety factor being that the electrosurgical current passage between the polypectomy site in the abdomen and patient plate (usually on the thigh) is reasonably remote from the pacemaker. If in doubt consult a competent cardiologist.

Because of deeply rooted fears about low-frequency house-

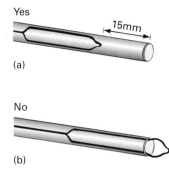

Yes

15mm

(a)

No

(b)

No

(c)

Fig. 10.4 (a) Snare closed 15 mm is right; (b) wire too loose; (c) wire too tight.

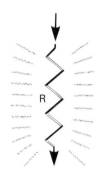

Fig. 10.5 Heat is generated by electricity (electrons) passing through resistance (R)—in this case tissue.

10^6 c/s

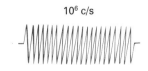

Fig. 10.6 An electrosurgical current alternates 1 000 000 times/s, producing heat but no shock.

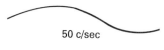

Fig. 10.7 A household current alternates 50–60 times/s, producing heat and shock.

hold currents, which shock because they alternate only 50–60 times per second (50 c/s) (Fig. 10.7), most people, including nurses and doctors, are unjustifiably nervous about high-frequency electrosurgical currents even though these are inherently safe. At the low power used in polypectomy, even the unlikely possibility of a direct thermal burn to the skin of a patient or operator is surprising but trivial, and actual burns are very rare because the heat resulting causes a strong protest long before actual damage occurs. The only danger from electrosurgical currents is that of the heat effect on the bowel wall at the site of the polypectomy.

Coagulating and cutting currents

It has already been mentioned that there is a theoretical difference between the pure coagulatin current normally used for polypectomy and cutting current, as used for surgical incisions.

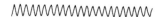

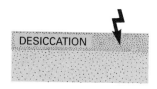

Fig. 10.8 Cutting current—continuous (high power) low-voltage pulses cannot pass desiccated tissue.

Cutting current (Fig. 10.8) has an uninterrupted waveform of relatively low voltage spikes. The interrupted current flow excites the air molecules into a charged 'ionic cloud', visible as high-temperature sparking which vaporizes the surface cell layer to steam. Because it is low voltage, however, cutting current is less able to cross desiccated tissue and to heat deeply.

Coagulating current (Fig. 10.9), by contrast, has intermittent higher-voltage spikes with intervening 'off periods' lasting for about 80% of the time. The higher voltage allows a deeper spread of current flow across desiccating tissue whilst the off periods reduce (except at high power settings) the tendency for gas ionization, sparking and local tissue destruction.

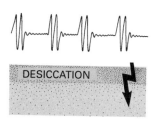

Fig. 10.9 Coagulating current—intermittent high-voltage pulses can pass desiccated tissue.

Blended current combines both waveforms (Fig. 10.10), some units providing the ability to select blends with relatively greater 'cut' than 'coag' characteristics. The differences in practice between the electrosurgical units of different manufacturers indicates that the output characteristics are more complex than this brief summary suggests, some appearing to provide more effective haemostasis than others. When changing from one unit to another it is essential to be cautious, to start with low power settings and, if possible, to try out the unit on a small lesion, or the periphery of a larger one, rather than to enter the big-time unrehearsed and then regret it.

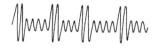

Fig. 10.10 Blended current combines the characteristics of both cutting and coagulating currents.

Monopolar or bipolar technique

For practical purposes all current endoscopic electrosurgery is by the *'monopolar'* approach with current flowing between the wire of the snare loop or jaws of the hot biopsy forceps and the patient plate; this principle and the means of handling it effectively and safely form the basis of this chapter. It is possible to use a *'bipolar'* electrosurgical technique with all current flowing from one side of the snare to the other, or from one jaw of a biopsy forceps to the other. This has the theoretical attraction that heating effects are extremely localized, a potential bonus for sessile polyps in particular, where bleeding is a lesser consideration than the potential for deep tissue damage or perforation. For most other applications the problem for the endoscopist is to be completely sure that there *has* been deep enough heating of the local vasculature before transection of a polyp head. There is thus limited interest in the bipolar approach, particularly the bipolar forceps, which will denature for histology any polyp tissue lying between the jaws. Bipolar generators ideally have 'intelligent' circuitry able to increase output as tissue desiccates and electrical resistance rises, although ordinary monopolar circuitry can be used with bipolar devices — preferably at a lower than usual power setting.

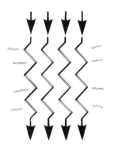

Fig. 10.11 Current flows more easily through larger areas of tissue resistance and so produces little heat.

Current density

Tissue heats because of its high electrical resistance, typically around 100 ohms, although this varies according to the particular tissue (fat conducts poorly and so heats little; water loss or desiccation during heating progressively decreases conductivity, but dry tissue is also mechanically harder to transect). If electric current is allowed to spread out and flow through a large area of tissue the overall resistance and heating effect falls (Fig. 10.11). To obtain effective electrocoagulation, the flow of current must be restricted through the smallest possible area of tissue—the principle of current density (Fig. 10.12). This principle is basic to all forms of electrosurgery and explains why no noticeable heat is generated at the broad area of skin contact with the patient plate, whereas intense heat occurs in the closed snare loop (Fig. 10.13). Even a relatively small area of contact

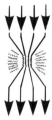

Fig. 10.12 Current density results from constricting tissue and greatly increases heating.

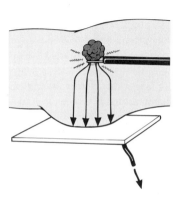

Fig. 10.13 Heating occurs at the closed snare but not at the plate.

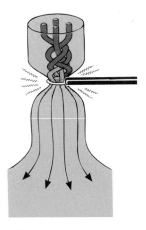

Fig. 10.14 The whole plexus of stalk vessels must be electrocoagulated before section.

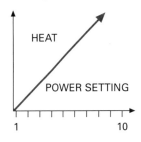

Fig. 10.15 Heat produced is directly proportional to power . . .

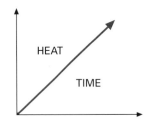

Fig. 10.16 . . . and directly proportional to time . . .

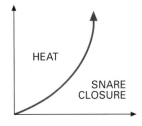

Fig. 10.17 . . . but increases as the *cube* of snare closure.

between the buttock or thigh and patient plate is adequate, and extra moisture or electrode jelly is unnecessary at the power used for polypectomy.

The problem in polypectomy is to be certain of coagulating the plexus of arteries and veins at the core of the polyp stalk before transection. Closing the snare loop both stops the blood flow (coaptation) and tends to concentrate current to flow through and heat coagulate the core (Fig. 10.14). The tightness of the loop is critical since the area through which the current is concentrated (current density) decreases as the square of snare closure (πr^2), thus causing a square law relationship between snare closure and increasing current density. The heat produced increases as the square of current density, so *heating increases as the cube of snare closure* (i.e. a slight increase of snare closure on a polyp stalk greatly increases the heat produced). Conversely, the fact that the closed snare loop is the narrowest part of the stalk means that the base of the stalk and the bowel wall should scarcely heat at all, which explains the rarity of bowel perforations during or after polypectomy.

Expressed graphically, the heat produced in a polyp stalk *increases directly with increased power settings* on the unit dial (Fig. 10.15). It also increases directly as time passes (ignoring complicating features such as heat dissipation) (Fig. 10.16); closure of the snare loop is much more important, resulting in a cubed increase of heat as the snare closes (Fig. 10.17). If the snare is too loose it will hardly heat the tissue at all; if too tight it will heat the tissue too fast. The soft stalk of a small polyp should, therefore, coagulate rapidly; a larger stalk, being less compressible, requires a slightly higher power setting and more time before visible tissue coagulation occurs. Visually it is difficult to be absolutely sure of the diameter and consistency of the stalk; the 'feel' of the stalk may also be inaccurate, especially with snares having a thin and compressible plastic sheath, so that the snare handle appears 'closed' when the stalk is not adequately narrowed (Fig. 10.18). It is to allow for this crumpling under pressure that a check for loop closure 15 mm within the sheath is so important before snaring a large polyp. Equally, it is to allow time to react to what is happening that the recommendation is to perform polypectomy using coagulating current only, and at a low power setting (corresponding to only 15–25 W). Only occasionally should it be necessary to increase the power if no visible coagulation has occurred; extra time will usually do the job.

'*Slow cooking*' is the essential principle of polypectomy, so as to electrocoagulate or cook an adequate length of stalk tissue before section. There should be visible whitening as the protein denatures, with swelling or even steam as the tissue boils. Remember that some tissue necrosis effect may extend beyond the zone of obvious electrocoagulation whitening, which is a particular consideration in avoiding mucosal ulceration and secondary bleeds after 'hot biopsy' in particular. However, if all the water boils off, electrons will no longer flow through the desiccated tissue of a polyp stalk and the wire may have to be pulled through mechanically—in principle a somewhat risky thing to do, because thick-walled vessels are usually the last part to sever. Inevitably it takes a little time at the safer lower current settings to heat the tissue but, if this takes more than 30–40 s, the risk of heat dissipation at a distance (and damage to the bowel wall) increases and it may be more realistic to increase the power setting so as to speed things up. The maximum power setting used should be equivalent to no more than 30–50 W.

Thick stalks of 1 cm or more in diameter carry a risk of inadequate central vascular electrocoagulation, particularly if the stalk is firm and relatively non-compressible and the vessels within it are large and thick-walled. However, a high power setting may be needed to start electrocoagulation peripherally and tight snaring may be needed to start electrocoagulation, with a rapid increase of heating and the unfortunate effect that, as the snare starts to transect and close down through the stalk, the heat produced increases very dramatically and results in electrocutting of the central core (which is precisely the part that needs slow and controlled coagulation). Additional factors such as current leakage may contribute and are discussed later. When no coagulation is occurring in a large polyp stalk despite a power setting of 35–50 W and bursts of current amounting to 20 s in total, all possible variables must be checked:

1 Are the circuitry and connections correct and the snare handle properly assembled and closed?
2 Has the stalk been correctly snared or is the head of the polyp trapped out of sight (see Fig. 10.3)?
3 Can the snare loop be re-positioned higher up the stalk where it is narrower?
4 Is the stalk very thick so that basal adrenaline injection should be considered before further snaring (or be available in case of immediate haemorrhage) (Fig. 10.19)?

If there is any fear of complications or the operator is inexperienced, this may be the moment to disengage the snare and leave the procedure to someone else (see below for how to disengage a 'stuck' snare).

Polypectomy

It can be difficult even for an expert to snare some polyps and easy for a beginner to miss them or to get inadequate views; it is therefore unwise to do polypectomies during the first 50 colonoscopies. Before starting, it is sensible to practise with the equipment under controlled conditions, such as with meat or a piece of resected bowel. Short strips of raw meat, cut to the diameter of a pencil, make good 'stalk substitutes', although the smell pro-

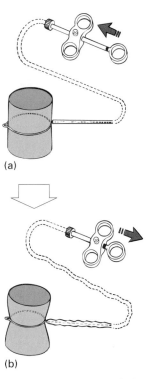

Fig. 10.18 When snaring a thick stalk (a) the plastic sheath may crumple before closure is adequate (b).

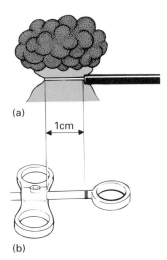

Fig. 10.19 (a) Thick stalks can bleed—think of pre-injection. (b) The distance to the closure mark indicates the stalk size.

duced can be unpleasant. The narrower end of the strip is held in the snare loop with the broader end wetted to make good contact and rested on the patient plate. Alternatively, a small portion of fresh colon resection specimen can be placed on the patient plate; a pseudopolyp of mucosa is lifted up with forceps and the snare loop closed onto it. The following steps and points should be undertaken.

1 *Check and mark the snare.* An overenthusiastic but inexperienced assistant can 'cheese-wire' through the polyp stalk before adequate electrocoagulation by closing the snare handle completely and too forcibly; this is particularly likely to occur if the snare wire is thin or the polyp stalk is small. There should be a mark on the snare handle to indicate the point at which the tip of the snare loop has closed down to the end of the outer sheath. This can be done visually beforehand or when the snare is already within the colon (see Fig. 10.2). When a thick stalk is snared the mark gives a useful approximate measure of its size and a warning that there may be problems (Fig. 10.19b).

2 *Get to know the electrosurgical unit.* When first using an electrosurgical unit, start with the lowest dial setting and use initial bursts of 2–3 s at each increased setting. Discover the lowest dial setting (usually 2.5–3) which will cause visible controlled electrocoagulation in the smallest stalk. Develop a standard routine or drill for each polypectomy and thereafter follow this routine. Check the connections, plate position and the electrosurgical unit setting before each polypectomy. Make sure that the foot pedal is in a convenient position, preferably where it can be felt with the foot without having to look down to search for it at the critical moment after the polyp is grasped, when the polyp can suddenly shift if the patient moves or coughs.

3 *Use the closed snare outer sheath to assess the base or stalk mobility* of larger polyps. Before polypectomy, try to assess whether the stalk is thin and soft or whether the stalk is thicker (when it may prove necessary to use a slightly higher power for a longer time). Visual assessment of the stalk size can be difficult due to the distorting effect of the wide-angle endoscope lens; compare the stalk size to the 2 mm width of the protruded plastic snare sheath; pushing it around to assess its length and mobility can be invaluable.

4 *Open the snare loop within the instrument channel* when snaring small or average-sized polyps. This avoids the need to manipulate the snare handle when the loop emerges from the endoscope. Lassooing the polyp head efficiently takes practice. It is usually best to have the loop fully open, and then to manoeuvre only with the instrument controls or shaft so that the snare loop is placed over the polyp head almost entirely by manipulation of the endoscope. It may help to open the snare in the colon beyond the polyp, and then to pull the colonoscope slowly back until the polyp head comes into the field of view and so into the open loop. Alternatively, the loop can be pushed backwards over a difficult polyp head (Fig. 10.20), or placed to one side or other of the polyp head and then swung over it by appropriate movements of the instrument. Rotatable snares have proved to be a disappointment in practice, since they are only fully torque-stable when the instrument is straight, whereas problem polypectomies usually occur when the tip is angled and the loop then will not torque predictably.

5 *Optimize the view and position of the polyp* before becoming committed, especially if the polypectomy looks as though it may be awkward—which is often only apparent after trying to place the loop over the polyp head. A change of patient position can improve the view of the stalk and rotation of the colonoscope shaft to exit the forceps or snare in a better position, at the bottom right of the field of view, means that the view is not lost during polypectomy (Fig. 10.21).

6 *Snare the polyp and push the snare sheath against the stalk* ('push' technique), which ensures that closing the loop will tighten it exactly at the same point. If the sheath is not pushed against the stalk, loop closure by the assistant will tend to move or even pull the wire off the polyp (Fig. 10.22) unless the endoscopist simultaneously advances the sheath (the 'pull' technique). If there is any doubt that the snare is properly over the polyp head, try shaking the snare or opening and closing the loop repeatedly so as to help it to slip down around the stalk, also try angling the colonoscope tip in the relevant direction, even if this means losing a proper view.

7 *Close the snare loop gently*, to the mark or by feel, until it is closed, ideally near the top of the stalk at its narrowest part and leaving a short segment of normal tissue to help pathological interpretation (Fig. 10.23). Initial snare closure should be gentle; the loop may be in the wrong place and once the wire has cut into polyp tissue it may be difficult to release and reposition it. With

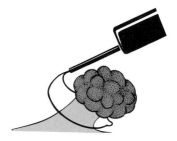

Fig. 10.20 Backward snaring is sometimes useful.

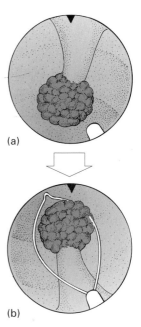

(a)

(b)

Fig. 10.21 (a) Bad position for snare placement? (b) Rotate the instrument to get a better working position and view.

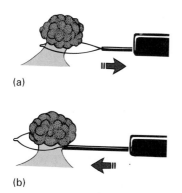

(a)

(b)

Fig. 10.22 (a) To avoid the snare pulling off during closure, (b) push the loop against the stalk before closing.

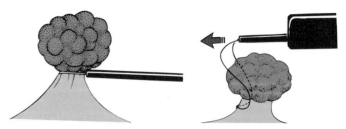

Fig. 10.23 Snare at the narrowest part of the stalk.

Fig. 10.24 To disengage a trapped snare, push it upstream over the polyp head.

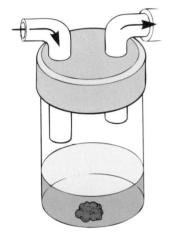

Fig. 10.25 (a) An old-style mucus trap.

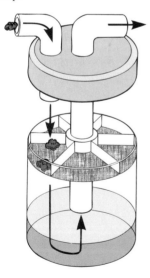

(b) A filtered polyp suction trap.

longer stalks, especially if there is any suspicion of malignancy, it may be possible and desirable to snare lower down to increase the chance of resecting all invasive tissue in the stalk.

8 *If the snare loop is stuck in the wrong position* or if it becomes apparent that the polyp cannot be safely transected, releasing the snare loop is made easier by lifting up over the polyp head and pushing it inwards—with the whole colonoscope if necessary (Fig. 10.24). Alternatively, if the loop is completely trapped, a second small-diameter instrument (gastroscope or paediatric colonoscope) can be inserted alongside the first scope and the biopsy forceps used to coax the trapped wire free. Remember that it is always possible (depending on type) either to dismantle the snare or to sacrifice it by cutting it with wire cutters, withdrawing the colonoscope and leaving the loop *in situ*. Either the polyp head will fall off or another attempt can be made with a new snare or, if necessary, a different endoscopist. It is never necessary to be 'committed' to a polypectomy just because it has been started.

9 *Electrocoagulate* using a low-power coagulating current (15 W or dial setting 2.5–3) with the snare loop kept *gently* closed to 'neck' the tissue and create favourable circumstances for electrocoagulation. Apply the current continuously for 10–15 s at a time, watching for visible swelling or whitening. When the snared part of the stalk or base is visibly coagulating, squeeze the handle more tightly whilst continuing electrocoagulation; transection will start.

10 *Watch where the polyp head falls*, or a lot of time can be wasted looking for it after severance. If it is lost, look for any fluid to indicate the dependent side of the colon where the head is likely to be. If none is visible squirt in some water with a syringe and watch where it flows; if the water simply refluxes back over the lens the polyp will also be behind the instrument tip and the endoscope will need to be withdrawn to find the specimen.

11 *Retrieval of the specimen* may be with the snare, one of the retrieval devices (such as the multiwire 'memory metal' Dormia basket) or by aspiration through the channel into a filtered suction trap (Fig. 10.25), onto a gauze placed where the suction tube joins the umbilical or onto the tip of the endoscope—which may mean having to reinsert the instrument if the view on withdrawal compromises examination. In the presence of numerous polyps it may be necessary to snare/transect some specimens of medium size to allow them to be aspirated and so save time.

Polyp management

Small polyps

During colonoscopy, particularly in patients with larger polyps, it is common to see one or more tiny polyps (2–5 mm diameter) which are below the normal resolution of the radiologist. Tiny polyps are just as awkward to snare as larger ones, and can be difficult to retrieve, even using the filtered suction trap. There has, therefore, been a tendency for some endoscopists to ignore small polyps or to describe them as 'hyperplastic', wrongly inferring that small polyps have no neoplastic potential. On biopsy, 70% of such small polyps prove to be adenomas, and only around 20% of those in the colon (as opposed to the rectum) are hyperplastic. Small polyps in the colon should therefore be destroyed or removed on sight. The best method of doing this is a matter of debate, for surprisingly large (1–2 unit) secondary bleeds can occur 1–12 days after removal or electrodestruction of a 1–2 mm polyp.

Snare or 'cold snare'

Snaring, with retrieval by aspiration into a suction trap, is a convenient way of managing many polyps 5–7 mm in diameter (larger polyps are unlikely to be able to be aspirated through the instrument channel unless fragmented by the snare or in the suction process). The mini-snare is slightly easier to control than the standard snare designed for large polyps. Snaring has the advantage over hot biopsy of squeezing the polyp base (coaptation), so markedly reducing the area and depth of electrocoagulation damage to the remaining mucosa and its underlying blood vessels. Some endoscopists go further and advocate 'cold snaring' without electrocoagulation, physically pulling through the base of the small snared polyp in order to avoid any risk of heat ulceration and delayed bleeds altogether.

The snag of snaring very small polyps is that it is sometimes time-consuming to snare and then find the snared specimen; the smallest specimens are not infrequently lost. Use of the filtered suction trap for retrieval is a significant improvement over the older mucus aspiration trap (designed for bronchoscopy or neonatal care), because each specimen is trapped in a separate numbered compartment and the incorporated filter prevents specimen loss even if excess fluid has to be aspirated.

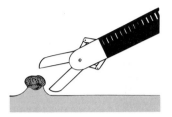

Fig. 10.26 (a) Hot biopsy forceps grasp the small polyp and pull up . . .

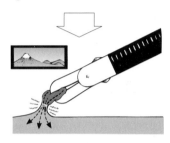

(b) . . . then coagulate until there is 'snow on Mount Fuji' . . .

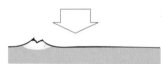

(c) . . . pull off the biopsy sample, leaving the coagulated polyp base.

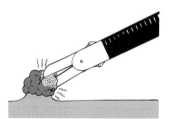

Fig. 10.27 Local burning at the forceps means the polyp is too large for hot biopsy.

'Hot biopsy'

Electrocoagulating hot biopsy forceps (Fig. 10.26a) are nonetheless a quick and effective alternative, with an over 95% yield of histology. Their use is now only considered appropriate for polyps up to 5 mm diameter and patients *not* taking aspirin (to avoid the significant risk in such patients of major delayed haemorrhage). Hot biopsy forceps have an electrically insulated plastic sheath and are connected to the electrosurgical unit. The patient plate is placed on the patient's thigh and connections made as for polypectomy. A similar 'coag' power setting is used to that for snaring a small polyp (15–25 W or equivalent) and the foot switch is placed so that it does not have to be looked for when required.

The polyp or part of its head is grasped in the jaws of the forceps, and the colonoscope angled or withdrawn slightly to pull up the grasped polyp away from the colon wall onto a pseudopedicle like a small mountain (Fig. 10.26b). Ensure that the black insulating plastic of the forceps is visible, so that the metal parts of the jaws do not contact the endoscope. Next apply the coagulating current for around 2–3 s. Since the pseudopedicle is the narrowest part, it will heat and coagulate. The extent of this coagulation is easily seen as whitening, which should only spread just over halfway down the 'mountain' — as in pictures showing snow on the summit of Mount Fuji (Fig. 10.26b; Plate 10.1). The idea is to destroy the narrow neck of tissue under the polyp but not to damage and ulcerate the bowel wall significantly. Pull off the biopsy at this point in the knowledge that, even if some of the head is left uncoagulated, its basal tissue and blood vessels will have been destroyed.

Providing that a high enough power setting is used to finish local electrocoagulation in around 2–3 s, the heat produced in the basal tissues will not conduct back to the metal parts of the forceps and the biopsy specimen protected within the jaws is therefore unharmed. Polyps over 5 mm in diameter are not suitable for hot biopsy removal; either the base will be broader than the area of contact of the forceps and so only a small burn will result at the surface of the polyp (Fig. 10.27) or the current fanning out from the point of contact of the hot biopsy forceps with a too-large polyp will heat tissue at a distance — invisibly and dangerously (Fig. 10.28). Coagulating for too long or attempting to destroy over-large polyps with the hot biopsy technique risks causing a deep ulcer with full-thickness heating and perforation (especially in the proximal colon) or delayed haemorrhage 24–48 h later. If a polyp proves to be too large for rapid and localized visible electrocoagulation, *stop*, take the biopsy, and remove the rest of the tissue by conventional snare polypectomy.

Problem polyps

Sessile polyps

Having appreciated the principles of current density in electro-coagulation, it should be obvious why removal of large sessile polyps (Fig. 10.29a) or broad-stalked polyps presents problems to the endoscopist. Fortunately, many so-called 'sessile' polyps are simply semipedunculated and can be pulled up by the snare onto an adequate and compressible pseudostalk. Having snared a polyp, the closed snare should always be moved to and fro; if the mucosa moves, but not the bowel wall, there is no danger; if the colon moves too, the full thickness of the wall has been 'tented' (Fig. 10.29b) and the snare should be repositioned to take only a smaller part. If a polyp base is over 1.5 cm in diameter, without a stalk, the safe course is to take the head piecemeal in a number of bits (Fig. 10.30); each bit can be cut through with no risk of full-thickness burns and little risk of bleeding since the vessels of the head are much smaller than those in the stalk. With the submucosal injection technique described below, however, it may be possible to remove flat sessile polyps up to 1.5–2 cm in diameter in a single specimen.

Sometimes a sessile polyp is better removed by surgery (or laparoscopy), but this should be a matter of expert opinion and clinical judgement; sessile polyps up to 5 cm in diameter can be removed, providing that the hazards and the trauma involved are appreciated by all concerned and that the endoscopist is very experienced. As a rule of thumb it has been suggested that sessile polyps occupying more than one-third of the colon circumference, or involving two haustral folds, are too big for safe endoscopic removal. If in doubt it is better to make repeated piecemeal attempts at different sessions to lessen the chance of full-thickness heat damage to the bowel wall, to give time for histological assessment (surgery will be indicated if any piece contains malignancy) and to allow the site to be checked for recurrent polyp tissue. The endoscopic approach is the obvious one in a patient who is a bad operative risk and is prepared to accept repeated endoscopy. In a younger patient, or if there are technical difficulties, it may be better sometimes to admit that the risks of surgery are not excessive compared to the trials of aggressive endoscopy, which may not remove all neoplastic tissue, or the use of a laser which destroys the evidence.

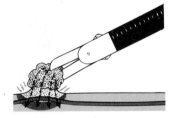

Fig. 10.28 Current fanning out from the point of contact will heat (invisibly) at a distance, risking delayed bleeding or perforation in polyps too large for hot biopsy.

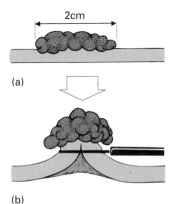

Fig. 10.29 (a) Sessile polyps can be risky to snare in one portion . . . (b) . . . because 'tenting' results.

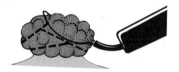

Fig. 10.30 Piecemeal removal is safer (although less satisfactory for the pathologist).

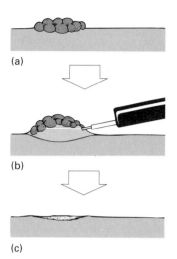

(a)

(b)

(c)

Fig. 10.31 Injection polypectomy.
(a) A small sessile polyp . . .
(b) . . . elevated by submucosal
saline injection . . . (c) . . . and
snared off in one piece.

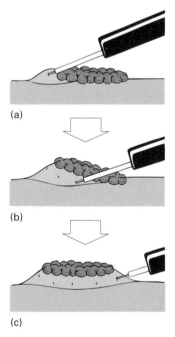

(a)

(b)

(c)

Fig. 10.32 (a) First inject
proximally to a larger sessile
polyp . . . (b) . . . then around the
periphery . . . (c) . . . to elevate it
completely before snaring.

Submucosal injection to elevate sessile polyps is common in proctology and was originally described for use in flexible endoscopy in 1973. It has been popularized by Japanese authors recently under the misnomer 'strip biopsy', with the object of obtaining small sessile polyps (flat adenomas) in a single histopathological specimen (Fig. 10.31). Injection polypectomy, as it has been called by several authors, can equally be used for removal of much larger polyps. When it works well the technique also has advantages in creating both an entirely bloodless transection and a 'safety cushion' of engorged submucosal stroma to protect the bowel wall from dissipated heat.

The solution used can be 1 : 10 000 adrenaline in 0.9% (N) saline, but this dissipates in 2–3 min whereas use of a hypertonic solution (2N saline or 20% dextrose, with or without adrenaline) makes the injected bleb last longer. With a 10 ml syringe the sclerotherapy needle is jabbed tangentially into the mucosal surface, and a very low-pressure injection made, if necessary withdrawing the needle slightly until a submucosal bleb is seen to be forming. An injection of 1–3 ml should be enough to raise the submucosa and a small polyp on top of it for immediate snaring. For larger lesions (Fig. 10.32) the trick is to make the first injection *proximal* to the polyp, and to insert the needle for each subsequent injection into the edge of the preceding bleb. There is no hazard involved if the needle passes into the peritoneum and no contraindication to injecting *through* the substance of a shallow sessile polyp if necessary, although usually the peripheral injections will coalesce centrally and make this unnecessary (unless there is invasion and fixation). A confluent ring of injections sufficient to raise a 4–5 cm sessile polyp may need up to 30 ml total injection volume. It is a mistake to start injecting distal to a larger lesion, as the resulting mound worsens the view of the proximal part of it.

Endoscopic gymnastics may be needed on occasion, such as when using a small-diameter instrument inverted to pre-inject in retroversion, or even to snare in this position as well. Standard polypectomy snares sometimes slip off the moist and domed pre-injected area and a 'spiked snare' is available, the barbs of which hook into the tissue satisfactorily. A stiffer thin monofilament snare can similarly be effective for cutting into the polyp (bleeding is not a significant risk in sessile polyps) and a needle-knife has been used by some to pre-cut at the margins. Another trick is to fix the tip of the snare into the mucosal surface at an appropriate point by brief electrocoagulation, which can make control of the loop easier. If a two-channel instrument is available a grasper can be used to elevate the polyp through a pre-placed snare, which is then closed and polypectomy performed.

Pain during polypectomy, unless due to overinsufflation, is a useful warning that full-thickness heating of the bowel wall is occurring and activating peritoneal pain receptors. Fortunately this occurs before there is any serious risk of damage. If pain occurs and deflation does not remove it (it is easy to be 'heavy' on the air button trying to keep a good view during a problematic polypectomy), the procedure should be abandoned until another session at least 3 weeks later — when healing should have occurred and the area can be properly assessed.

Large rectal polyps

Large sessile polyps in the rectum within 12 cm of the anal verge, are usually better and more safely removed by local proctological techniques under anaesthesia, with anal dilatation and a two-handed approach, including ligature or suture if necessary. Partial electrocoagulation or attempted laser photodestruction of such rectal polyps by the endoscopist forms scar tissue which greatly complicates the method of submucosal adrenaline injection and scissor excision used by skilled proctologists. Only 1 : 100 000 adrenaline solution is used in the rectum (compared to 1 : 10 000 solution in the colon) because of the possibility of communication to the systemic circulation and danger of cardiac dysrhythmias. Sessile polyps more than 12 cm above the anal margin can be reached with a Buess stereoptic microsurgical operating sigmoidoscope where this is available, but will more often be managed by the flexible endoscopist using injection and piecemeal removal, argon beam electrodestruction or laser photocoagulation. Smaller rectal polyps, situated close to the 'dentate line' of anal canal squamous epithelium, can be snared in retroversion using prior injection of local anaesthetic unless the polyp is very small; the distal part of the rectal ampulla can otherwise be difficult to visualize properly and is also richly supplied with sensory nerves.

Large-stalked polyps

Extra electrocoagulation is needed to minimize the chance of bleeding from the relatively large plexus of vessels in a large stalk. Start at a mechanical advantage, take time and care to place the snare optimally on the narrowest part of the stalk, having palpated with the closed snare and, if needs be, rotated the endoscope or patient to get the best possible view (Figs 10.21 & 10.33). Have an adrenaline-filled injection cannula available in case of bleeding, and consider pre-injection at the base. Be prepared to use a slightly higher than usual current setting, and to electrocoagulate for a much longer than usual time before swelling and whitening indicate that it is safe to start transection. If, in the process of transection, the core desiccates and the snare will not make the final cut, resist the urge to 'pull through' the snare because the thickest arteries are the last to sever; it is

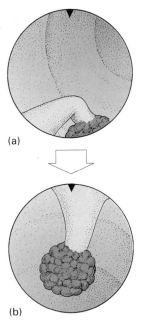

(a)

(b)

Fig. 10.33 (a) Bad view of a polyp? (b) Change the patient's position to let gravity help.

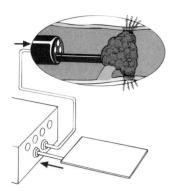

Fig. 10.34 'Leak' current can result in contralateral burns.

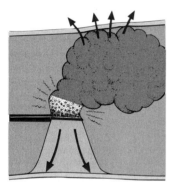

Fig. 10.35 A large area of contact reduces the risk of contralateral burn, but also reduces current flow and heat coagulation in the lower stalk.

better to raise the current setting still further. After the polyp head separates, the thick stalk remnant sometimes shows little visible electrocoagulation, in which case it may be wise to re-snare lower down, squeeze gently and electrocoagulate further (without transection) before removing the loop.

Contralateral burns have been a matter of (largely unwarranted) concern. During snaring of a large-stalked polyp, the head will flop about, inevitably touching the bowel wall in several places. 'Leak' currents flow at each point of contact, which results in inefficient heating of the stalk (Fig. 10.34) and the possibility of a contralateral burn—often out of the field of view. The burn hazard is more theoretical than real but any possibility can be avoided by moving the whole polyp around during coagulation so that no one point gets all the heat, or by making sure that the area of point of contact is larger than that of the stalk. During a difficult polypectomy of a large polyp, try to keep a view of the snared stalk to ensure that adequate visible coagulation occurs below the snare loop. If leak currents flow up the stalk, electrocoagulation can occur primarily above the snare (Fig. 10.35) and bleeding can result from inadequately coagulated vessels in the lower part of the stalk.

Stalk pre-injection or sclerotherapy is a possible preventive measure before snaring and transection of large-stalked polyps (Fig. 10.36a). The technique is exceedingly easy. Adrenaline (1–10 ml 1:10 000 dilution in 0.9–1.8% (N or 2N) saline) is injected at one or more sites into the base of the polyp (Plate 10.2) and causes visible blanching from vessel contraction within a minute or so; employing hypertonic saline slows dissipation from the site. The endoscopist sees blanching and swelling of the stalk and finally mauve coloration of the ischaemic head. Transection can then be made through the upper part of the stalk or above the injected area in the certain knowledge that there will be no bleeding at all.

Addition of sclerosant to the injection may be relevant for some long-stalked polyps, especially in a patient on aspirin, non-steroidal anti-inflammatory drugs (NSAIDs) or other

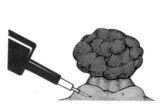

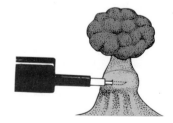

Fig. 10.36 (a) Inject broad-stalked polyps with adrenaline before snaring to avoid bleeding. (b) For long-stalked polyps with a risk of bleeding inject sclerosant and adrenaline.

platelet-coating agents, or when anticoagulants cannot be withdrawn. The sclerosant solution (ethanolamine, sodium tetra-
decyl sulphate or ethoxysclerol) is made up in equal volume to
the adrenaline; inject only 1–3 ml (Fig. 10.36b) This injection
causes aggressive long-lasting local vascular coagulation and
oedema in the stalk which should remove any risk of delayed
haemorrhage. Because of the obvious risk of causing bowel
wall damage, addition of sclerosant is only indicated for
stalked polyps where the risk of haemorrhage is thought to be
significant.

Nylon safety loop or metal clipping devices are available to
control or prevent stalk bleeding, and the use of rubber-band
placement (as for variceal therapy) has been similarly described.
This is particularly relevant to large-stalked polyps or smaller
polyps in patients on anticoagulants or aspirin as a way of
placing strangulating accessories onto the remaining stalk. The
most certain method for larger stalks is the nylon self-retaining
loop (Fig. 10.37), usually placed *after* polypectomy on the stalk
remnant because the loop is difficult to manoeuvre over a head
of 2 cm or more. For smaller stalks, one or more metal clips can
be placed easily before or after snaring; the clips are also said to
be effective in controlling local bleeding after polypectomy in
any size polyp.

Snare-loop intussusception or 'pull-down' polypectomy is a rare
possibility for co-operative management between the endoscopist and surgeon of very large broad-stalked polyps in the
distal sigmoid colon. Such polyps situated 30–35 cm from the
anus occasionally present spontaneously to the anus and can,
providing that there are no pericolic adhesions (diverticular
disease, pelvic surgery, etc.), often be snared and pulled down
by snare-loop intussusception (Fig. 10.38) for local removal by a
colorectal surgeon under general anaesthesia. A thick monofilament nylon loop (Fig. 10.39) (passed through a catheter and
opened by pulling on one end whilst pushing on the other) is
ideal for this purpose, since it is unlikely to cut through the
polyp stalk and has no handle. After snaring the stalk, the
colonoscope is withdrawn altogether, leaving the snare *in situ*
and held closed with an artery forceps. If the intussuscepted
head can be felt by digital palpation the extra pelvic relaxation of
general anaesthesia will allow it to be delivered to the anus.
After the patient is anaesthetized with muscle relaxants the
polyp can be pulled down with gentle traction to the dilated
anus, grasped, locally excised and the base sutured for extra safety.

Recovery of very large polyps, 3 cm or more in diameter, can
be difficult, particularly through tonic anal sphincters. The
polyp will often fragment if excessive traction is needed on the
snare or retrieval forceps, although the multiwire Dormia basket
or polyp-retrieval net may avoid this. Ask the patient to bear
down 'as if to pass wind' in order to relax the sphincters; at the

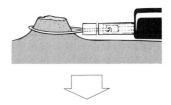

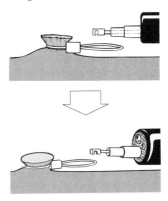

Fig. 10.37 (a) A nylon self-
retaining loop can be placed over
a large stalk . . .

(b) . . . and its self-retaining cuff
tightened and the loop unhooked.

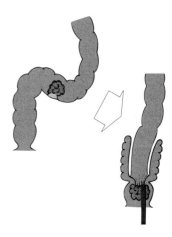

Fig. 10.38 Snare-loop
intussusception can be used for
very large polyps in the distal
sigmoid.

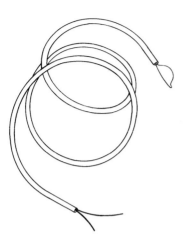

Fig. 10.39 A homemade (handleless) snare or retrieval loop.

same time traction is applied to produce the polyp (cover the perineal area to avoid explosive surprises!). If withdrawal fails in the left lateral position, asking the patient to squat on the floor or sit on a commode seat and expelling the polyp while traction is maintained on the retrieval device is more physiological; the minor embarrassment of the manoeuvre is well worthwhile, for rapid polyp delivery invariably results. Alternatively, a split overtube can be inserted into the rectum over the colonoscope, the polyp pulled into the end of the tube and the whole assembly removed together; a large rigid proctoscope and tissue-grasping or sponge-holding forceps can be similarly used to pull out the polyp and instrument together.

For removal of a large single polyp, putting a volume of air and water through the endoscope, some enema solution in the rectum and then waiting for self-expulsion is a reasonable last resort, albeit with some risk of autolysis of the specimen.

Multiple polyps

Fortunately 90% of adenoma patients have only one or two polyps and it is very uncommon to find more than five polyps. Some multiple polyps (hyperplastic, Peutz–Jeghers, juvenile, lymphoid, lipomatous or inflammatory) are non-neoplastic, so that it may sometimes be preferable to await results of standard biopsies before undertaking heroic multiple polypectomies. In the rare circumstance that a patient has six or more obvious polyps, it is essential to examine the whole colon before snaring to be certain that multiple other smaller polyps are not present, with the possibility of a diagnosis of polyposis coli. Looking for tiny reflective nodules in the 'light reflex' off the transparent mucosal surface shows up polyps down to 1 mm in diameter which are invisible to direct vision. Melanosis coli (more properly pseudomelanosis) also shows up tiny non-pigmented polyps or lymphoid follicles very well (Plate 10.3).

Dye spray, sometimes called 'chromoscopy', is a way of enhancing the endoscopist's accuracy of view even further, to nearly dissecting microscopic level (Plate 10.4). The principle is to use a spray of surface dye (such as 10% dilution of washable blue fountain-pen ink or 0.1% indigo carmine) (see p. 262) which will emphasize any small polyps down to under 0.5 mm in size as pale islands on a blue background facilitate accurate biopsy. Dye is most accurately applied using a washing or purpose-made dye-spray catheter. An alternative is to use the syringe washing attachment of the colonoscope to introduce more concentrated dye, the water button being used to eject the dye close-up onto the mucosa. A small amount of silicone particle antifoam can be added to the dye if bubbles create a problem by simulating tiny polyps. Histology is essential because lymphoid follicles can resemble adenomas to the untutored eye and hyperplastic polyposis is indistinguishable from adenomatous polyposis, but does not need surgery.

Retrieval of multiple polyps is potentially tedious since it can mean passing the colonoscope several times; even this is preferable to surgery and can be facilitated by a number of means including the use of a split overtube (see above) for quicker reintroduction of the instrument. Accessories such as the multi-wire Dormia basket or the polyp-retrieval net will retrieve up to three to five moderately large polyps, but one or two polyps may be more easily picked up in the polypectomy snare. Any smaller polyps present can be hot biopsied or snared and then aspirated through the suction line into the filtered polyp suction trap (see Fig. 10.25).

The 'wash-out' technique is a reasonable compromise after the snare removal of a large number of non-neoplastic polyps (Peutz–Jeghers syndrome, juvenile or inflammatory polyposis) or if the colonoscopy has been too difficult to justify repeated withdrawal and reinsertion. All snared polyps are first retrieved to the descending colon or below; the colonoscope is then passed to the splenic flexure and 500 ml of warm tap water is syringe-injected through the instrument channel. The proximal colon is air-insufflated until the patient feels some distension and, just before the colonoscope is withdrawn from the anus, a disposable or phosphate enema can be injected through the endoscope to ensure passage of most of the polyps or polyp fragments into a commode within a few minutes.

Inflammatory polyps, sometimes called pseudopolyps, characteristically appear as shiny tags of healthy and non-neoplastic tissue after the healing of previous severe colitis of any kind (Plate 10.5). Only those of 1 cm or greater need be removed, partly because of their tendency to bleed but also because of the difficulty in distinguishing them from adenomas; if in doubt a single forceps biopsy will confirm the trivial nature of the lesion. Larger post-inflammatory polyps can be composed of disorganized tissue remarkably similar to that of a hamartomatous (juvenile) polyp or of granulation tissue. They can bleed surprisingly after snaring, partly because they tend to have soft bases which 'cheese-wire' through too quickly compared to the more muscular pedicle of other polyps, but also because they can be very vascular. Sessile polyps after ulcerative colitis must be treated with suspicion, since they may represent the most visible part of a 'field change' of high-grade dysplasia; take mucosal biopsies around the base before snaring to discount this possibility.

Malignant polyps

It is sometimes not obvious at the time of snaring that a polyp is malignant. Malignancy may be suspected if a polyp is irregular, ulcerated, firm or has a particularly thick stalk; firmness to palpation is probably the best single discriminant. If malignancy is possible, it is important to be certain that transection has been made low down the stalk (to give the pathologist a proper assessment) and to ensure that all visible polyp tissue has been removed, although without risking perforation. The endoscopist should report whether or not the polyp has been completely removed. If necessary an early repeat examination can be made, preferably within 2 weeks since at a longer interval there may be no visible ulcer to indicate the polypectomy site. Because of the possibility of malignancy, each polyp must be retrieved and identified separately on an anatomical polyp map. It is inadequate to say that a polyp was removed at '70 cm from the anus' since this might represent the mid-sigmoid colon or caecum.

Tattooing, using a 1 ml aliquot of diluted India ink injected intramucosally at the time of polypectomy, is an excellent way to mark the site of a suspicious or partially removed polyp. Sterile black India ink is used. The carbon particles of the ink remain in the submucosa for many years (probably for life), and are easily visible to the endoscopist as a blue-grey stain for follow-up purposes. The permanency of the tattoo reflects the lack of local lymphatics to remove the inert particles—and parallels the tendency of colonic malignant cells also to stay localized. The *non*-waterproof variety of painter's brushing India ink is appropriate (as used for water colours), rather than pen ink (which contains noxious materials such as shellac, and solvents which can result in inflammation or peritoneal irritation). Ideally the ink should be diluted 1 : 100 and autoclaved before injection; use of an 0.22 µl syringe-mounted bacterial filter has been said to be an effective alternative means of sterilization. Injection is made using a sclerotherapy needle inserted just under the mucosal surface (Fig. 10.40; Plate 10.6) the frequent problem of leakage and 'black-out' of the endoscopic view can be avoided by first gently injecting a small saline bleb submucosally, then changing syringes so that the 1 ml India ink aliquot enters the preformed space. If surgery is a possibility rather than endoscopic follow-up, it is best to make three to four larger tattoos around the circumference for easy serosal identification.

The dilemma of 'adequate' removal of malignancy is a recurrent problem when a polyp is reported as malignant by the pathologist, and not infrequently a surprise to the endoscopist as well because (other than the non-specific features of large size, induration or irregular surface) the macroscopic appearance can be unremarkable. The clinician or the endoscopist is then faced with a dilemma, but happily one which can usually be resolved in favour of conservatism, certainly for pedunculated polyps. If the cancer is reported histologically as 'well' or 'averagely well' differentiated, with a margin between the limit of invasion at

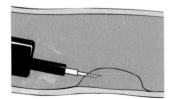

Fig. 10.40 A 1 ml India ink tattoo marks a polypectomy site permanently.

least 2 mm from the electrocoagulated tissue at the transection line, most experts would not recommend surgery, assuming that endoscopic removal also appeared complete. The likelihood of there being resectable lymph node involvement under these circumstances is extremely small (as opposed to the even smaller possibility of unresectable distant metastases), whereas the mortality of surgery is significant.

If the malignant polyp is sessile or invasion extends histologically to the resection line, involves lymphatic vessels or is poorly differentiated (anaplastic), the likelihood of involved lymph nodes is significant and most would favour operation, unless the patient is a poor surgical risk. Clinical judgement is involved, balancing risks and clinical factors. It may be difficult not to operate in a young patient, mainly for emotional reasons. In older patients the decision is not so obvious; very few patients have been found at operation to have locally involved resectable lymph nodes or residual tumour even when the histology appears unfavourable, but some with no residual cancer have died as a result of unnecessary surgery.

Complications

Bleeding. Bleeding is the most frequent complication which, when it occurs, is usually visible immediately after section, but sometimes not until many days later. Bleeding should complicate under 1% of polypectomies, the previous problems with haemorrhage from large polyp stalks having been largely removed by awareness of the need for maximum electrocoagulation and adjuncts such as adrenaline injection and nylon-loop or clip strangulation. *Secondary haemorrhage* may occur 1–14 days after polypectomy, particularly after the removal of large-stalked polyps or the use of hot biopsy on over-large polyps or in patients on aspirin, which should be stopped 7–10 days beforehand. Patients who have had polypectomy should know of the possibility of delayed bleeding and the need to report to an emergency department for observation should any occur. Delayed haemorrhage normally stops spontaneously but transfusion may occasionally be required.

An *immediate haemorrhage* is usually a slow ooze but can be an arterial spurt of frightening proportions, as viewed endoscopically. Every possible attempt should be made to stop an arterial bleed immediately as any delay can result in the view being lost or in clot formation. Quickly re-snare the remaining stalk or inject up to 5–10 ml of 1:10000 adrenaline solution submucosally into or adjacent to the stalk remnant. If the stalk has been re-snared, simple strangulation alone, with taping of the snare handle closed for 10–15 min is usually sufficient without further electrocoagulation. If bleeding recurs on releasing the snare, attempts to stop it can be made with further electrocoagulation or by injection, if necessary using a second instrument (paediatric colonoscope or gastroscope) passed up alongside the first. In the unlikely event that arterial bleeding persists in spite of all efforts, the most elegant solution is to perform selective arterial catheterization and embolization or infusion of pitressin (success has been reported using pitressin or somatostatin by intravenous infusion alone). A surgical team must be alerted and adequate supplies of blood ensured.

If blood does obscure the view of the bleeding point, the most effective action is to infuse large volumes of water containing dilute topical adrenaline (5 ml 1 : 10 000 adrenaline per 50 ml water) in the region of the bleeding. This helps to prevent the formation of clots, which are impossible to aspirate and, with posturing to the right side if necessary to visualize the distal colon, should allow location of the polypectomy site. Persistent or secondary haemorrhage in the left colon will be indicated by repeated calls to stool and the passage of fresh clots, whereas in the right colon the rate of bleeding is more difficult to assess because of the long delay before volumes of altered blood are expelled.

The 'post-polypectomy syndrome' or 'closed perforation' of full-thickness heat damage to the bowel wall is an occasional sequel to a difficult polypectomy, such as the piecemeal removal of a sessile polyp. The patient experiences localized abdominal pain and fever for 12–24 h following polypectomy, without free gas on X-ray or signs of generalized peritonitis. This is due to the inflammatory reaction of the peritoneum and is followed by adherence to the omentum or small bowel; it is therefore self-limiting. Conservative management with bed rest and systemic antibiotics is indicated, but surgical consultation is wise if the symptoms and signs do not abate rapidly.

Frank perforation with an electrosurgical snare is fortunately a rare occurrence. Its management may often be conservative, but this depends on the area of the polyp base. A small polyp removed by snare or hot biopsy in a well-prepared bowel is obviously a low risk, whereas signs of perforation after a larger or sessile lesion in a poorly prepared colon mandates surgery. A surgeon should always be alerted and, if in doubt, it is safest to operate.

Safety

It cannot be overemphasized that polypectomy is potentially hazardous and that rigorous adherence to all possible safety factors is essential. Assuming that the correct equipment has been acquired, it must be carefully handled and maintained. Never bend or coil the connecting leads tightly or they will fracture; if a lead looks or feels partially fractured, replace it or have it mended at once. If polypectomy is not proceeding according to plan, check the connections, patient plate and circuitry before anything else.

As already explained, the greatest single safety factor lies in a strict routine regularly repeated for each polypectomy, because human error is much more likely than failure of the equipment. A military-type approach has much to commend it: any request from the endoscopist being repeated out loud by the assistant so that each knows what the other is doing. The assistant and the endoscopist must check on each other to watch that all is in order during the procedure, having checked the equipment (including marking the snare handle at the point of closure) beforehand.

Good bowel preparation is needed to give a good view and a dry field in which to work. If bowel preparation is poor, as during flexible sigmoidoscopy, use carbon dioxide instead of air to prevent the possibility of explosive combinations of oxygen (from inflated air) with methane (from bacterial metabolism of protein residues) or hydrogen (from bacterial fermentation of carbohydrates). Alternatively take great care to insufflate and then aspirate repeatedly to dilute any gas present. In a well-prepared bowel (other than with mannitol) there is no explosion hazard and air can be safely used (see the caveat on mannitol bowel preparation, p. 195).

The patient's medications should be checked. To minimize the risk of delayed haemorrhage, patient medication with aspirin, NSAIDs and other medications affecting platelet adhesion should ideally be withdrawn 7–10 days before (to allow a new generation of 'sticky' platelets to form), and for 14 days after, the procedure. Only a very experienced operator should undertake polypectomy in a patient still taking anticoagulants; the patient should be warned of the need for immediate repeat endoscopy should bleeding occur, and careful precautions should be taken for effective coagulation during polypectomy and perhaps safety loops or clips placed afterwards. Often, with the approval of the relevant clinician, anticoagulants can be stopped for the 10–12-day period needed to cover the likelihood of immediate or delayed bleeding after polypectomy. Some favour admitting the patient to hospital and transfer to heparin for the immediate post-polypectomy period, but the major risk of (delayed) bleeding comes later, often after discharge from hospital.

Polypectomy outside the colon

Although the principles and techniques described refer primarily to polypectomy in the colon, they are essentially the same for gastric polypectomy or polypectomy in the small intestine and the same rules can be followed. There may be a higher risk of bleeding when snaring gastroduodenal polyps compared with those in the colon. Snare-loop biopsy for diagnostic purposes (Ménétrièr's disease, etc.) is useful in the stomach but some caution is needed since it is easy to take a much bigger bite than intended when using a wide-angled instrument in a large viscus. We suppress gastric acid for 1 week afterwards to reduce the likelihood of delayed haemorrhage after gastric electrosurgery. Gastric polyps are easily lost after snaring so that antispasmodics and a quick eye and hand are desirable; a Dormia basket is the ideal means for safe retrieval of specimens.

The wall of the duodenum and small intestine is thin and there is a corresponding need for caution in snaring and electrosurgery. Apart from patients with Peutz–Jeghers polyps, which are usually thin-stalked and easy to snare, the major indication for duodenal polypectomy is in patients with familial adenomatous polyposis. The large sessile polyps that occur in about 10% of these patients are too hazardous to remove, whereas the tiny polyps or dysplastic areas that can be seen in almost all the remainder can be ignored. The endoscopist's role in their surveillance currently seems to be limited to 1–3-yearly observation with representative biopsies and potential for using ultrasound probes; severe dysplasia histologically or worrying macroscopic appearances occasionally indicate open surgery, mucosectomy or excision being performed as appropriate.

Other therapeutic procedures

Balloon dilatation

Balloon dilatation of short colonic strictures, particularly postoperative anastomoses, has been made easy by through the scope (TTS) balloons made of non-distensible polyethylene (as used in the upper gastrointestinal tract). Balloons of at least 18 mm diameter give the best long-term results — often with relief of symptoms for a year or more. Those that are 5 cm long are easiest to 'dumb-bell' in a stricture, whereas 3 cm long balloons tend to slip in or out of the narrowing on distension. Ideally a large (4.2 mm) channel should be used for TTS balloons in the proximal colon to allow easy passage through the angled instrument and to avoid expensive breakages. For similar reasons it is important that any TTS balloon is completely deflated and silicone-lubricated before insertion, and that the instrument shaft should be straightened as much as possible to minimize insertion force. Balloons should always be fluid-distended, using either water or dilute contrast material. A pressure-gun and manometer are essential, for it is impossible to generate and to sustain the recommended distension pressure by hand for the 2 min needed to dilate effectively, especially as the balloon itself slowly stretches a little. Check carefully on the pressure for the particular balloon (larger balloons need less pressure) so as not to overdistend and burst it unnecessarily.

Colonic strictures are frequently found at an angulation, which may make the passage of a balloon difficult; there can therefore be a place for initial passage of a flexible guidewire followed by a suitable balloon. In the left colon, endoscopic insertion of a guidewire can be followed either by a balloon or bougie. Wire-guided dilators can be used under fluoroscopic control or with the instrument also inserted for visual control.

Tube placement

Colonoscopic placement of drainage tubes or recording devices is possible as far as the ileocaecal region, ideally with an internal removable stiffening wire to stop early tube displacement. The technique is particularly important in prolonged postoperative ileus or episodic pseudo-obstruction of the colon (Ogilvie's syndrome), where endoscopic deflation avoids the need for surgery. The easiest technique is the 'piggy-back' method in which a loop attached to the leading end of the tube is grasped by forceps (Fig. 10.41). A variation which allows better suction during the procedure (the colon may be unprepared and foul) is to use a thin loop of cotton thread at the end of the tube, held by a loop of strong monofilament nylon passed through the suction channel; once in the proximal colon a sharp tug on the nylon breaks the cotton loop and the tube is free.

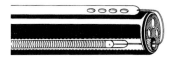

Fig. 10.41 A deflation tube can be carried up alongside the colonoscope.

Derotation of the volvulus

If the passage of a rectal tube will not deflate a sigmoid volvulus and allow it to derotate, the colonoscope can be passed as a steerable flatus tube. Large-channel colonoscopes allow a deflation tube (with a stiffening guidewire) to be inserted through the instrumentation channel. After the tube or endoscope tip is passed gently into or through the twisted segment, deflation alone is usually sufficient for the torsion to reverse spontaneously; actual endoscopic manipulation is usually unnecessary. However, if the segment appears blue-black and gangrenous, surgery is indicated because of the high risk of perforation.

Use of the colonoscope to reduce *intussusception* in the proximal colon is generally unrewarding, because not enough inward push can be transmitted around the looped colon.

Angiodysplasia

The electrocoagulation of angiodysplasia (Plate 9.14) has been mentioned previously. Since they occur mainly in the thin-walled proximal colon, great care should be taken with whichever modality is used — electrocoagulation (mono- or

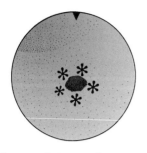

Fig. 10.42 Point coagulation around angiodysplasia before heating the centre.

bipolar, contact or argon beam), heater probe and, especially, laser. The object of the exercise is to damage the superficial part of the lesion (which extends also into the submucosa) in such a way as both to coagulate the vessels nearest the surface which are most liable to trauma and to produce re-epithelialization thereafter by normal mucosa. It is preferable to cause a ring of local heating points around the periphery of a larger lesion, followed by one or more applications near the centre, rather than to apply excessive heat in one area alone (Fig. 10.42). Err on the side of too little heat; even minor whitening and oedema will progress to produce remarkable local ulceration within 24 h. It is easy enough to repeat the examination a few weeks later to check results, but difficult to justify perforation from over-aggression during the first procedure. The careful use of hot biopsy forceps is particularly effective with smaller lesions, which can be grasped, the mucosa tented up and selectively heated. It is unnecessary to take a biopsy, the jaws being simply re-opened after minimal visible coagulation. Larger lesions should be tackled last because mechanical trauma can cause them to bleed and obscure other lesions which may be present. For the same reason the most dependent lesions are treated first. Protuberant cavernous haemangiomas (blue rubber bleb naevus syndrome) are better managed by sclerotherapy.

Tumour destruction

Use of laser photocoagulation to vaporize inoperable or obstructing tumour tissue is described in Chapter 5. A similar effect can be achieved, more laboriously but very cheaply, by multiple injections of 100% ethanol using a sclerotherapy needle, the procedure being repeated every day or two until the desired clearance is achieved. In many circumstances piecemeal snare de-bulking is a useful and quick preliminary to 'pare down' tumour tissue. In the rectum the use of a wire resectoscope loop, similar to that employed during transurethral prostatectomy, under glycine solution or in air, has also been described.

The argon beam electrocoagulator allows non-contact superficial tissue destruction, like a laser but at a more moderate price. A catheter with an integral wire allows current flow to ionize the argon gas forming an intensely hot local plasma discharge. This causes tissue necrosis to a predictable depth of 2–3 mm, sufficient for some sessile lesions or superficial residual tumour.

Further reading

Polypectomy techniques

Barlow, DE. Endoscopic applications of electrosurgery: a review of basic principles. *Gastrointest Endosc* 1982;**28**:73–6.

Karita M, Tada M, Okita K, Kodama T. Endoscopic therapy for early colon cancer: the strip biopsy resection technique. *Gastrointest Endosc* 1991;**37**:128–32.

Mathus-Vliegen EMH, Tytgat GNJ. Laser ablation and palliation in colorectal malignancy. *Gastrointest Endosc* 1986;**32**:393–6.

McNally PR, DeAngelis SA, Rison DR, Sudduth RH. Bipolar polypectomy device for removal of colon polyps. *Gastrointest Endosc* 1994;**40**:489–91.

Nivatvongs S. Complications in colonoscopic polypectomy. An experience with 1555 polypectomies. *Dis Colon Rectum* 1986;**29**:825–30.

Shatz BA, Thavorides V. Colonic tattoo for follow-up of endoscopic sessile polypectomy. *Gastrointest Endosc* 1991;**37**:59–60.

Shirai M, Nakamura T, Matsuura A. Safer colonoscopic polypectomy with local submucosal injection of hypertonic saline-epinephrine solution. *Am J Gastroenterol* 1994;**89**:334–8.

Tappero G, Gaia E, DeGiuli P *et al.* Cold snare excision of small colorectal polyps. *Gastrointest Endosc* 1992;**38**:310–13.

Wadas DD, Sanowski RA. Complications of the hot-biopsy forceps technique. *Gastrointest Endosc* 1987;**33**:32–7.

Waye JD. Endoscopic treatment of adenomas. *World J Surg* 1991;**15**:14–19.

Waye J, Geenen J, Fleischer D. *Techniques in Therapeutic Endoscopy.* Philadelphia: WB Saunders, 1987.

Wu D, Silverstein FE. Principles of electrosurgery. In: Raskin JB, Nord HJ, eds. *Colonoscopy: Principles and Technique.* Tokyo: Igaku-Shoin, 1995:83–93.

Clinical aspects of polypectomy

Bond JH. Polyp guideline: diagnosis, treatment and surveillance for patients with nonfamilial colorectal polyps. *Ann Int Med* 1993;**119**:836–43.

Cranley JP, Petras RE, Carey WD, Paradis K, Sivak MV. When is endoscopic polypectomy adequate therapy for colonic polyps containing invasive carcinoma? *Gastroenterology* 1986;**91**:419–27.

Giardiello FM, Welsh SB, Hamilton SR *et al.* Peutz–Jeghers syndrome: perhaps not so benign. *N Engl J Med* 1987;**316**:1511–14.

Haggitt RC, Glotzbach RE, Soffer EE, Wruble LD. Prognostic factors in colorectal carcinomas arising in adenomas: implications for lesions removed by endoscopic polypectomy. *Gastroenterology* 1985;**89**:328–36.

Hoff G. Colorectal polyps. Clinical implications: screening and cancer prevention. *Scand J Gastroenterol* 1987;**22**:769–75.

Jass JR. Do all colorectal carcinomas arise in pre-existing adenomas? *World J Surg* 1989:**13**:45–51.

Ransohoff DF, Lang CA, Kuo HS. Colonoscopic surveillance after polypectomy: considerations of cost effectiveness. *Ann Int Med* 1991;**114**:177–81.

Rex DK, Lehman GA, Hawes RH, Ulbright TM, Smith JJ. Screening colonoscopy in asymptomatic average-risk persons with negative fecal occult blood tests. *Gastroenterology* 1991;**100**:64–7.

Williams CB, Bedenne L. Quadrennial review: management of colonic polyps — is all the effort worthwhile? *Hepatogastroenterology* 1990;**5**(Suppl.):144–65.

Williams CB, Price AB. Colon polyps and carcinoma. In: Sivak MV, ed. *Gastroenterologic Endoscopy*. Philadelphia: WB Saunders, 1987: 921–45.

Williams CB, Saunders PB. The rationale for current practice in the management of malignant colonic polyps. *Endoscopy* 1993;**25**:469–74.

Winawer SJ, Zauber AG, May Nah Ho MS *et al*. Prevention of colorectal cancer by colonoscopic polypectomy. *N Engl J Med* 1993;**329**:1977–81.

Winawer SJ, Zauber AG, O'Brien MJ, May Nah Ho MS, Gottlieb L. Randomised comparison of surveillance intervals after colonoscopic removal of newly diagnosed adenomatous polyps. *N Engl J Med* 1993;**328**:901–6.

Endoscopy of the Small Intestine

11

Standard upper gastrointestinal (GI) endoscopes can be passed into the *distal duodenum*. The major application (apart from ERCP) is to diagnose or rule out mucosal abnormality (e.g. coeliac disease) in the context of malabsorption; details of endoscopic 'jejunal' biopsy are given in Chapter 4. The *terminal ileum* can be examined by passing a colonoscope through the ileocaecal valve (see Chapter 9). The remainder of the small intestine has proved rather resistant to endoscopy. Fortunately, small intestinal diseases are relatively rare. However, there has recently been greater interest in enteroscopy, particularly in the context of obscure GI bleeding and symptoms suggestive of inflammatory bowel disease.

There are three methods for endoscopic examination of the small bowel—push, sonde and intraoperative enteroscopy.

Push enteroscopy

This examination is done with a dedicated video-endoscope 170–250 cm in length which incorporates enhanced tip flexibility to facilitate deep intubation of the proximal small intestine. A standard (properly disinfected) colonoscope can be used when the specialized enteroscope is not available. The enteroscopes have working channels which allow tissue sampling and therapeutic interventions in the proximal small intestine. The instrument can be passed approximately 30–150 cm into the jejunum, with careful manipulation, depending on the experience of the operator. The use of a stiffening overtube to reduce gastric looping (the main cause of patient discomfort and failure to advance the enteroscope) can facilitate deep intubation of the proximal small intestine (Fig. 11.1). However, these stiffening techniques have not proved universally popular due to patient intolerance. Complications of gastric mucosal stripping and pancreatitis have been reported. Keeping air insufflation to a minimum and avoiding drugs that reduce bowel motility until immediately before withdrawal (thereby making use of peristalsis), allows similar depths of insertion to be achieved without overtubes. If biopsy forceps are needed or haemostasis is anticipated, the instrument may be 'preloaded'; the passage of forceps and therapeutic probes at a later stage can be difficult when the instrument is looped acutely. Average procedure duration is 30–45 min, depending on whether therapeutic intervention is required, and mucosal views are excellent.

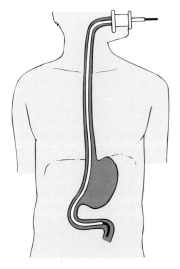

Fig. 11.1 A long overtube may facilitate jejunoscopy.

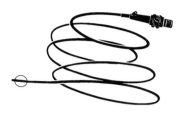

Fig. 11.2 A sonde-type small intestinal endoscope with a terminal weighted balloon.

Sonde enteroscopy

The sonde enteroscope is essentially a passive fibreoptic bundle 270 cm in length without tip deflection or a therapeutic channel (Fig. 11.2). A balloon on the distal tip of the instrument is inflated once the endoscope is in the duodenum. This method utilizes the passive propulsive effect of peristalsis to pull the instrument into the distal jejunum and ileum.

The sonde instrument is passed through the nose under light sedation, after applying topical anaesthesia to the nasal mucus membranes (cocaine 4–10% solution is particularly effective). The enteroscope can be allowed to pass spontaneously through the pylorus but this lengthens the procedure significantly. Most experts prefer to pass a standard upper GI endoscope *alongside* the enteroscope, and use grasping forceps to place the sonde tip into the duodenum. The patient is then kept comfortable and the progress of the instrument monitored by fluoroscopy. Prokinetic drugs have not proven beneficial in enhancing distal transit, but a single dose of metoclopramide (10 mg i.v.) may help initially in the distal duodenum. The patient may walk around once sedation has worn off (under nursing supervision); this may speed instrument advance. It usually takes 6–8 h for the enteroscope to reach the ileum.

Examination is performed on withdrawal. Water instillation and bimanual palpation, along with intermittent balloon inflation, can enhance the luminal views. Balloon inflation should be minimized to prevent a 'concertina' effect — rapid unfolding of compressed bowel loops during withdrawal. Unfortunately, due to the small bowel anatomy and inability to control tip deflection fully, only 40–70% of small bowel mucosa is viewed adequately by this technique. Few complications of sonde enteroscopy have been described; these include epistaxis and perforation of small bowel ulcers during the 'blind' intubation part of the examination.

Clinical indications

The duration of the procedure, and the need for continuous nursing care and fluoroscopy, make it unlikely that this technique will be attractive outside a few specialized centres. However, there is a significant role in selected patients.

Push and sonde enteroscopy should be seen as complementary in the investigation of patients with suspected small bowel disease. The commonest indication for enteroscopy is obscure GI bleeding which has not been explained by standard endoscopic and radiological investigations. These patients account for 5–15% of all patients presenting with GI bleeding. The yield is substantial, and enteroscopy should replace barium radiology and isotope studies in this context. Since it is possible to treat lesions (e.g. angiodysplasia) through the push enteroscope, and because the examination is much simpler for the patients, this technique is used first in patients with obscure GI bleeding. Sonde enteroscopy is used only when that examination is normal. Haemostasis can be carried out using either a heat probe or a BICAP probe passed via the push enteroscope. In general, lower energy settings are required in the small intestine compared to the upper GI tract. Typically, 1–2 s pulses of 15–30 J are utilized to minimize the risk of perforation in the thin wall of the small bowel. Enteroscopy has highlighted the problems of ulcers and enteropathy induced by non-steroidal anti-inflammatory drugs in the small bowel. The procedure has also been used to evaluate patients presenting with abnormal small bowel radiology. Enteroscopic examination and biopsy are justified to aid diagnosis in patients where Crohn's disease or tumours are suspected.

Intraoperative enteroscopy

The small intestine can be examined endoscopically during laparotomy; the surgeon guides the endoscope through the small bowel with the abdomen open (or at laparoscopy). The new push enteroscopes are ideal in this setting, but colonoscopes can be used. Intraoperative enteroscopy is indicated particularly in the context of obscure GI bleeding when push and sonde enteroscopy are unavailable or unrevealing.

There are three possible approaches for intraoperative enteroscopy:

1 *Via the mouth.* The endoscopist passes the endoscope as far as possible into the duodenum/jejunum. Intubation of the duodenum is easier if it is done before the abdomen is opened and the tamponade effect of the abdominal wall is lost.

2 *Via a surgical enterotomy.* Opening the bowel for intraoperative endoscopy has historical precedent but should rarely be required; in general it should be avoided since it carries an infection risk.

3 *Via the anus.* The colonoscopy takes up about 70 cm of instrument, leaving less for examination of the small bowel.

The endoscope used for enteroscopy should be fully disinfected before the procedure, and the bowel is prepared by standard techniques. Intraoperative enteroscopy must be managed carefully and methodically, with special care taken to avoid overinsufflation and rough handling of the intestine. Counterpressure is applied by the surgeon to straighten out acute angles and to prevent loops from forming in the stomach and duodenum (Fig. 11.3) — or in the colon during a transanal approach.

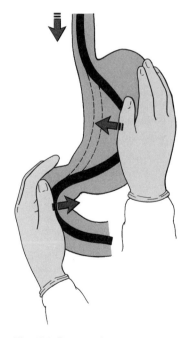

Fig. 11.3 Peroperative straightening of the stomach and duodenum.

The instrument tip is advanced by the surgeon, slowly feeding the bowel over the tip of the enteroscope whilst the endoscopist inspects the mucosa, keeping air insufflation to a minimum. It is particularly important that the surgeon and endoscopist should be aware of the risk of torsion or tear in the mesentery during the procedure. Utilizing this technique, the entire small intestine can be fed over the enteroscope with little difficulty. Surgical mobilization of the duodenum (the Kocher manoeuvre) is usually not necessary.

If enteroscopy is being performed for occult bleeding, it is important to view the bowel during advancement, so as not to be confused by haematomas caused by instrument trauma and suction. Angiomas can be seen by transillumination, performed simply by switching off the operating room lights. Sometimes, reverse transillumination is also helpful; the bowel is viewed endoscopically, using only the operating room lights for illumination. Lesions are marked by the surgeon with a suture. The decision whether to over-sew or resect is taken only after the examination is completed.

Intraoperative endoscopy appears to be a remarkably safe procedure when performed by an expert. It is preferable to 'blind' segmental resections such as empirical right hemicolectomy due to the frequency of recurrent bleeding in such situations.

The following points are the most important things for the beginner to appreciate and to perform:

1 Review the technique with the surgeon preoperatively. Agree that a complete examination should be carried out before the decision on the surgical approach is made.

2 Always advance under direct vision, but keep air insufflation to a minimum. This requires constant dialogue with the surgeon.

3 Examine the mesentery frequently. Do not allow tension on it to become excessive.

4 All but the distal 10–20 cm of small bowel is usually easily examined from above. The distal ileum can be intubated after passage of the endoscope through the colon.

5 Decompress the bowel completely before withdrawal with the enteroscope.

Complications

Complications of intraoperative enteroscopy are rare. Prolonged postoperative ileus and both mucosal and serosal tears have been described. This is a procedure which requires excellent co-operation between endoscopists and surgeons. Published results have been encouraging with a site-specific source of bleeding identified in up to 70% of patients. Unfortunately, many patients re-bleed following surgery, since lesions such as angiodysplasia may recur in previously unaffected areas of the bowel.

Future developments

There have been a number of innovative approaches to endoscopy of the small bowel recently. These include laparoscopy-assisted panenteroscopy, intraoperative sonde enteroscopy and the development of sonde instruments with tip deflection and biopsy facilities. It remains to be proven whether these innovations will prove useful in the clinical arena.

Further reading

Berner JS, Mauer K, Lewis BS. Push and sonde enteroscopy for the diagnosis of obscure gastrointestinal bleeding. *Am J Gastroenterol* 1994;**89**:2139–42.

Lewis BS, Waye JD. Chronic gastrointestinal bleeding of obscure origin: role of small bowel enteroscopy. *Gastroenterology* 1988;**94**:1117–20.

Morris AJ, Wasson LA, McKenzie JF. Small bowel enteroscopy in undiagnosed gastrointestinal blood loss. *Gut* 1992;**33**:887–9.

Ress AM, Benacci JC, Sarr MG. Efficacy of intra-operative enteroscopy in diagnosis and prevention of recurrent, acute gastrointestinal bleeding. *Am J Surg* 1992;**163**:94–9.

12

Outcomes, Documentation, Quality and Training

Outcomes

Adverse outcomes (complications) have been discussed in general in Chapter 3, and in relation to specific procedures in relevant chapters. We pointed out the importance of careful definition and objective assessment. The same provisos are equally important when attempting to assess the 'success' of our procedures. These are the tools of 'outcomes research', which has recently become more fashionable.

Whether a procedure succeeds or fails can be judged only if the intent is stated clearly beforehand. Our traditional list of *indications* are essentially symptoms or brief clinical scenarios, e.g. haematemesis, post-cholecystectomy pain, jaundice or heartburn. We know that endoscopy may be helpful in these circumstances, but cannot use such terms to define success or failure. In the acutely bleeding patient, we may or may not find a bleeding lesion, and may or may not attempt (or succeed) to treat it effectively. End-points need to be defined more carefully. One method, which lends itself to computer documentation and analysis, is to define the elements of the clinical situation separately. We document the presence or absence of a series of clinical *facts*, i.e. symptoms, prior established diagnoses, prior interventions, aetiological factors, risk factors for malignancy and test results. In that context, we define whether the aim of the endoscopy is: (i) to make (or clarify) a diagnosis; (ii) to check on the progress of a known disease (or the results of recent treatment); or (iii) to provide treatment. Complexity is added by the realization that a single endoscopic procedure may be both diagnostic and therapeutic — or only therapeutic if a diagnosis is made. In a patient with haematemesis, our goal will usually be to make a diagnosis, and to apply therapy if this is technically appropriate and feasible.

There is plenty of room for wishful thinking if we do not define our objective precisely and up-front. Even if we do so, defining a 'success rate' is complex, for this depends on many factors, including (hopefully) the expertise of the endoscopist. The *quality* of the indication is also important, and varies across groups of patients and certainly between reported series. For example, a referral centre may expect to have more 'difficult' cases e.g. a larger proportion of difficult stones or patients with Billroth II gastrectomy for ERCP. Definitions of success also depend on the audience. Endoscopists tend to be preoccupied with *technical* success rates (and complications). As clinicians we

308

should define success as a procedure which is *more effective* than other available alternatives (as judged by carefully controlled research studies). However, there are other arbiters of success, not least the patient. Herein lies the importance of attempting to assess the effect of an intervention on the patient as a whole, which has led to the development of *quality of life indices*. Another measure of success is *value*, or *cost-benefit*. For those who pay the bills, this may appear to be the most important criterion.

One other problem is the *timescale* of outcome measurement, particularly in relation to therapeutic procedures. Stenting for malignant biliary obstruction looks very good during the first few weeks (e.g. compared with surgery), but the advantages diminish as time passes (and stents clog).

These complexities and others emphasize the importance of using established scientific methods in trying to evaluate our procedures.

Documentation

The importance of careful documentation should be self-evident. There should be a 'paper trail' for any patient undergoing endoscopy which covers the whole process from initial referral (on paper or via the telephone), pre-procedure preparation, examination and checklists, the endoscopy report, the nurses' procedure report, documentation of the recovery phase and discharge, and of the final disposition, advice and follow-up recommendations. The trail should also encompass 'delayed' information such as pathology reports and complication data.

Like many other aspects of endoscopy, the degree to which these aspects of documentation are standardized and regulated varies enormously. In some healthcare systems, payment is dependent upon specific documentation criteria — which is a powerful stimulus to compliance. But proper documentation is nothing more than an illustration of quality care. It is certainly excellent defence against speculative lawsuits. The lawyers tell us 'if it is not written down, it was not done'.

Quantity is not the same as *quality*. Some endoscopy reports are so verbose that it is also almost impossible to find the few crucial pieces of clinical information. Thus, structuring of the data is important.

In most institutions the 'paper trail' is still indeed a trail of paper. It will be a series of sheets, including freehand writing, checklists (e.g. for risk factors), printed forms (e.g. consent forms) and typed procedure reports and recommendations. Paper records are inefficient, usually in the wrong place and easily lost. It is certainly time to leap from the notepad to the keypad. Desktop (and handheld) computers provide an excellent medium for this documentation. With appropriate networking, all of the information can be available to anyone who wishes to see it it at numerous sites — including at home or a distant office. Endoscopy reports can be faxed directly without going through a paper report, or transmitted electronically to another location (Fig. 12.1).

We have been particularly interested in computer databases for almost 20 years. The equipment is no longer a problem. The power of desk and laptop instruments is now sufficient to deal with all of our data (and images). The problem has been to define the content and structure of endoscopy-related databases and, in particular, to agree on some standards for content and terminology.

The efforts of many individuals and some national endoscopy societies has resulted in a document entitled *Minimum Common Terminology*, recently published jointly by the European, US and Japanese endoscopy societies. This is essentially a method for describing what we may see or do. Version 1.0 is not perfect, but it is a good start.

Commercial endoscopy databases are in evolution; several function effectively already. One practical question is whether the data are entered by secretarial staff alone, or also by nursing and medical staff (directly or via printed checklists). In our units, the patient details and administrative data are entered by a secretary/receptionist; doctors then enter all the medical data, which immediately generates reports for the medical record and referring doctors. A goal is to have each data entry take no longer than dictating a report. However, dictation is only part of the doctor's work if computers are not used; there are delays involved in correcting and signing typed documents. With a little practice and suitable programs, all of the data can be entered in 3–5 min.

There are many advantages of computer databases over other forms of record-keeping. The structure can be defined carefully, with safeguards so that key questions must be answered before the program will proceed or the report record is complete. Only appropriate answers are accepted, and irrelevant keys made non-operative. It is easy to produce and modify automatically word-processed forms, listings and reports — although most systems do allow some free text sections so that the format is not restrictive. Computers can deal with large amounts of data for analysis, but can also be individualized so that relevant points (e.g. drug sensitivities, previous technical problems, sedation requirements) for particular patients are automatically presented for any subsequent visit. Multi-user operation or a network system means that several screens can work simultaneously, and all of the data are instantly available (or can be entered) in different places (e.g. reception/secretary/endoscopy room) without the problems of physical transfer of paper. Computer management is virtually indispensable for any unit offer-

GASTROENTEROLOGY

ERCP REPORT (10/10/___)

Name: Mrs Smith
MRN: 890856
DOB: 04/08/45   Age: 51 yrs
SEX: Female
Attending MD: R. Jones

Mrs Smith...... presented with pain and jaundice, with a diagnosis of GB stone/disease (574.2).

Prior treatment: No relevant surgery; no endoscopic therapy.

Health status: Mild problem (ASA II). Co-morbidities were not noted. Risk factors for endoscopy were not identified.

Recent diagnostic studies: US scan (abnormal).

Laboratory results: Haematocrit normal, platelets normal, WBC normal, PTT normal, prothrombin ratio normal, albumen normal, AST normal, ALT normal, alkaline phosphatase 196, bilirubin normal, amylase normal, lipase normal.
Results in <u>attacks</u>: LFTs abnormal, amylase normal, lipase normal.

Indication: To clarify diagnosis and to treat. Cholecystectomy is planned.

Procedure: Endoscopy was performed in the X-ray dept as an inpatient/consult, on an urgent (on schedule) basis by Dr. Jones, assisted by Dr. Brown, after fully informed consent was obtained. The patient was sedated and was given prophylactic antibiotics; vital signs and oxygenation were carefully monitored (for details see nurses' report). The procedure started at 15:02 and lasted 31 minutes. It was very well tolerated, and views were excellent.

Radiological findings

```
   Oesophagus : normal
      Stomach : normal
      Pylorus : normal
Duodenal bulb : normal
   Post bulbar : normal
  Main papilla : normal
 Minor papilla : not sought
```

Endoscopic survey

```
    Bile duct : Stone (common duct)
                distal duct size was 7mm, drainage was not checked
                there was 1 stone, max diameter 5mm
  Gall bladder : did not fill
    Pancreatic : main orifice filled; minor orifice not attempted
         Duct : normal
```

Special diagnostic techniques: Biopsies were not taken; cytology was not taken; cultures were not taken.

Endoscopic treatments: Biliary stone extraction was performed with success. (43264) Stones were removed by basket. Balloon dilator to 8mm.

Complications: None immediate.

Comments: PT WITH KNOWN STONE DISEASE, EPISODIC BILIARY PAIN, ADMIT FROM SURGERY CLINIC WITH JAUNDICE, NO F/C/S. SINGLE STONE REMOVED, UNABLE TO FILL CYSTIC DUCT. REC. CHOLECYSTECTOMY AS SOON AS POSSIBLE.

Diagnosis after Endoscopy: GB stone/disease (574.2).

Follow-up plan: Clinic review within one month.

Signed ....

report to attending MD, patient file. (printed: 10/11/___)
Copy to Dr. Local (fax: 904 8763)

Fig. 12.1 Computer-generated endoscopy report.

ing proper follow-up and surveillance services, not only because of the need to spot non-attenders and follow correct schedules, but because the sheer volume of correspondence becomes overwhelming without the ability to print batches of letters automatically, correctly addressed and dated.

With these advantages come some constraints—the need for immediate technical help, regular data backup and a fool-proof security system.

Image documentation

Photographic slides and cine and video recording have been part of endoscopy since its beginning. These records were mainly used for teaching, and their physical mass often defied attempts at efficient storage and retrieval.

The fact that all of our information is now digital opens wonderful new possibilities. Colour prints can be produced immediately at the touch of a button for inclusion in the patient record and report. We are rapidly moving towards comprehensive 'image management' so that vast amounts of image data can be captured, stored and retrieved electronically. Automatic storage of full motion videos will follow.

Digital storage opens up the possibility of image analysis and enhancement (possibly for enhanced diagnosis), and also *image transmission*. This allows the sharing of images (and related data) at distant sites through telephone lines. Endoscopy (and its related images from radiology and histology) lends itself to 'telemedicine'. We can already supervise and advise our trainees from a distance (through TV links) in our units. Soon we will be giving advice and teleconsultations across the country on a routine basis.

Data analysis

Computerization of data collection and storage provides tremendous opportunities for analysing our activities (Figs 12.2 and 12.3). Essentially these are of two types: housekeeping and research.

1 *Housekeeping* means keeping track of who is doing what and why (including costs). We can monitor patients who need to come back, e.g. for stent exchange or polyp follow-up. With appropriate input, this becomes an important management tool, e.g. providing data about procedure room and equipment usage, turn-around times and staff requirements.

2 *Research* is enormously enhanced by computerization. Provided the right questions are asked prospectively, we can look at important correlations and outcomes. Standardization of databases will allow sharing of data from multiple institutions.

Run date: 11/03/96 | Statistics of procedures with Exam date 01/01/96 – 30/06/96
Run time: 14:20:08
Run by: | Doctor:

| | Diag-nostic | Thera-peutic | Sub-total | Rel. value | Emergency | | Public | Out-patient | In-patient | |
					In hr	Out hr			GI	Consult
UPPER	372	141	513	654	74	37	92	273	109	131
COLON	189	75	264	603	32	14	35	147	48	69
FLEX	128	15	143	79	8	3	13	99	20	24
ERCP	98	257	355	1,836	39	14	45	200	103	52
TOTAL	787	488	1,275	3,172	153	68	185	719	280	276

Fig. 12.2 Computer-generated report of endoscopy activities.

Quality improvement

Knowing accurately what we are doing (using housekeeping data) is the essential basis for improvement. We measure the process, institute new policies and measure the result. 'Quality assurance' or 'audit' used to be presented or at least perceived in a negative light: somebody was checking up on us, expecting to find deficiencies or complications. 'Quality (or process) improvement' gives this context a positive spin, which is attractive to most doctors. Essentially it is a way of helping us to do a better job—and of documenting the process.

Training

Flexible endoscopy is a manual technique like driving a car or playing a musical instrument; some people learn more quickly than others and some may never become particularly adept. Practice is essential, but it helps if correct habits are instilled at an early stage. Because patients are involved, some form of apprenticeship is essential, with an experienced endoscopist overseeing the early examinations during which patients (and instruments) are at risk. As well as performing endoscopies under supervision, a trainee should make use of available written, slide or video material, practice under supervision on teaching models, attend teaching courses and see several different endoscopy centres. All of these methods have their advantages.

It should be emphasized that—like driving a car or playing a musical instrument—the technical aspects of the procedures are not an end in themselves, merely a way of getting somewhere or making good music. Thus, learning endoscopy should be inte-

Run date: 03/11/95 Run time: 14:24:46 Run by:		Summary of ERCP procedures with follow-up due date between 01/01/95 – 30/06/95 Endo attending: Follow up plan: stent removal/exchange				
					Follow up	
Exam date	MRN/Full Name	Endo doctor(s)	Endoscopic treatments	Final diagnosis	Plan by	Realized
06/10/95	891294		Biliary sphincterotomy / Pancreatic stent insertion	Papillary stenosis/spasm / Pancreatitis	06/11/95	11/10/95
11/10/95	892359		Minor papilla sphincterotomy / Minor papilla orifice dilation / Minor papilla stent insertion	Pancreas divisum / Pancreatitis	11/11/95	
14/7/95	022149743		Biliary sphincterotomy / Biliary stricture dilation / Biliary stent insertion	? Biliary cancer (hilar)	14/11/95	
15/09/95	876131		Pancreatic sphincterotomy / Pancreatic stricture dilation / Pancreatic stent insertion	Pancreatitis/stone / Pancreatic leak	15/11/95	
25/10/95	893162		Biliary sphincterotomy / Pancreatic stent insertion	Papillary stenosis/spasm / GB stone/disease	25/11/95	27/10/95
30/08/95	091284		Biliary sphincterotomy / Biliary stent insertion	Pancreatitis / Biliary other	30/11/95	
30/10/95	868868		Pancreatic sphincterotomy / Pancreatic stent insertion	GB stone/disease / Pancreatitis / Papillary stenosis/spasm	30/11/95	
10/06/95	887061		Pancreatic stricture dilation / Pancreatic stent insertion	Pancreatitis / Pancreatitis/stone / ? Biliary other	06/12/95	
09/10/95	352574		Biliary stent extraction / Biliary stent extraction / Biliary stent insertion	Pancreatitis/stone / Biliary other	09/12/95	
08/10/95	807092		Biliary stent extraction / Biliary stent insertion / Biliary stone extraction	Bile duct stone(s) / Dilated bile duct ?cause	10/12/95	
13/10/95	890902		Minor papilla stent insertion / Minor papilla orifice dilation	Pancreas divisum / Pancreatitis/stone	13/12/95	
13/10/95	863907		Biliary sphincterotomy / Pancreatic sphincterotomy / Pancreatic stone extraction	Pancreatitis/stone / Papillary stenosis/spasm	13/12/95	27/10/95
16/08/95	882718		Biliary sphincterotomy / Pancreatic stent insertion	Pacreatitis / Papillary stenosis/spasm	16/12/95	
18/08/95	854491		Pancreatic sphincterotomy / Pancreatic stent insertion	Pancreatitis/stone	18/12/95	

Total number of procedures:

Fig. 12.3 Computer-generated report for follow-up of ERCP stents.

grated into training in gastroenterology, with full appreciation of its clinical application (indications, risks and alternatives).

Apprenticeship

Watching an expert is useful, providing that the expert actively explains what he is doing and seeing. In countries where endoscopy is a well-established speciality with numerous staff, trainees may be expected to watch many procedures on video monitors before going 'hands-on'. In other places, the beginner may be thrown in at the deep end. He finds himself being asked to use an expensive instrument he does not understand in an organ with unfamiliar anatomy, and gets a poor view of appearances he cannot interpret. One answer is to 'phase' trainee introduction to a set period (e.g. 5–10 min) or a defined part of the examination (e.g. insertion to the cardia or the proximal sigmoid colon), with the extent of examination and responsibility being gradually lengthened. The trainee can be entrusted with some of the routine duties in the endoscopy room, helping the nurses and learning correct techniques in handling and cleaning the endoscopes. An old or broken instrument available in partly stripped-down form can help to demonstrate the complexity of the equipment and the need to treat it with respect.

The teacher needs considerable patience and the ability to adapt to the different physical and personality traits of different pupils. Some need calming down, to learn to be more cerebral and more humane in their actions; others need to be speeded up to become gradually more positive and fluent. Generally speaking, a slow, thoughtful endoscopist with integrity can learn to excel, whereas the aggressive and erratic often remain so.

Endoscopic technique builds up by learning to combine visual interpretation with the correct mechanical response. Attention to the detail of finger movements, shaft twist and even body position are all important. The teacher may need, for instance, to hold his own hand over that of the trainee on the shaft of the instrument to demonstrate the requisite amounts of to-and-fro or twisting movements, or to check that when the pupil intends to angle either up or down he is actually moving the control knob in the correct direction first time. Regrettably, there are too few experienced endoscopists combining the necessary skills themselves with the amount of time and interest required to teach successfully.

There is a range of teaching material which can be used between endoscopic sessions. A collection of books, atlases and selected reprints can be assembled with little effort. Teaching video tapes and education slide tapes liven up the topic and help to show that there are different approaches to endoscopy. Homemade slide–tape sequences are also not difficult to produce and help the teacher to avoid tedious repetition. National endoscopic societies can ensure availability of teaching material (e.g. the American Society for Gastrointestinal Endoscopy (ASGE) Teaching Library).

Models and simulators

No model can simulate exactly the varying and variable anatomy of the human gastrointestinal (GI) tract, especially its combination of elasticity and contractility. None the less, half an hour spent working on a stomach or colon model under expert guidance, followed by some practice alone, is very helpful in understanding spatial relationships and co-ordinating the view down the endoscope with the correct movements of the controls. It is easy to see, explain and practice on a model how to perform retroversion at the cardia, why the pylorus must be correctly positioned with a side-viewer, why upwards angling approximates to the papilla, or why clockwise rotation undoes an alpha loop. Once seen and understood, these things are never forgotten and with the opportunity to practice them repeatedly without involving a patient, the trainee develops self-confidence and better understanding of correct instrument handling.

A newer approach, not yet either fully developed or evaluated, is the use of electronic endoscopy simulators. The severe constraints of the limited budgets available for medical teaching mean that the sophisticated but enormously expensive simulators available to train pilots in aviation are regrettably not applicable to endoscopy. The prototypes available currently for endoscopy teaching make use either of video-disc technology to show actual endoscopic images or computer-graphic techniques to produce a cruder image simulated mathematically in real time. The trainee handles a dummy endoscope, the steering controls, shaft movements and air/water/suction buttons which are converted by transducers and switches into electrical outputs so as to modify the image display according to the handling of the instrument. The computer, in addition to controlling the image, will produce screen prompts and a 'score' to give interactive teaching without the presence of an expert teacher, and can also evaluate the progress of the trainee in different simulated circumstances on an objective basis without patient trauma or danger of instrument damage.

Certification of competence

Professional organizations in many countries have struggled with the need to certify when endoscopists are competent. This is an issue with complex ramifications, and it is pertinent sometimes to remember that most specialities (including surgery) do not certify competence specifically by procedure. In addition, certification is only meaningful if there is any disadvantage in not being certified.

Both the UK and US national organizations with which we are familiar have discussed these issues repeatedly. The perspectives are different. In the UK, the relative lack of medical staff means that most trainees gain a lot of experience, but often with relatively little supervision. The British Society of Gastroenterology (BSG) is setting up a mechanism for certifying trainees in four different groups of techniques: diagnostic upper GI endoscopy, therapeutic upper GI endoscopy, colonoscopy and ERCP. Certification will be done by accredited trainers, who have to prove their own competence and the adequacy of their facilities. In the USA, fellows may do less procedures, but the much shorter period of training and both medicolegal and financial concerns mean they are fully supervised. They keep a log book of all endoscopies, and expect to be certified as competent at the end of the training (now 3 years). This is the responsibility of a designated 'endoscopy training director'. It is not one to be undertaken lightly, for heads of gastroenterology and endoscopy departments have actually been held partly responsible for complications of procedures performed by people they have certified to be competent. The ASGE has published 'threshold' numbers, below which it is judged unlikely that any endoscopist will be fully competent in any particular procedure. The training director is expected to make an informed judgement once these threshold numbers have been achieved, and to advise trainees when (and what) further instruction is required. It is self-evident that learning should be a life-long process, and that competence is a relative term. Defining minimal or threshold numbers is controversial, and requires a compromise between reality and idealism. There has been a tendency for professional societies to agree on the lowest common denominator. This tendency should be resisted; it is our responsibility to define appropriate training and to insist that guidelines are followed. We also have the responsibility to provide that training, which can be time-consuming and frustrating.

In practice, the crucial question is whether the particular hospital (or healthcare system) to which attachment is sought will award 'privileges' for performing these procedures. The issues here become even more complex, since they involve not only the question of competence but also the perceived needs of the community and also of the established specialists.

Levels of training

It must be recognized that not all trainees can expect to become competent in all of the GI procedures. Furthermore, at least in the USA, the number of specialists within a single community may be such as to dilute the work load for any individual below the threshold for continuing competence. It is therefore logical to consider different levels of endoscopic training. Most clinical gastroenterologists will be trained in upper endoscopy and colonoscopy with their standard therapeutic applications (polypectomy, sclerotherapy and endoscopic haemestasis). This level can be called *standard* training. Some family practitioners may wish to be trained only in flexible sigmoidoscopy; some surgeons and research gastroenterologists may need only to perform diagnostic upper GI endoscopy and flexible sigmoidoscopy. A small proportion of trainees will go on after standard to *advanced* training in more specialized (rarer and more dangerous) procedures, including ERCP and its therapeutic applications, laser therapy, laparoscopy, etc. Restricting advanced techniques to a selected group of trainees is not universally popular, since many wish to keep their options open. However, such selection is inevitable if quality is to be maintained and if we are to produce experienced trainers for the next generation. Another emphasis is that (with rare exceptions at the basic level) no one should be taught diagnostic procedures without learning the therapeutic applications. It is illogical to do a colonoscopy without being able to perform polypectomy, and equally so (as well as potentially hazardous) to undertake ERCP in a patient with jaundice without the skills to provide drainage. It follows that these endoscopic trainees will spend additional time in attaining competence — whilst their colleagues may obtain specialized training in other directions, such as clinical or laboratory research.

Endoscopy is a valuable tool; it is worth doing well.

Further reading

American Society of Gastrointestinal Endoscopy. *Principles of Training in Gastrointestinal Endoscopy*. ASGE Guideline. Manchester: American Society of Gastrointestinal Endoscopy, 1991.

American Society of Gastrointestinal Endoscopy. *Defining the Endoscopy Report*. Manchester: American Society of Gastrointestinal Endoscopy, 1992.

American Society of Gastrointestinal Endoscopy. *Guideline for Enhancement of Endoscopic Skills*. Manchester: American Society of Gastrointestinal Endoscopy, 1993.

American Society of Gastrointestinal Endoscopy. *Minimum Common Terminology*. Manchester: American Society of Gastrointestinal Endoscopy, 1995.

Baillie J, Williams CB. Simulators for teaching endoscopy. In: *Annual of Gastrointestinal Endoscopy*. London: Current Science, 1990:5–6.

Benson JA, Cohen S. Evaluation of procedural skills in gastroenterologists. *Gastroenterology* 1987;**92**:254–7.

Cotton PB. Therapeutic gastrointestinal endoscopy. Problems in proving efficacy. *N Engl J Med* 1992;**326**:1626–8.

Cotton PB. Outcomes of endoscopy procedures: struggling towards definitions. *Gastrointest Endosc* 1994; **40**:514–18.

Cotton PB, Schmitt C. Quality of life in palliative management of malignant obstructive jaundice. *Scand J Gastroenterol* 1993;**28**(Suppl. 199):44–6.

Myren J, Hellers G. The OMGE recommendations for education and training in gastroenterology, adapted to the major areas of the world. *Scand J Gastroenterol* 1991;**26**(Suppl. 189).

Provenzale D. Endoscopic technology assessment in the 1990s; the role of decision analysis. In: *Annual of Gastrointestinal* Endoscopy. London: Current Science, 1995:1–8.

Sivak MV, Vennes JA, Cotton PB *et al*. Advanced training programs in gasrointestinal endoscopy. *Gastrointest Endosc* 1993;**39**:462–4.

Zuccaro G. *Electronic Endoscopy*. Gastrointestinal Endoscopy Clinics of North America, Vol. 2(2) (series ed. Sivak MV). Philadelphia: WB Saunders, 1992.

Proctoring and hospital endoscopy privileges; guideline. *Gastrointest Endosc* 1991;**37**:666–7.

13 Endoscopy 2000: Postscript

Our attempts at forecasting in previous editions of this book have met with mixed success. We have predicted that some new procedures would be described (but not by us), and that some of them would prove to be worthwhile. However, most of our comments have been targeted elsewhere—at the practical difficulties involved in getting the message out and the job done. We stated 'toys have turned into tools, and the excitements of conception have inevitably engendered the obligations of parenthood'. These issues continue to dominate, and have come into somewhat closer focus.

However, it does no harm to speculate first on some of the technical trends. The imperatives of disinfection, always logical but recently driven by the acquired immune deficiency syndrome (AIDS) pandemic, have caused manufacturers to give ease of cleaning and disinfection a high priority in design, and has even spawned the first (partially) disposable endoscopes. These are beginning to prove popular for flexible sigmoidoscopy in some isolated units which do not wish to gear up fully for formal chemical disinfection. The search for better cleaning and disinfection machines and effective, safe disinfectants continues. The demand for less costly procedures has led to increasing interest in sedation-free endoscopy which reduces the need for monitoring and recovery. Smaller 'screening' endoscopes and transnasal passage are being re-evaluated. The opposite trend is for more complex therapeutic instruments, for example a large-channel 'bleeding' endoscope. Double-channel instruments have particular application but have not become widely popular. Developments in enteroscopy are to be anticipated, particularly a sonde-type instrument with tip deflection and a therapeutic capability. Control body ergonomics will be improved; self-steering and 'lumen-seeking' instruments are in prototype development. Automatic scope location (without fluoroscopy) is being developed using electromagnetic sensors; the endoscopic image and the scope position in the body are viewed simultaneously on the video monitor.

Diagnostic devices will be improved. Surely it is possible to develop a biopsy instrument which would provide multiple samples without repeated passage down the channel? The marriage of endoscopy and ultrasound will generate better devices for sampling submucosal and adjacent organs. Focused ultrasound may become a therapeutic tool for the destruction of tumours and stones. Tumour therapy should improve in other ways. The pioneering efforts of Japanese endoscopists in resection of early tumours (mucosectomy) will gradually be adopted in the West—with endoscopic ultrasound defining the target and the result. Photodynamic therapy will become more popular as more convenient and safer photosensitizers are developed. Endoscopic gene therapy is already being explored. Engineering skills being used in the laparoscopic revolution will have some spin-off in flexible endoscopy. We will be able to sew, and to leave clips and loops. Current stent research will yield an increasing harvest. Expandable, covered and removable stents will improve existing applications and open new ones.

Other new perspectives will be opened with the 'digital key'. The change from fibreoptic to charged couple device (CCD) image capture has been a terrific boost for teaching, and reduces the risk to endoscopist's eyes (and necks). But the real gold is in the potential for image capture, enhancement, analysis and transmission. Spectroscopy may well yield important clinical information. Image transmission opens up all the potential of 'telemedicine'.

Evaluation and documentation

The simplicity of electronic databases and the increasing interest in 'outcomes research' provide the tools and an environment in which we can evaluate our procedures in a meaningful way. We need to track defined patients, lesions, goals and outcomes—and demand that other specialties undergo the same discipline. What we do nowadays is so complex that we cannot possibly keep track without accurate and detailed recordings, including representative images stored from every examination. Without documentation there is no measurement. Without repetitive measurement (audit) we cannot improve the process. For this is the essence of our task — to do the job better. Comparisons of endoscopic treatments with surgery and interventional radiology are not possible unless we develop a common database, and particularly a method for recording realistic risk factors. Increasing interest in quality of life indices is a welcome development since it swings the focus back to the object of our profession—the patient.

Delivery problems

Some endoscopy procedures are undoubtedly worthwhile. Others need to be tested. Whatever is good (or at least better than the current alternatives) has to be made available as widely as possible, and at high quality. This requires a functional health-care system and effective methods for teaching and funding the necessary professionals (doctors, nurses, support staff). In the last edition of this book, we spoke of the different arrangements in the UK and USA. At that time, budgets were fixed annually in the UK, and there was pressure to do *fewer* procedures, or at least to prioritize stringently. The pressures were quite different in the fee for service sector of the USA. Doctors and institutions both had a vested interest in maximizing endoscopic activity. There was less scrutiny of indications, and more opportunity for abuse. Gastroenterologists and endoscopy units proliferated. It is a fascinating irony that these polarities are being (somewhat) reversed. The UK is moving to a system with some competition, at the same time that the USA is flirting with capitation. These trends will have an enormous impact.

We have also spoken before about the relationship between surgery and gastroenterology. In the USA, the endoscope has been used as a weapon in an academic turf battle. Whether endoscopes 'belong' to gastroenterologists or to surgeons is a sterile issue. It is surely more productive to think of therapeutic endoscopy simply as a new form of surgery, and to attempt to break down the artificial barriers which may interfere with its best use. The laparoscopic revolution has substantially changed the surgical mind set, providing more flexibility and greater mutual respect across the disciplines. The opportunity to develop a multidisciplinary Digestive Disease Centre was the reason why one of us (PBC) has moved recently to the Medical University of South Carolina, in Charleston. The plan is to blur the distinction between surgeons and gastroenterologists to the extent that these differences no longer interfere with streamlined specialty care. There are joint facilities, goals and documentation, and a common springboard for clinical research. These collegial principles have long been espoused at St Marks Hospital in London, where CBW does most of his endoscopic 'surgery'. This small hospital specializing in colorectal disease is renowned for its team spirit, and has spawned numerous alumni devoid of interprofessional paranoia. St Marks Hospital has also moved recently to join a large community hospital with a new endoscopic centre and renewed commitment to teaching.

We sincerely hope that our book provides some guidance as we approach the 21st century. The next time we meet will probably be in cyberspace.

General Reading

Books

Baillie J. *Gastrointestinal Endoscopy. Basic Principles and Practice.* Oxford: Butterworth-Heinemann, 1992.

Barkin J, O'Phelan CA. Advanced therapeutic endoscopy. New York: Raven Press, 1990 (1st edn) and 1995 (2nd edn).

Brooks LC. *Current Techniques in Laparoscopy.* Philadelphia: Current Medicine, 1994.

Greene FL, Ponsky JL. *Endoscopic Surgery.* Philadelphia: WB Saunders, 1994.

Silvis SE, Rohrmann CA, Ansel HJ. *Text and Atlas of Endoscopic Retrograde Cholangiopancreatography.* Tokyo: Igaku-Shoin, 1995.

Sivak MV. *Gastroenterologic Endoscopy.* Philadelphia: WB Saunders, 1987.

Wilcox CM. *Atlas of Clinical Gastrointestinal Endoscopy.* (Companion to Sleisinger and Fortran, *Gastrointestinal Disease.*) Philadelphia: WB Saunders, 1995.

Annuals of Gastrointestinal Endoscopy

Edited by Cotton PB, Tytgat GNJ, Williams CB; published by Current Science, London, 1988–95.

These include reviews of the previous year's literature by international experts, covering all aspects of gastrointestinal endoscopy.

Gastrointestinal Endoscopy Clinics of North America

Series editor Sivak MV; published by WB Saunders, Philadelphia, 1991–96.

Quarterly editions with guest editors. Each edition focuses on a particular endoscopic topic.

Endoscopy Society Publications

Many endoscopy societies produce guideline documents and technology assessment evaluations. We recommend particularly those produced by the British Society of Gastroenterology and American Society for Gastrointestinal Endoscopy (often in collaboration with other digestive disease societies).

British Society of Gastroenterology, 3 St Andrews Place, London, NW1 4LB UK.

American Society for Gastrointestinal Endoscopy, 13 Elm Street, Manchester, MA 01944 USA.

Endoscopy Web Sites

American Society for Gastrointestinal Endoscopy
http://WWW.ASGE.COM
Medical University of South Carolina Digestive Disease Center
http://WWW.DDC.MUSC.EDU

Index